Network Science

Ernesto Estrada · Maria Fox · Desmond J. Higham ·
Gian-Luca Oppo

Editors

Network Science

Complexity in Nature and Technology

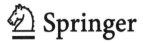 Springer

Editors

Prof. Ernesto Estrada
University of Strathclyde
Department of Mathematics and Statistics
   and Department of Physics
G1 1XH Glasgow
UK
ernesto.estrada@strath.ac.uk

Prof. Maria Fox
University of Strathclyde
Department of Computer and
   Information Sciences
G1 1XH Glasgow
UK
maria@maths.strath.ac.uk

Prof. Desmond J. Higham
University of Strathclyde
Department of Mathematics and Statistics
G1 1XH Glasgow
UK
djh@maths.strath.ac.uk

Prof. Gian-Luca Oppo
University of Strathclyde
Department of Physics
G4 0NG Glasgow
UK
gianluca@phys.strath.ac.uk

ISBN 978-1-4471-6034-2   ISBN 978-1-84996-396-1 (eBook)
DOI 10.1007/978-1-84996-396-1
Springer London Dordrecht Heidelberg New York

British Library Cataloguing in Publication Data
A catalogue record for this book is available from the British Library

Cover design: deblik

Printed on acid-free paper

Springer is part of Springer Science+Business Media (www.springer.com)

Preface

This book of invited, edited chapters arose from the six month programme **Complex Networks across the Natural and Technological Sciences**, held in 2009 at the *Institute for Advanced Studies*, Glasgow.

The motivation for the program was the emergence of a new interdisciplinary activity, sometimes called *Network Science*, that focuses on the patterns of interactions that arise between individual components of natural and engineered systems. The programme had several key objectives:

- To identify commonality across very different areas of application;
- To advance one area by injecting ideas and techniques from another;
- To allow *practitioners* (those who collect and use data) to pose challenges to *theoreticians* (those who develop concepts and derive analytical and computational tools);
- To allow *theoreticians* to bring *practitioners* up to speed on the state of the art.

The programme included three one-week workshops, featuring invited presentations by internationally-renowned researchers.

Workshop 1: Static Networks, organised by Ernesto Estrada and Des Higham, focused on the classic network science of fixed connectivity structures: empirical studies, mathematical models and computational algorithms.

Workshop 2: Dynamic Properties of Complex Networks, organised by Maria Fox, looked at (a) the study of time-dependent processes that take place over networks and modern topics such as *synchronisation*, and *message passing algorithms*, and (b) the study of time-evolving networks such as the World Wide Web and shifts in *topological properties* (connectivity, spectrum, percolation).

Workshop 3: Applications of Complex Networks, organised by Gian-Luca Oppo, emphasised the physical and engineering sciences, and looked ahead to new developments in the field.

In addition to these three international workshops, the six month programme featured tutorials, public lectures and an outreach event for children at the Glasgow Science Centre.

Having organised the programme and witnessed the remarkably wide applica-
bility of the research themes, we feel that the time is ripe for an interdisciplinary,
cross-cutting view of the state-of-the-art in network science. We therefore invited
a cross-section of the participants to contribute to this book, encouraging them to
review recent developments in a specific area of relevance to complex networks, discuss challenging open problems and, where possible, indicate how the field is likely
to develop over the next few years. We were delighted with the uniformly enthusi-
astic response from these authors, and we were equally pleased that the publisher
Springer shared our vision. These chapters, which have been brought together with
a unified index, appear in an order that reflects the sequence of topics considered in
the three workshops.

It is our hope that this resulting book will appeal to a wide range of scientists and
stimulate new lines of research.

Acknowledgements   This book would never have appeared without the funding and administrative support of the Institute for Advanced Studies, for the programme *Complex Networks across
the Natural and Technological Sciences*. We thank the Institute's officers at that time, Nigel Mot-
tram, Jane Morgan and Jason Reese for strategic advice and moral support, and also the Institute's
manager, Patricia Krus, for her expert assistance.

Further financial support was provided by the *Institute of Complex Systems at Strathclyde.*

We are extremely grateful to Mary McAuley in the Department of Mathematics and Statistics
at the University of Strathclyde for efficiently converting three of the submitted chapters from
Microsoft Word format into Springer-style LaTeX.

Finally, we are, of course, hugely indebted to the authors of these chapters for sharing their
expertise and insights.

Strathclyde, Glasgow   Ernesto Estrada
                                                                       Maria Fox
                                                               Desmond J. Higham
                                                               Gian-Luca Oppo

Contents

Contributors

Gabriella Baranyi Institute of Environmental Studies, Eötvös University, Budapest, Hungary.
Gabriella Baranyi is an environmental scientist with research interests in conservation biology and habitat planning, aided by habitat network analysis.

Stefano Battiston Systemgestaltung, ETH-Zentrum, Zurich, Switzerland, sbattiston@ethz.ch.
Stefano Battiston has a background in physics and neuroscience and has research interests in the modelling and empirical study of economic and social networks.

Guido Caldarelli Centre SMC, and ISC CNR, Dip. Fisica, University "Sapienza", Piazzale Aldo Moro 5, Rome, Italy, Guido.Caldarelli@roma1.infn.it.
Guido Caldarelli has interests in fractal growth, self-organised criticality and the analysis of scale-free networks.

Federica Ciocchetta Centre for Computational and Systems Biology, The Microsoft Research–University of Trento, Povo-Trento, Italy, ciocchetta@cosbi.eu.
Federica Ciocchetta has a background in biomathematics and information/communication technology, and has research interests in modelling and analysis of biological systems, process calculi and state-space reduction techniques.

Ernesto Estrada Department of Mathematics and Statistics, University of Strathclyde, Glasgow, UK; Department of Physics, University of Strathclyde, Glasgow, UK, ernesto.estrada@strath.ac.uk.
Ernesto Estrada has research interests in spectral graph theory, complex networks and their applications in chemistry, biology and many other areas in the physical, social and technological sciences.

Maria Fox Department of Computer and Information Sciences, University of Strathclyde, Glasgow, UK, maria.fox@cis.strath.ac.uk.
Maria Fox has research interests in automated planning, scheduling and constraint satisfaction and their application in solving combinatorial search and optimisation problems.

Diego Garlaschelli Said Business School, University of Oxford, Oxford, UK.
Diego Garlaschelli has research interests in complex networks and statistical
mechanics, with applications to biological and socio-economic systems.

James B. Glattfelder Systemgestaltung, ETH-Zentrum, Zurich, Switzerland,
jglattfelder@ethz.ch.
James Glattfelder develops ideas from complexity science and agent-based
modelling to study large databases of international companies and ownership
networks.

Naomichi Hatano Institute of Industrial Science, University of Tokyo, Tokyo
153-8505, Japan, hatano@iis.u-tokyo.ac.jp.
Naomichi Hatano develops and analyses models from the perspective of statistical
and mathematical physics, to capture the essence of complicated physical
phenomena.

Desmond J. Higham Department of Mathematics and Statistics, University of
Strathclyde, Glasgow, UK, d.j.higham@strath.ac.uk.
Des Higham is an applied/computational mathematician with interests in matrix
computations, stochastic modelling and simulation, and applications in biology and
neuroscience.

Ferenc Jordán Centre for Computational and Systems Biology, The Microsoft
Research-University of Trento, Povo-Trento, Italy, jordan@cosbi.eu.
Ferenc Jordán is a researcher at CoSBi with MSc in biology and PhD in genetics
who has research interests that span across all organisational levels of biological
networks, ranging from molecular to landscape graphs.

Holger Kantz Max Planck Institute for the Physics of Complex Systems,
Dresden, Germany, kantz@pks.mpg.de.
Holger Kantz has research interests that are centred around understanding,
modelling, and predicting the complex temporal evolution of real world systems.

Rowland R. Kao Faculty of Veterinary Medicine, University of Glasgow,
Glasgow, UK, r.kao@vet.gla.ac.uk.
Rowland Kao has research interests that include modelling and parameter
estimation for the transmission of livestock diseases using network analysis,
differential equations, statistics and computer simulations, principally funded
through a Wellcome Trust Senior Research Fellowship.

Vito Latora Dipartimento di Fisica ed Astronomia, Universitá di Catania and
INFN Sezione di Catania, Catania, Italy, latora@ct.infn.it.
Vito Latora uses his background in theoretical physics and nonlinear dynamics to
look into biological problems, to model social systems, and to find new solutions
for the design of technological networks.

Fabrizio Lillo Dipartimento di Fisica e Tecnologie Relative, Università di
Palermo, Palermo, Italy, lillo@unipa.it; Santa Fe Institute, Santa Fe, USA.
Fabrizio Lillo has research interests that focus on the application of methods and
tools of statistical physics to economic, financial, and biological systems.

Stefano Luccioli Consiglio Nazionale delle Ricerche, Istituto dei Sistemi Complessi, 50019 Sesto Fiorentino, Italy; Centro Studi Dinamiche Complesse, Sesto Fiorentino, Italy.
Stefano Luccioli has a background in nonlinear dynamics and statistical mechanics with interests in modelling and simulating biological systems (proteins and neural networks).

Gian-Luca Oppo Department of Physics, University of Strathclyde, Glasgow, UK, gianluca@phys.strath.ac.uk.
Gian-Luca Oppo, who is director of the Institute of Complex Systems at Strathclyde, has research interests that include complexity and spatial structures in nonlinear optics, and nonlinear dynamics of laser devices

Antonio Politi Consiglio Nazionale delle Ricerche, Istituto dei Sistemi Complessi, 50019 Sesto Fiorentino, Italy; Centro Studi Dinamiche Complesse, Sesto Fiorentino, Italy, antonio.politi@isc.cnr.it.
Antonio Politi is a physicist who works on the dynamics of neural networks, heat conductivity in low-dimensional systems and chaotic behaviour in systems with many degrees of freedom.

Sergio Porta Urban Design Studies Unit, Department of Architecture, University of Strathclyde, Glasgow, UK, sergio.porta@strath.ac.uk.
Sergio Porta has research interests that span from urban morphology, adaptive space and spatial analysis to public space design, urban design and traffic management.

Nataša Pržulj Department of Computing, Imperial College London, London, UK, natasha@imperial.ac.uk.
Nataša Pržulj is a computer scientist with research interests in applications of graph theory, mathematical modelling, and computational techniques to solving large-scale problems in computational and systems biology, especially planar cell polarity, proteomics, cancer informatics, and chemo-informatics.

V. Anne Smith School of Biology, University of St Andrews, St Andrews, Fife KY16 9TH, UK, anne.smith@st-andrews.ac.uk.
V. Anne Smith uses computational methods to analyse complex biological networks, and evaluates the computational methods with both computer simulation and biological intervention.

Emanuele Strano Urban Design Studies Unit, Department of Architecture, University of Strathclyde, Glasgow, UK, emanuele.strano@gmail.com.
Emanuele Strano has research interests that include urban studies, informal settlements, land titling, urban morphology, complex system theory applied to urban studies, urban sociology.

Alan Taylor Department of Mathematics and Statistics, University of Strathclyde, Glasgow, UK, a.taylor@strath.ac.uk.
Alan Taylor has a background in mathematics and computer science, and his research interests lie in computational algorithms for network science.

Chapter 1
Complex Networks: An Invitation

**Ernesto Estrada, Maria Fox, Desmond J. Higham,
and Gian-Luca Oppo**

Abstract Most of us recognize that connections are important. The *science* of connectivity has formalized and quantified this broad truism and produced a collection of concepts and tools that have proved to be remarkably useful in practice. With this brief opening chapter, we aim to prepare the reader for the cutting-edge and application-specific material to be found in the rest of the book by providing some motivation and background material. We also hope to give a taste of the excitement and the challenges that this area has to offer.

E. Estrada (✉) · D.J. Higham
Department of Mathematics and Statistics, University of Strathclyde, Glasgow, UK
e-mail: ernesto.estrada@strath.ac.uk

D.J. Higham
e-mail: d.j.higham@strath.ac.uk

E. Estrada · G.-L. Oppo
Department of Physics, University of Strathclyde, Glasgow, UK

G.-L. Oppo
e-mail: gianluca@phys.strath.ac.uk

M. Fox
Department of Computer and Information Sciences, University of Strathclyde, Glasgow, UK
e-mail: maria.fox@cis.strath.ac.uk

E. Estrada et al. (eds.), *Network Science*,
DOI 10.1007/978-1-84996-396-1_1, © Springer-Verlag London Limited 2010

Network: Any thing reticulated or decussated, at equal
distances, with interstices between the intersections.
Samuel Johnson
A Dictionary of the English Language,
First Edition, 1755

Network: A large system consisting of many similar parts that
are connected together to allow movement or communication
between or along the parts or between the parts and a control
centre.
Cambridge Advanced Learner's Dictionary,
on-line, 2010

1.1 Complex Networks: Introduction

In its most basic form, a *network* simply records

- a list of individuals, and
- a list of connections between pairs of these individuals.

Information of this type appears across a vast range of disciplines. In Table 1.1, we
offer a representative range of examples; many more can be found throughout this
book. From a mathematical perspective, a network of this type takes the form of
a *graph* (more precisely, an undirected, unweighted graph). To the left in Fig. 1.1,
we illustrate a very simple case. There we have seven individuals, more formally
known as *nodes* or *vertices*, and eight *edges* connecting pairs of them. The nodes
are labelled $1, 2, \ldots, 7$ and in this way we could also refer to the edges as $(1, 2)$,
$(1, 3)$, $(1, 6)$, $(1, 7)$, $(2, 3)$, $(2, 4)$, $(2, 5)$ and $(3, 4)$. We emphasize that the physical

Table 1.1 Examples of networks

Individuals	Connections based on	Reference
Hollywood actors	co-appearance in a movie	[1]
proteins	physical interaction	[61]
mobile phone users	act of communication	[14]
products in an on-line store	co-purchased by a customer	[48]
web pages	hyperlink	[58]
on-line social network users	friendship declaration	[28]
electrical power stations	physical power line	[68]
brain regions	anatomical connection	[38]
company board members	co-membership	[12]
cities	direct airline flight	[26]
researchers	publication co-authorship	[52]
computer networks	direct internet link	[25]
lasers	optical fibres	[4]

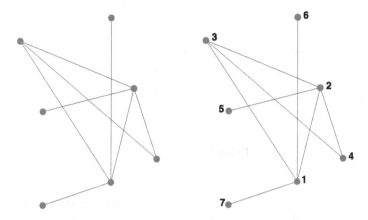

Fig. 1.1 *Left*: a graph, consisting of nodes (circles) joined by lines (edges). *Right*: the same graph, with the nodes labelled from 1 to 7

location of the nodes in Fig. 1.1 is not significant—the graph is completely specified by listing the nodes and the edges. To make this point clear, let us mention that we could equally well define the graph through the *adjacency matrix*

$$A = \begin{bmatrix} 0 & 1 & 1 & 0 & 0 & 1 & 1 \\ 1 & 0 & 1 & 1 & 1 & 0 & 0 \\ 1 & 1 & 0 & 1 & 0 & 0 & 0 \\ 0 & 1 & 1 & 0 & 0 & 0 & 0 \\ 0 & 1 & 0 & 0 & 0 & 0 & 0 \\ 1 & 0 & 0 & 0 & 0 & 0 & 0 \\ 1 & 0 & 0 & 0 & 0 & 0 & 0 \end{bmatrix},$$

so that a_{ij}, the element in the ith row and the jth column, takes the value $a_{ij} = 1$ if nodes i and j are connected and $a_{ij} = 0$ otherwise.

At the risk of disappearing into a recursive spiral, we present in Fig. 1.2 a snapshot of a thesaurus-based network, where edges join words with related meanings. This picture, produced from the Visual Thesaurus published by Thinkmap, Inc. at http://www.visualthesaurus.com/ zooms in on a small region centred at the word `network`.

Of course, in any particular application there may be more information available than simply the nodes and edges; for example, the nodes may have characteristics such as size, height or colour that place them into distinct categories, and the edges may be quantifiable in terms of length, age or processing power, and hence there are many ways to generalize this basic framework. However, abstracting to the simple network level has proved to be a surprisingly useful device: the loss of information is often outweighed by the convenience and elegance of the resulting data structure.

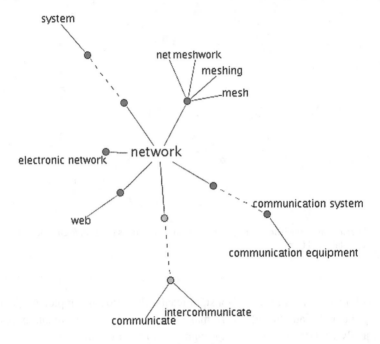

Fig. 1.2 A sub-network of words relating to the word network

1.2 Complex Networks: Origins

The mathematical idea of a graph can be traced back at least as far as the 1730s, when Leonhard Euler posed, and answered, the question of whether it is possible to walk through the city of Königsberg crossing each of its seven bridges only once [51]. Graph theory has subsequently become a mainstream activity in pure mathematics and the notion of a graph has a long history of applications in areas such as chemistry [65], physics [31], the social sciences [67] and computer science [43].

In the pre-digital era, the development of graph theory as an applied subject was hampered by the difficulty of obtaining and processing large data sets. A pioneering, and hugely influential, effort in the 1960s by the experimental psychologist Stanley Milgram [46] exploited the US postal service in an effort to understand important features of a large social acquaintance network, where nodes are people and edges connect those who know each other on a first name basis. One lasting consequence of Milgram's work is the "Six Degrees of Separation" principle, which has evolved into many different forms, but loosely conjectures that almost any pair of individuals in the world can be connected in at most six steps, where each step follows an acquaintanceship link.

Although the work of Milgram and many other notable social scientists laid the foundations for the study of real networks, it was not until the widespread availability of scientific computing resources that large-scale studies could be used to test

out ideas and refine them accordingly. Nowadays, in the era of high-throughput biological experiments, on-line trading information, smart-meter utility supplies and
pervasive telecommunications and surveillance technologies, we can store, manip-
ulate and compute with a plethora of network data sets, and visualize our results at
high resolution. Studying large, realistic networks, has given us the opportunity to
develop common concepts and tools, framed in a well-defined language. This has
led to the emerging discipline of *network science*, a field that is now represented
by its own conference series (NetSci) that has run each year since 2006, a number
of research monographs and lay science texts [10, 11, 63], and various highlighted
articles and special issues of magazines and journals [2, 6, 13, 36, 53, 54, 62].

The networks that we are now able to study are not only large, in many cases
they qualify for the more exotic title of *complex*. The field of *complexity science* has developed alongside network science, without enjoying the same clear-
cut set of principles. The Engineering and Physical Science Research Council—
the main UK government agency for funding research and training in engineering and the physical sciences—describes complexity science at its website
http://www.epsrc.ac.uk/about/progs/cdi/complex/Pages/whatwemean.aspx through
four principles, which we quote here:

Emergent properties Properties at system level consist of interaction-
induced co-operative emergence. Interacting components lead to hierarchical structures with different causations at different levels.
Adaptation A multiple-component system evolves and adapts as a consequence of internal and external dynamic interactions. The system keeps becoming a different system, and the demarcation between the system and its
surroundings evolves.
Many levels Complexity science bridges the gap between the individual and
the collective, for example, from psychology to sociology, from organism to
ecosystems, from genes to protein networks, from atoms to materials, from
the PC to the World Wide Web, and from citizens to society.
Feedback to manipulation When a multiple-component system is manipu-
lated, it reacts. The manipulator and the complex system inevitably become
entangled, for example, as a farmer harvests what he sows and cultivates.
Complexity research attempts to understand the sum of the multiple causes.

We emphasize here that, by definition, *emergent properties* are understood to be
neither predictable from nor reducible to the original elements of the complex system under investigation. Complexity is indeed different from complication. Complex is the opposite of independent, while complicated is the opposite of simple.

1.3 Complex Networks: Models and Algorithms

The modern era of network science was given a huge impetus by the publication in 1998 of an article by Watts and Strogatz [68]. This work, inspired by the efforts of Milgram [46] and others, contributed on at least three separate levels.

- It characterized the "small world phenomenom" as the combination of small *pathlength* (a typical pair of nodes can be connected by following relatively few edges) **and** a high *clustering coefficient* (if node A is connected to both nodes B and C, then it is very likely that B and C will also be connected).
- It measured a number of real life networks and showed that they exhibited the small world phenomenon.
- It demonstrated through computational experiments that the small world phenomenon can be created artificially by connecting nodes according to a simple set of rules.

Watts and Strogatz argued that real life networks do not coincide with two of the standard modelling paradigms:

(1) Completely random graphs [8, 15–17, 27], much studied by pure mathematicians, where either

  - for each pair of nodes, an edge is inserted according to the toss of a (possibly biased) coin, or
  - a graph with a prescribed number of nodes and edges is chosen uniformly at random from the collection of all such graphs.

  These classical random graphs can possess short typical pathlengths ($O(\log N)$ for a graph with N nodes) but do not have a high clustering coefficient.

(2) Regular lattices, where nodes are placed in a geometric pattern and connections are determined by geographical proximity. These graphs can have a high clustering coefficient but pathlengths will typically be long.

However, by combining elements of both model types—taking a lattice and adding extra links at random that offer opportunities for short-cuts—it was shown via computational experiments in [68] that the small world phenomenon can emerge.

The Watts–Strogatz article, which at the time of writing has over 9,500 citations on Google Scholar, led to a plethora of experiments where networks were measured and labelled as small worlds. Around the same time, Barabási and Albert [2] observed another seemingly universal network property. That work focused on the nodal *degree*; that is, the number of edges possessed by a node. Barabási and Albert found that networks typically display a power law relation, so that

$$\text{number of nodes with degree } k \propto k^{-\gamma},$$

where γ is a constant in the range $2 < \gamma < 3$. This is also referred to as a *scale free* degree distribution [10]. A consequence of this property is that very few nodes have high degree and very many have low degree—this effect has been likened to the *Pareto Principle*, or *80–20 rule*, according to which, for example, 80% of a nation's wealth lies in the hands of 20% of its population. Furthermore, Barabási and Albert showed that a scale-free network may be grown from an initial seed according to a *preferential attachment* or *rich-get-richer* process. New nodes are added one at a time, and each new node is connected into the network at random, but with a bias towards existing nodes of high degree. So new nodes tend to link to the popular nodes, which then become even more popular. With over 7,500 citations currently on Google Scholar, this work has been highly influential, with many subsequent studies discovering scale-free patterns. However, it should be noted that the complete universality of small world and scale free properties is now being called into question [39, 42, 61].

The models of Watts and Strogatz, Barabási and Albert, and related versions [56], have the benefit of simplicity, but they do not attempt to capture the fine details involved in any particular scenario. Other models have been proposed that assign links in a probabilistic manner. Some of these have been designed to mirror realistic features. Examples include

- *duplication/attachment/detachment models*, where evolutionary processes such as point mutation and gene duplication are incorporated into a model for protein interactions [7, 24, 66],
- *range-dependent random graphs*, where nodes are placed on a lattice and short-range edges are more likely than long-range [29, 30, 33, 41],
- *fitness or stickiness networks*, where nodes are assigned a value, and a connection is more likely between a pair of high-valued nodes [9, 60],
- *lock-and-key graphs*, where different types of locks and keys are assigned to nodes at random, and connections are made between matching lock-and-key pairs [50, 64],
- *geometric random graphs*, where nodes are strewn at random in Euclidean space and connected if they land close by [32, 44, 59, 61].

All such models inevitably possess parameters that must be calibrated against existing data in order to produce a useful explanatory and predictive tool. This type of parameter estimation can be extremely challenging, yet it forms only a sub-task of the easily posed yet deceptively tricky *model selection* problem: which of these generic random graph models best describes my particular network?

1.4 Complex Networks: Quantitative Features

In addition to the global issues of network modelling and comparison, many interesting questions may be asked at the local level. For example,

- Are there clusters of well-connected *communities* [23, 28]?
- Are there common subpatterns, sometimes called *motifs* or *graphlet signatures*, that form the basic building blocks of the network [3, 35, 45, 47]?
- Do some nodes or links have a key role in the network, forming *hubs*, *authorities* or having special *centrality* or *betweenness* [19, 20, 22, 23, 40, 55] and is the

network vulnerable to the removal of nodes or edges by *targeted* or *random attack* [37, 69]?

• Are there any special subpatterns of connectivity, such as *assortativity* where high-degree nodes tend to link to other high-degree nodes [5, 57] or *bipartivity* where two groups of nodes have weak inter-group but strong cross-group connectivity [18, 21, 34]?

Perhaps the most compelling application of this type of network analysis is the PageRank algorithm developed by Larry Page and Sergey Brin, co-founders of Google Inc., who were then Ph.D. students in computer science at Stanford University. This algorithm assigns a "centrality" or "importance" level to every page on the web by studying the overall structure of hyperlinks. The monthly Pageranking exercise, or *Google Dance*, has been dubbed *The World's Largest Matrix Computation* [49]. According to Google's Technology Department http://www.google.co.uk/intl/en_uk/technology/index.html

> "The heart of our software is PageRank, a system for ranking web pages ... And while we have dozens of engineers working to improve every aspect of Google on a daily basis, PageRank continues to provide the basis for all of our web search tools."

1.5 Complex Networks: Chapters in this Book

The invited chapters in this book cover a range of disciplines where concepts and tools from network science have begun to reveal their potential. The emphasis is on networks that arise in nature—including examples such as food webs, protein interactions, gene expression, and neural connections—and in technology—including examples such as finance, airline transport, urban development and global trade.

We commend these chapters as excellent markers for the state-of-the-art and pointers to future hot topics.

References

1. Albert, R., Barabási, A.L.: Topology of evolving networks: local events and universality. Phys. Rev. Lett. **85**(24), 5234–5237 (2000)
2. Albert, R., Barabási, A.L.: Statistical mechanics of complex networks. Rev. Mod. Phys. **74**, 47–97 (2002)
3. Alon, U.: An Introduction to Systems Biology. Chapman & Hall/CRC Press, London (2006)
4. Amann, A., Pokrovskiy, A., Osborne, S., O'Brien, S.: Complex networks based on discrete-mode lasers. J. Phys. Conf. Ser. **138**, 012001 (2008)
5. Badham, J., Stocker, R.: The impact of network clustering and assortativity on epidemic behaviour. Theor. Popul. Biol. **77**(1), 71–75 (2010)
6. Barabási, A.L., Oltvai, Z.N.: Network biology: Understanding the cell's functional organization. Nat. Rev. Genet. **5**, 101–113 (2004)
7. Berg, J., Lassig, M., Wagner, A.: Structure and evolution of protein interaction networks: A statistical model for link dynamics and gene duplications. BMC Evol. Biol. **4**, 51 (2004). arXiv:cond-mat/0207711

8. Bollobas, B.: Random Graphs. Academic Press, London (1985)
9. Caldarelli, G., Capocci, A., De Los Rios, P., Munõz, M.A.: Scale-free networks from varying vertex intrinsic fitness. Phys. Rev. Lett. **89**, 258702 (2002)
10. Caldarelli, G.: Scale-Free Networks: Complex Webs in Nature and Technology. Oxford Finance Series. Oxford University Press, Oxford (2007)
11. Christakis, N.A., Fowler, J.H.: Connected: The Surprising Power of Our Social Networks and How They Shape Our Lives. Little, Brown and Company, London (2009)
12. Conyon, M.J., Muldoon, M.R.: The small world of corporate boards. J. Bus. Finance Account. **33**, 1321–1343 (2006)
13. Durrani, M.: Complexity made simple. Phys. World **23**, 15 (2010). Special issue on complex affairs: Challenges in network science
14. Eagle, N., Pentland, A., Lazer, D.: Inferring social network structure using mobile phone data. Proc. Natl. Acad. Sci. USA **106**, 15274–15278 (2009)
15. Erdős, P., Rényi, A.: On random graphs. Publ. Math. **6**, 290–297 (1959)
16. Erdős, P., Rényi, A.: On the evolution of random graphs. Publ. Math. Inst. Hung. Acad. Sci. **5**, 17–61 (1960)
17. Erdős, P., Rényi, A.: On the strength of connectedness of a random graph. Acta Math. Acad. Sci. Hung. **12**, 261–267 (1961)
18. Estrada, E.: Protein bipartivity and essentiality in the yeast protein–protein interaction network. J. Proteome Res. **5**, 2177–2184 (2006)
19. Estrada, E., Hatano, N.: Statistical-mechanical approach to subgraph centrality in complex networks. Chem. Phys. Lett. **439**, 247–251 (2007)
20. Estrada, E., Rodríguez-Velázquez, J.A.: Subgraph centrality in complex networks. Phys. Rev. E **71**, 056103 (2005)
21. Estrada, E., Higham, D.J., Hatano, N.: Communicability and multipartite structures in complex networks at negative absolute temperatures. Phys. Rev. E **77**, 026102 (2008)
22. Estrada, E., Higham, D.J., Hatano, N.: Communicability betweenness in complex networks. Physica A **388**, 764–774 (2009)
23. Estrada, E., Hatano, N.: Communicability in complex networks. Phys. Rev. E **77**(3), 036111 (2008). doi:10.1103/PhysRevE.77.036111
24. Evlampiev, K., Isambert, H.: Modeling protein network evolution under genome duplication and domain shuffling. BMC Syst. Biol. **1**, 49 (2007)
25. Faloutsos, M., Faloutsos, P., Faloutsos, C.: On power-law relationships of the internet topology. Comput. Commun. Rev. **29**, 251–262 (1999)
26. Gautreau, A., Barrat, A., Barthelemy, M.: Microdynamics in stationary complex networks. Proc. Natl. Acad. Sci. USA **106**, 8847–8852 (2009)
27. Gilbert, E.N.: Random graphs. Ann. Math. Stat. **30**, 1141–1144 (1959)
28. Girvan, M., Newman, M.E.: Community structure in social and biological networks. Proc. Natl. Acad. Sci. USA **99**(12), 7821–7826 (2002)
29. Grindrod, P.: Range-dependent random graphs and their application to modeling large small-world proteome datasets. Phys. Rev. E **66**, 066702 (2002)
30. Grindrod, P., Higham, D.J., Kalna, G.: Periodic reordering. IMA J. Numer. Anal. **30**, 195–207 (2010)
31. Harary, F., Palmer, E.M.: Graph Theory and Theoretical Physics. Academic Press, New York (1968)
32. Higham, D.J., Rašajski, M., Pržulj, N.: Fitting a geometric graph to a protein–protein interaction network. Bioinformatics **24**(8), 1093–1099 (2008)
33. Higham, D.J.: Unravelling small world networks. J. Comput. Appl. Math. **158**, 61–74 (2003)
34. Holme, P., Liljeros, F., Edling, C.R., Kim, B.J.: Network bipartivity. Phys. Rev. E **68**, 056107 (2003)
35. Itzkovitz, S., Milo, R., Kashtan, N., Ziv, G., Alon, U.: Subgraphs in random networks. Phys. Rev. E **68**, 026127 (2003)
36. Jasny, B.R., Zahn, L., Marshall, E.: Connections. Science **325**, 405 (2009). Special issue on complex systems and networks

37. Jeong, H., Mason, S.P., Barabási, A.L., Oltvai, Z.N.: Lethality and centrality in protein networks. Nature **411**(6833), 41–42 (2001)
38. Kamper, L., Bozkurt, A., Rybacki, K., Geissler, A., Gerken, I., Stephan, K.E., Kötter, R.: An introduction to CoCoMac-Online. The online-interface of the primate connectivity database CoCoMac. In: Kötter, R. (ed.) Neuroscience Databases: A Practical Guide, pp. 155–169. Kluwer Academic, Norwell (2002)
39. Khanin, R., Wit, E.: How scale-free are gene networks? J. Comput. Biol. **13**(3), 810–818 (2006)
40. Kleinberg, J.: Authoritative sources in a hyper-linked environment. In: Proceedings of the 9th ACM Conference on Hypertext and Hypermedia. ACM Press, New York (1998)
41. Kleinberg, J.M.: Navigation in a small world. Nature **406**, 845 (2000)
42. Kleinfeld, J.S.: Could it be a big world after all? The 'six degrees of separation' myth. Society **39**, 61–66 (2002)
43. Knuth, D.E.: The Art of Computer Programming, Volume 4, Fascicle 4: Generating All Trees—History of Combinatorial Generation. Addison-Wesley, Reading (2006)
44. Kuchaiev, O., Rasajski, M., Higham, D., Pržulj, N.: Geometric de-noising of protein–protein interaction networks. PLoS Comput. Biol. **5**, 1000454 (2009)
45. Milenković, T., Pržulj, N.: Uncovering biological network function via graphlet degree signatures. Cancer Inform. **6**, 257–273 (2008)
46. Milgram, S.: The small world problem. Psychol. Today **2**, 60–67 (1967)
47. Milo, R., Shen-Orr, S.S., Itzkovitz, S., Kashtan, N., Chklovskii, D., Alon, U.: Network motifs: simple building blocks of complex networks. Science **298**, 824–827 (2002)
48. Min, H.-K., Hwang, C.-S.: Comparison on the high school girls' purchasing pattern of fashion products at online and offline markets. The Korean Society of Fashion Business **12**, 124–137 (2008)
49. Moler, C.: The world's largest matrix computation. MATLAB News and Notes (October 2002)
50. Morrison, J.L., Breitling, R., Higham, D.J., Gilbert, D.R.: A lock-and-key model for protein–protein interactions. Bioinformatics **2**, 2012–2019 (2006)
51. Newman, J.: Leonhard Euler and the Königsberg bridges. Sci. Am. **189**, 66–70 (1953)
52. Newman, M.E.: Scientific collaboration networks: I. network construction and fundamental results. Phys. Rev. E **64**, 016131 (2001)
53. Newman, M.E.J.: Models of the small world: a review. J. Stat. Phys. **101**, 819–841 (2000)
54. Newman, M.E.J.: The structure and function of complex networks. SIAM Rev. **45**(2), 167–256 (2003)
55. Newman, M.E.J.: A measure of betweenness centrality based on random walks. Soc. Netw. **27**, 39–54 (2005)
56. Newman, M.E.J., Moore, C., Watts, D.J.: Mean-field solution of the small-world network model. Phys. Rev. Lett. **84**, 3201–3204 (2000)
57. Newman, M.: Assortative mixing in networks. Phys. Rev. Lett. **89**, 208701 (2002)
58. Page, L., Brin, S., Motwani, R., Winograd, T.: The PageRank citation ranking: Bringing order to the web. Technical report, Stanford Digital Library Technologies Project (1998). http://www.citeseer.nj.nec.com/article/page98pagerank.html
59. Penrose, M.: Geometric Random Graphs. Oxford University Press, London (2003)
60. Pržulj, N., Higham, D.J.: Modelling protein–protein interaction networks via a stickiness index. J. R. Soc. Interface **3**, 711–716 (2006)
61. Pržulj, N., Corneil, D.G., Jurisica, I.: Modeling interactome: Scale-free or geometric? Bioinformatics **20**(18), 3508–3515 (2004)
62. Strogatz, S.H.: Exploring complex networks. Nature **410**, 268–276 (2001)
63. Strogatz, S.H.: SYNC: The Emerging Science of Spontaneous Order. Hyperion, New York (2003)
64. Thomas, A., Cannings, R., Monk, N.A.M., Cannings, C.: On the structure of protein–protein interaction networks. Biochem. Soc. Trans. **31**, 1491–1496 (2003)
65. Trinajstić, N.: Chemical Graph Theory. CRC Press, Boca Raton (1992)

66. Wagner, A.: How the global structure of protein interaction networks evolves. Proc. R. Soc. Lond. B, Biol. Sci. **270**, 457–466 (2003)
67. Wasserman, S., Faust, K.: Social Network Analysis. Cambridge University Press, Cambridge (1994)
68. Watts, D.J., Strogatz, S.H.: Collective dynamics of 'small-world' networks. Nature **393**, 440–442 (1998)
69. Ye, P., Peyser, B.D., Pan, X., Boeke, J.D., Spencer, F.A., Bader, J.S.: Gene function prediction from congruent synthetic lethal interactions in yeast. Mol. Syst. Biol. (2005). doi:10.1038/msb4100034

Chapter 2
Resistance Distance, Information Centrality, Node Vulnerability and Vibrations in Complex Networks

Ernesto Estrada and Naomichi Hatano

Abstract We discuss three seemingly unrelated quantities that have been introduced in different fields of science for complex networks. The three quantities are the resistance distance, the information centrality and the node displacement. We first prove various relations among them. Then we focus on the node displacement, showing its usefulness as an index of node vulnerability. We argue that the node displacement has a better resolution as a measure of node vulnerability than the degree and the information centrality.

2.1 Introduction

The study of complex networks is a truly multidisciplinary subject which covers many areas of nature, technology, and society [1, 27, 30]. These networks are graph-theoretic representations of complex systems in which the nodes of a graph represent the entities of the system and the links represent the relationship between them [1, 27, 30]. The use of the graphs for studying complex systems is not new. For instance, the study of social networks is a discipline with a long tradition of using graphs [19] and has provided many theoretical tools that are now used in the analysis of networks in many disciplines. In the physical sciences, graph analysis of relatively small systems has also been in use for long time. Some well known examples include the entire area of chemical graph theory [31] and the use of the graphs in

E. Estrada (✉)
Department of Mathematics and Statistics, University of Strathclyde, Glasgow, UK
e-mail: ernesto.estrada@strath.ac.uk

E. Estrada
Department of Physics, University of Strathclyde, Glasgow, UK

N. Hatano
Institute of Industrial Science, University of Tokyo, Tokyo 153-8505, Japan
e-mail: hatano@iis.u-tokyo.ac.jp

E. Estrada et al. (eds.), *Network Science*,
DOI 10.1007/978-1-84996-396-1_2, © Springer-Verlag London Limited 2010

statistical mechanics [20]. Then, it is not rare that concepts arising in one discipline are rediscovered and used in another with success. For instance, the concept of node centrality [18, 32], which arises in the study of social networks, is now widely used in the analysis of biological, ecological, and infrastructural networks [5, 7, 9, 11, 13, 21, 22]. Another example is given by the Wiener index, which was introduced in 1947 [34] and defined as the sum of the distances of all shortest paths in the graph representing hydrocarbon molecules. This index has proved to be useful in describing the boiling points and other physico-chemical properties of organic molecules [10]. The mean Wiener index is nowadays known as the average shortest-path distance and it has been instrumental in the definition of the concept of 'small-world' networks [33]. Here we are interested in analysing three concepts arising from different scientific disciplines, in the new context of complex networks. The first of these concepts is the resistance distance introduced in mathematical chemistry by Klein and Randić in 1993 [25] on the basis of electrical network theory. The resistance distance is defined as the effective resistance between two nodes in a graph when a battery is connected across them and the links are considered as unit resistors. The second concept is the information centrality developed by Stephenson and Zelen in 1989 [29], which tries to capture the information that can be transmitted between any two points in a connected network. The third, seemingly unrelated concept is the one of physical vibrations in a network [14, 15]. We consider the displacement of every node in a network due to vibrations/oscillations as a measure of the perturbations that are caused by external factors such as social agitation, economic crisis and physiological conditions. The main objective of this work is to show that these three seemingly unrelated concepts are mathematically connected. Then, we can consider the physically appealing concept of the node vibration as a fundamental concept for complex networks, which is useful in defining: (i) a topological metric, e.g. the resistance distance; (ii) a node centrality, e.g. the information centrality; and (iii) a measure of node vulnerability.

2.2 Resistance Distance in Networks

Let us associate a connected network with an electrical network in such a way that we replace each link of the network with a resistor of electrical resistance equal to one ohm. Then we can calculate the resistance Ω_{ij} between any pair of nodes i and j in the network by the Kirchhoff and Ohm laws. Such resistance is known to be a distance function [25] and called the resistance distance. It was introduced in a seminal paper by Klein and Randić a few years ago [25] and has been intensively studied in mathematical chemistry [14, 15, 25, 29, 35]. The Moore–Penrose generalised inverse (or the pseudo-inverse) $\mathbf{L}^+$ of the graph Laplacian $\mathbf{L}$, which has been proved to exist for any connected graph, gives the following formula [15, 25, 29] for computing the resistance distance:

$$\Omega_{ij} = \left(\mathbf{L}^+\right)_{ii} + \left(\mathbf{L}^+\right)_{jj} - \left(\mathbf{L}^+\right)_{ij} - \left(\mathbf{L}^+\right)_{ji} \qquad (2.1)$$

Fig. 2.1 Simple graph used
for illustration of the concepts
of the shortest path and the
resistance distance

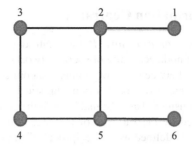

for $i \neq j$, where $\mathbf{L} = \mathbf{D} - \mathbf{A}$ with $\mathbf{D}$ the diagonal matrix of degrees k_i and $\mathbf{A}$ the adjacency matrix of the network.

Let $\mathbf{L}(i)$ be the matrix resulting from removing the ith row and column of the Laplacian and let $\mathbf{L}(i, j)$ the matrix resulting from removing both the ith and jth rows and columns of $\mathbf{L}$. Then, it has been proved that the resistance distance can be also calculated as

$$\Omega_{ij} = \frac{\det \mathbf{L}(i, j)}{\det \mathbf{L}(i)}. \tag{2.2}$$

The resistance matrix $\mathbf{\Omega}$ is the matrix whose non-diagonal elements are the resistance distance Ω_{ij} with the diagonal elements $\Omega_{ii} = 0$ [25]. In Fig. 2.1, we illustrate a simple graph having six nodes whose resistance distance matrix is given below. For the sake of comparison, we also give the topological-distance matrix in which the element d_{ij} is given by the number of links in the shortest path between the nodes i and j.

$$\mathbf{\Omega} = \begin{bmatrix} 0.00 & 1.00 & 1.75 & 2.00 & 1.75 & 2.75 \\ & 0.00 & 0.75 & 1.00 & 0.75 & 1.75 \\ & & 0.00 & 0.75 & 1.00 & 2.00 \\ & & & 0.00 & 0.75 & 1.75 \\ & & & & 0.00 & 1.00 \\ & & & & & 0.00 \end{bmatrix}, \quad \mathbf{D} = \begin{bmatrix} 0 & 1 & 2 & 3 & 2 & 3 \\ & 0 & 1 & 2 & 1 & 2 \\ & & 0 & 1 & 2 & 3 \\ & & & 0 & 1 & 2 \\ & & & & 0 & 1 \\ & & & & & 0 \end{bmatrix}.$$

It is straightforward to realise that for networks that contain no cycles, i.e. trees, both matrices coincide. However, the presence of cycles reduces the resistance distance in comparison with the topological distance. The semi-sum of all entries of the $\mathbf{D}$ matrix is known as the Wiener index $W(G)$. Then, the average path length $\bar{l}$ is given by $\bar{l} = 2W(G)/n(n-1)$. The analogue of the Wiener index in the context of the resistance distance matrix is known as the Kirchhoff index Kf and is defined as $Kf = \sum_{i<j} \Omega_{ij}$ [6, 25, 35, 36, 38]. It is known that Kf can be expressed in terms of the Laplacian eigenvalues as follows [35]:

$$Kf = n \sum_{j=2}^{n} \frac{1}{\lambda_j} = n \operatorname{Tr} \mathbf{L}^+. \tag{2.3}$$

The Wiener and Kirchhoff indices for the graph illustrated in Fig. 2.1 are 20.75 and 27, respectively.

2.3 Information Centrality

The *information centrality (IC)* was introduced by Stephenson and Zelen [29] as a measure of node centrality of social networks. It is based on information that can be transmitted between any two points in a connected network. The motivation for this measure comes from the theory of statistical estimation. Here a path connecting two nodes is considered as a "signal", while the "noise" in the transmission of the signal is measured by the variance of this signal. The information measure I_{ij} between two nodes is defined as the reciprocal of the topological distance d_{ij} between the corresponding nodes, $I_{ij} = 1/d_{ij}$. Stephenson and Zelen [29] proposed to define I_{ii} as infinite for computational purposes, which makes $1/I_{ii} = 0$. The information centrality of the node i is then defined by using the harmonic average:

$$IC(i) = \left[\frac{1}{n} \sum_j \frac{1}{I_{ij}} \right]^{-1}. \tag{2.4}$$

If $\mathbf{A}$ is the adjacency matrix of a network, $\mathbf{D}$ a diagonal matrix of the degree of each node and $\mathbf{J}$ a matrix with all its elements equal to one, then IC is defined by inverting the matrix $\mathbf{B} \equiv \mathbf{D} - \mathbf{A} + \mathbf{J} = \mathbf{L} + \mathbf{J}$, from which the information matrix is obtained as follows:

$$I_{ij}^{-1} = \left(\mathbf{B}^{-1} \right)_{ii} + \left(\mathbf{B}^{-1} \right)_{jj} - 2 \left(\mathbf{B}^{-1} \right)_{ij}. \tag{2.5}$$

The information centrality for the nodes of the graph illustrated in Fig. 2.1 is $IC(1) = IC(6) = 0.649$, $IC(2) = IC(5) = 1.143$ and $IC3 = IC(4) = 0.960$.

2.4 Vibrations in Complex Networks

We now introduce a recently proposed measure of node vulnerability, namely the node displacement [14, 15]. For the purpose, we regard the nodes of the complex network as balls of a common mass and the links as springs of a common spring constant k. We immerse this system of balls and springs in a thermal bath of inverse temperature β and observe the amplitude of thermal fluctuation of each ball. The thermal bath simulates an external stress to the network, such as economical crisis, social agitation, environmental pressure or physiological conditions. The amplitude of thermal fluctuation of a ball tells us how vulnerable the corresponding node is to such stresses.

The vibrational potential energy of the network can be expressed as

$$V(\mathbf{x}) = \frac{k}{2} \mathbf{x}^T \mathbf{L} \mathbf{x}, \tag{2.6}$$

where the ith component x_i of the vector $\mathbf{x}$ denotes the displacement of the node i from its static position due to thermal fluctuation and $\mathbf{L}$ is the same graph Laplacian as used in (2.1). The probability distribution of the displacement of the nodes may be given by the Boltzmann distribution according to the potential energy:

$$P(\mathbf{x}) = \frac{e^{-\beta V(\mathbf{x})}}{Z} = \frac{1}{Z} \exp\left(-\frac{\beta k}{2} \mathbf{x}^T \mathbf{L} \mathbf{x} \right), \tag{2.7}$$

where Z is the partition function of the network:

$$Z \equiv \int d\mathbf{x} \exp\left(-\frac{\beta k}{2} \mathbf{x}^T \mathbf{L} \mathbf{x}\right). \tag{2.8}$$

The mean square displacement of a node i is given by

$$(\Delta x_i)^2 \equiv \langle x_i^2 \rangle = \int x_i^2 P(\mathbf{x}) \, d\mathbf{x} \tag{2.9}$$

and the correlation between the displacements of nodes i and j is given by

$$\langle x_i x \rangle_j = \int x_i x_j P(\mathbf{x}) \, d\mathbf{x}, \tag{2.10}$$

where $\langle \cdots \rangle$ denotes the average with respect to $P(\mathbf{x})$.

We can calculate these quantities by diagonalising the graph Laplacian $\mathbf{L}$. Here we should take care of the fact that the Laplacian of a connected network has a spectrum of the form $0 = \lambda_1 \leq \cdots \leq \lambda_n$; i.e. it has one zero eigenvalue apart from positive eigenvalues. In fact, we should not let the zero eigenvalue contribute in the calculation because the mode $\mu = 1$ represents the motion of the centre of mass and hence its vibrational energy is zero; see [14, 15] for details of the calculation. Here we simply list the results of the calculation. We can represent the results in the following unified form [14, 15]:

$$\langle x_i x \rangle_j = \sum_{\mu=2}^{n} \frac{(\boldsymbol{\psi}_\mu)_i (\boldsymbol{\psi}_\mu)_j}{\beta k \lambda_v} = \frac{1}{\beta k} \left(\mathbf{L}^+\right)_{ij}, \tag{2.11}$$

where $\boldsymbol{\psi}_\mu$ is the eigenvector of the mode μ and $\mathbf{L}^+$ is again the Moore–Penrose generalised inverse of the graph Laplacian [35]. The case $i = j$ gives the mean square displacement $(\Delta x_i)^2 \equiv \langle x_i^2 \rangle$ in (2.11). This quantity is obviously related to the resistance distance defined by (2.11), which we will elucidate in the next section. Meanwhile, (2.11) is followed by the thermal average of the vibrational potential energy (2.6) in the form

$$\langle V(\mathbf{x}) \rangle = \frac{1}{2} \sum_{i=1}^{n} k_i \langle x_i^2 \rangle - \sum_{i,j \in E} \langle x_i x_j \rangle = \frac{1}{\beta k} \sum_{i=1}^{n} k_i \left(\mathbf{L}^+\right)_{ii} - \sum_{i,j \in E} \left(\mathbf{L}^+\right)_{ij}. \tag{2.12}$$

2.5 Node Displacements and Resistance Distance

Hereafter we set $\beta k \equiv 1$ for simplicity. By using (2.11) in (2.1), we have

$$\Omega_{ij} = \left[\langle x_i^2 \rangle + \langle x_j^2 \rangle - \langle x_i x_j \rangle - \langle x_j x_i \rangle\right] = \langle (x_i - x_j)^2 \rangle. \tag{2.13}$$

Roughly speaking, the right-hand side of (2.13) is small if the nodes i and j vibrate coherently in the same direction and large if they move in the opposite directions.

More rigorously, let us focus on the mode $\mu = 2$ of the graph Laplacian $\mathbf{L}$. Then the corresponding eigenvector $\boldsymbol{\psi}_2$ is called the Fiedler vector [17]. This vector is known to define a partitioning of the graph [17] in the following way. The nodes of a graph are partitioned into two sets $V_1 = \{i | (\boldsymbol{\psi}_2)_i < 0\}$ and $V_2 = \{i | (\boldsymbol{\psi}_2)_i \geq 0\}$. Therefore, two nodes in the same partition according to the Fiedler vector vibrate in the same direction and ones in different partitions vibrate in the opposite directions, when we restrict ourselves to the mode $\mu = 2$. Then, (2.13) gives us a plausible observation that two nodes i and j that are close in terms of the resistance distance Ω_{ij} tend to be in the same partition of the Fiedler vector, whereas ones that are far tend to be in different partitions.

We can also express the Kirchhoff index defined by (2.3) in terms of the node displacements as

$$Kf = n \sum_{i=1}^{n} (\Delta x_i)^2 = n^2 \overline{(\Delta x)^2}, \qquad (2.14)$$

where the bar on the right-hand side denotes the average over the nodes. Equation (2.14) tells us that the Kirchhoff index of a molecular graph is proportional to the sum of the squared atomic displacements due to molecular vibrations. Since the Kirchhoff and Wiener indices are known to coincide for acyclic networks, i.e. trees, we also have

$$W(T) = n \sum_{i=1}^{n} (\Delta x_i)^2 = n^2 \overline{(\Delta x)^2}. \qquad (2.15)$$

We now consider the average potential energy in (2.12). For this purpose, let us calculate the quantity

$$R_i = \sum_{j=1}^{n} \Omega_{ij}, \qquad (2.16)$$

the sum of all resistance distances from atom i to any atoms in the molecule. By combining expression (2.1) with the general fact $\sum_{j=1}^{n} (\mathbf{L}^+)_{ij} = 0$, we have

$$R_i = n (\mathbf{L}^+)_{ii} + \mathrm{Tr}\,\mathbf{L}^+ = n(\Delta x_i)^2 + n\overline{(\Delta x)^2} = n(\Delta x_i)^2 + \frac{Kf}{n}. \qquad (2.17)$$

This shows that $(\Delta x_i)^2$ and R_i are linearly related for all nodes of a given network. Using then (2.13), we also have

$$\Omega_{ij} = \frac{R_i + R_j}{n} - 2\frac{Kf}{n^2} - 2\langle x_i x_j \rangle. \qquad (2.18)$$

The average potential energy is then given by

$$\langle V(\mathbf{x}) \rangle = \frac{1}{2n} \sum_{i=1}^{n} k_i R_i - \frac{1}{2n} \sum_{i,j \in E} (R_i + R_j - n\Omega_{ij}). \qquad (2.19)$$

The first term on the right-hand side of (2.19) was first introduced by Estrada et al. [16] as a topological index for trees obtained from the quadratic form $\langle \mathbf{v} | \mathbf{D} | \mathbf{u} \rangle$, where $\mathbf{v}$ is a vector of node degrees, $\mathbf{D}$ is the distance matrix and $\mathbf{u}$ is a vector of ones of length equal to the number of nodes in the graph.

2.6 Node Displacement and Information Centrality

In the present section, we explore the relation between the node displacement and the information centrality (2.4). Let us first prove that the inverse of $\mathbf{B} = \mathbf{L} + \mathbf{J}$ exists and is given by

$$\mathbf{B}^{-1} = \mathbf{L}^{+} + \frac{1}{n^2}\mathbf{J}. \tag{2.20}$$

Let $\boldsymbol{\psi}_\mu$ denote the μth eigenvector of the graph Laplacian $\mathbf{L}$, which has the spectrum $0 = \lambda_1 < \lambda_2 \leq \cdots \leq \lambda_n$ for a connected network. Note here that $\boldsymbol{\psi}_1 = \frac{1}{\sqrt{n}}\mathbf{1}$. For $\mu \neq 1$, we have

$$\mathbf{B}\boldsymbol{\psi}_\mu = \mathbf{L}\boldsymbol{\psi}_\mu + \mathbf{J}\boldsymbol{\psi}_\mu = \mathbf{L}\boldsymbol{\psi}_\mu = \lambda_\mu \boldsymbol{\psi}_\mu \tag{2.21}$$

because

$$(\mathbf{J}\boldsymbol{\psi}_\mu)_j = \sum_{i=1}^{n}(\boldsymbol{\psi}_\mu)_i = \sqrt{n}\boldsymbol{\psi}_1 \cdot \boldsymbol{\psi}_\mu = 0 \quad \text{for } \mu \neq 1.$$

For $\mu = 1$, we have

$$\mathbf{B}\boldsymbol{\psi}_1 = \mathbf{L}\boldsymbol{\psi}_1 + \mathbf{J}\boldsymbol{\psi}_1 = n\boldsymbol{\psi}_1. \tag{2.22}$$

The above means that the eigenvalues of the matrix $\mathbf{B}$ are $n, \lambda_2, \lambda_3, \ldots, \lambda_n$, which are all positive. The matrix $\mathbf{B}$ is thereby invertible. Indeed, we can confirm (2.20) as

$$(\mathbf{L} + \mathbf{J})\left(\mathbf{L}^{+} + \frac{1}{n^2}\mathbf{J}\right) = \mathbf{I} - \frac{1}{n}\mathbf{J} + \frac{n\mathbf{J}}{n^2} = \mathbf{I}, \tag{2.23}$$

because $\mathbf{L}\mathbf{L}^{+} = \mathbf{L}^{+}\mathbf{L} = \mathbf{I} - \frac{1}{n}\mathbf{J}$, $\mathbf{L}\mathbf{J} = \mathbf{J}\mathbf{L} = \mathbf{L}^{+}\mathbf{J} = \mathbf{J}\mathbf{L}^{+} = 0$, and $\mathbf{J}^2 = n\mathbf{J}$. This proves that the matrix in (2.20) is the inverse of $\mathbf{B}$.

Equation (2.20) then transforms (2.5) into the form

$$I_{ij}^{-1} = (\mathbf{B}^{-1})_{ii} + (\mathbf{B}^{-1})_{jj} - 2(\mathbf{B}^{-1})_{ij} = (\mathbf{L}^{+})_{ii} + (\mathbf{L}^{+})_{jj} - 2(\mathbf{L}^{+})_{ij} = \Omega_{ij}. \tag{2.24}$$

Therefore, the information centrality (2.4) is now given by

$$IC(i) = \left(\frac{1}{n}\sum_j \frac{1}{I_{ij}}\right)^{-1} = \left(\frac{1}{n}\sum_j \Omega_{ij}\right)^{-1} = \frac{n}{R_i} = ((\Delta x_i)^2 + \overline{(\Delta x)^2})^{-1}. \tag{2.25}$$

2.7 Node Displacement as a Measure of Node Vulnerability

Most of the studies on vulnerability of complex networks consider how resilient the whole network is to random failures and intentional attacks. In these studies, it is assumed that we can attack any node by simply removing it from the graph. The primary removal of these nodes can give rise to the secondary disconnection of other nodes from the main connected component of the network. The most resilient network is the one that, after many removals, still keeps the functioning size of the main connected component.

Here we are interested in the vulnerability of a node rather than the vulnerability of the whole network to targeted attacks. Intuitively, a node is highly vulnerable if there are many other nodes whose individual removal disconnects the node in question from the main connected component of the network. The information centrality $IC(i)$ can be an index of the node vulnerability; we may be able to say that a node i with a larger information centrality is less vulnerable. The resistance distance can provide an equivalent index; as was shown in the previous section, the quantity R_i is inversely proportional to the information centrality. Hereafter, we will suggest that the node displacement Δx_i can be another index of the vulnerability and actually has a better resolution than the information centrality.

Let us first explain in terms of the Fiedler vector why the node displacement can measure the node vulnerability. Recall that we have ordered the eigenvalues of the Laplacian as $0 = \lambda_1 < \lambda_2 \leq \cdots \leq \lambda_n$. The eigenvector of the second mode (the first non-zero mode) is the Fiedler vector [17]. Let us consider the particular case $\lambda_2 < \lambda_3$. Then (2.11) implies that the term $(\psi_2)_i^2/\lambda_2$ of the Fiedler vector has the largest contribution to Δx_i. Among the nodes, a node with $(\psi_2)_i$ close to zero does not strongly belong to either of the two partitions V_1 and V_2 defined by the Fiedler vector. Such nodes are located in between the partitions; in other words, they tend to have ties with many other nodes and hence may be less vulnerable to external stresses. Then a small value of $(\psi_2)_i^2/\lambda_2$ can indeed indicate little node vulnerability.

In the seminal paper by Albert, Jeong and Barabási [2], they chose the nodes with the highest degree for their targets of the primary removals. This is based on an empirical observation that the nodes with the lowest degree are the most vulnerable. Consider the case where a node i has only one connection, i.e. $K_i = 1$. Then, we can isolate it from the network by removing the node to which i is connected. A measure of the node vulnerability in complex networks should be consistent in some way with the above observation that low-degree nodes are more vulnerable than high-degree ones. As we discussed above, the term $(\psi_2)_i^2/\lambda_2$ indeed has such a property.

In fact, the node displacement (2.11) takes account of the higher modes, too. As the Fiedler vector defines a bipartition of the network, the eigenvectors of higher modes can define partitions into a larger number of groups. These partitions may identify the clusters and the nodes in between them in a more appropriate way. The use of the eigenvectors of higher modes also helps avoiding the problem that can arise when $\lambda_2 = \lambda_3$. This degeneracy can happen in square grids and complete graphs, for example. In this degenerate case, it has been reported that the convergence of partitioning algorithms can be poor.

Let us demonstrate that the node displacement can be indeed a measure of the node vulnerability in the sense that it tends to give higher vulnerability to low-degree nodes than to high-degree nodes. For the purpose, we use the trade network of miscellaneous manufactures of metal (MMM) among 80 countries in 1994. The data was compiled by de Nooy [8] and the reader is refereed to this work to obtain

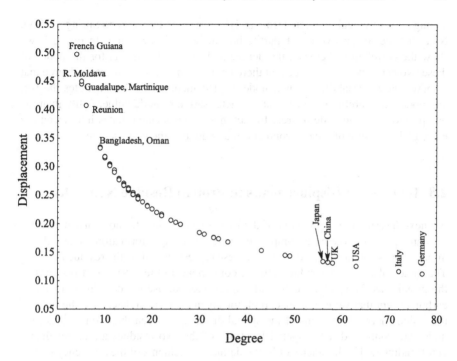

Fig. 2.2 Illustration of the relationship between the node displacement and the node degree for the trade network of miscellaneous manufactures of metal among 80 countries in 1994

the details of this dataset. We consider here only the undirected and unweighted version of this network. Here, the nodes represent the countries and a link exists between two countries if one of them imports MMM from the other.

We show in Fig. 2.2 the relation between the node degree and the node displacement for the above trade network. The node displacement decreases with the node degree under a power law. Interestingly, the countries with the largest node displacements are mostly the poorest countries in the network, whereas the richest countries are among the ones with the smallest node displacements. Choosing the node displacement as a measure of the node vulnerability, we can say that the poorest countries are the most vulnerable to changes in economical situations such as a financial crisis.

Having said this, we emphasise here that the node degree accounts only for the nearest neighbours of a node. In other words, the influence of more distant nodes is not taken into account if we use the node degree as a measure of the node vulnerability. This can be seen in the fact that many networks have several nodes with the same degree but with different values of the node displacement.

For an illustrative example, let us study two networks of sexual contacts collected by Lind et al. [26]. One of them is composed solely of heterosexual contacts among 82 people, which was extracted from the Cadham Provincial Laboratory during a period of six months. The other is formed by sexual contacts (mainly homosexual) among 250 individuals collected from an HIV test study in Colorado Springs (USA). Note that the first network is bipartite but the second one is not. In Fig. 2.3, we show the correlations between the degree and the displacements for the nodes of these two networks. We can see that there are many nodes with the same degree that display a large variability of their node displacements. This demonstrates the fact that node vulnerability is a different characterisation of node vulnerability than the one provided by the node degree. In fact, node displacement takes into account a more global picture of the environment of a node than the node degree.

2.8 Topological Displacements in Protein Residue Networks

We next describe the application of the node displacement to molecular networks. We can represent proteins as complex networks by using information on their three-dimensional structures. One example of these representations is the residue network. The nodes of a spatial residue network correspond to the amino acid residues of the protein; as the spatial location of the residue, we use the coordinate of its β-carbon except that we use the α-carbon for glycine. We then determine the links of the residue network in terms of the spatial distance between the two residues; two nodes are connected if the spatial locations of the two residues are closer than a cutoff radius r_C [3]. In other words, we define the elements of the adjacency matrix of the residue network as

$$A_{ij} = \begin{cases} \Theta(r_C - r_{ij}) & \text{for } i \neq j, \\ 0 & \text{for } i = j, \end{cases}$$

where $\Theta(x > 0) = 1$ and $\Theta(x \leq 0) = 0$. We can thus represent a protein as a graph $G = (V, E)$, where V is the set of the amino acid residues and E is the set of the connections between them. The residue network of the protein with PDB code 1ash, for example, is shown in Fig. 2.4 [3, 12].

It is then natural to suppose that the node displacement Δx_i calculated for a node of the residue network displays linear correlation with an experimental measure of how much a residue oscillates or vibrates around its equilibrium position. One such experimental measure is the B-factor, or the temperature factor provided by X-ray experiments. It represents the reduction of coherent scattering of X-rays due to thermal motion of the atoms.

The B-factors are important for the study of protein structures as they contain valuable information on the dynamical behaviour of proteins. Several methods have been designed for the prediction of the B-factors [28]. Regions with large B-factors are known to be flexible and functionally important. Bahar et al. have used the atomic displacements to describe thermal fluctuations in proteins [4]. Note that we use here Bahar et al.'s representation of a residue network in the sense that we use the β-carbons instead of the α-carbon for the spatial locations of the amino acids.

In Fig. 2.5, we show the profiles of the normalised B-factors and the node displacements of the residue networks for the spinach ferredoxin reductase (top) at 1.7 angstroms resolution (1fnc) and for the human uracil-DNA glycosylase (1akz) at

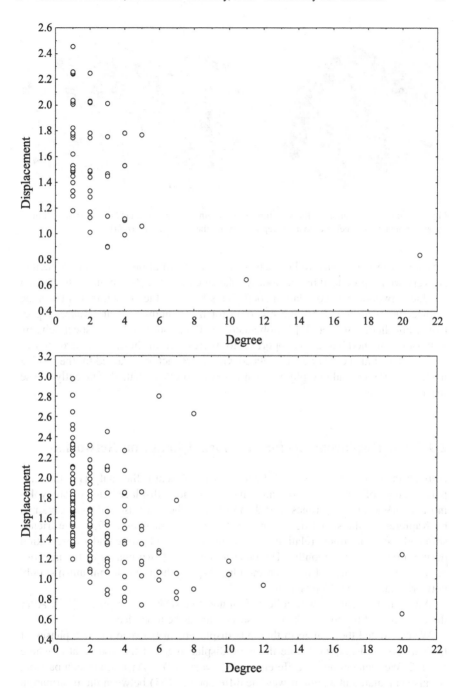

Fig. 2.3 Illustration of the relationship between the node displacement and the node degree for two networks of sexual contacts. (*Top*) A network formed solely by heterosexual contacts. (*Bottom*) Network of sexual contacts (mainly homosexual) among 250 individuals in Colorado Springs (USA)

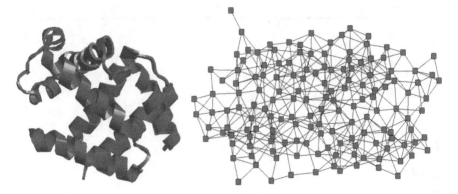

Fig. 2.4 3D representation of the structure of a protein (*left*) and the network representation of physical contacts between amino acids represented by their β-carbons (*right*)

1.57 angstroms (bottom). In both cases, the experimental profiles of the B-factors are very well reproduced by the node displacements of the β-carbons in the protein residue networks. The correlation coefficients between the B-factors and the node displacements are $r = 0.56$ and $r = 0.65$ for the proteins 1fnc and 1akz, respectively. For them, Yuan et al. [37] obtained $r = 0.48$ and $r = 0.72$, respectively, by a statistical method based on support vector regression. In short, the node displacements of a residue network are correlated with the B-factors obtained for the residue itself by X-ray crystallography in a similar way to other methods currently in use for this purpose.

2.9 Node Displacements for Temporal Change on Networks

Another interesting application of the node displacement is the analysis of the temporal change of a network. We can compare the node displacements of an evolving network at different times. For demonstration, here we use a dataset obtained by Kapferer for the social ties among 39 tailor shops in Zambia [23]. The friendship and socio-emotional relationship among the 39 tailors were under observation during a period of ten months. The dataset consists of two phases of the network recorded with an interval of seven months [23]; see http://vlado.fmf.uni-lj.si/pub/networks/data/Ucinet/UciData.htm.

After the first dataset was collected an abortive strike was reported [23]. After the collection of the second dataset, a successful strike took place.

We calculated the change in the node displacement between the two phases of the network. Let $\Delta x_i(t)$ denote the node displacement of the node i at t, where $t = 1, 2$. We then define the difference $\Delta\Delta x_i = \Delta x_i(2) - \Delta x_i(1)$. For comparison, we also calculated in a similar way the difference $\Delta IC(i)$ between the information centralities of the node i at the two phases.

In order to analyse the differences in the ranking of nodes in terms of $\Delta\Delta x_i$ and $\Delta IC(i)$, we use a nonparametric measure of correlation known as the *Kendall*

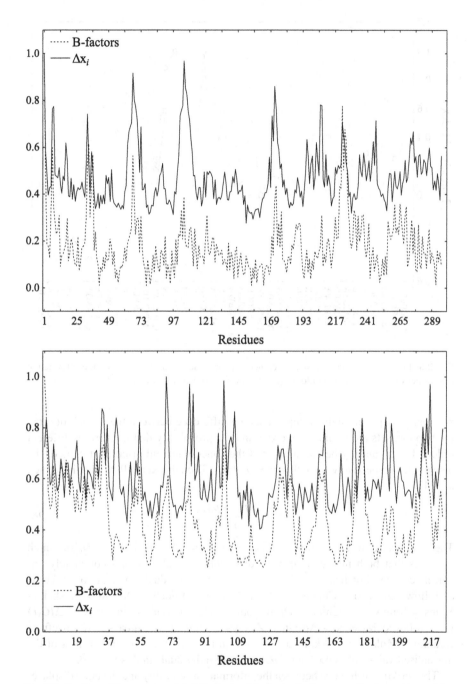

Fig. 2.5 Profiles of the experimental B-factors and the node displacements for the residues of the spinach ferredoxin reductase, PDB: 1fnc, (*top*) and for the human uracil-DNA glycosylase, PDB: 1akz, (*bottom*) represented by their residue networks

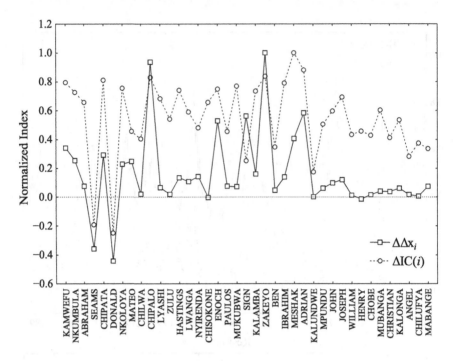

Fig. 2.6 Profiles of the normalised differences of the nodes displacements and the information centralities of the nodes in the tailor shop network observed at two different times

τ statistic [24]. This statistic represents the difference between the probability that the two datasets are in the same order and the probability that they are in different orders. Let p_c and p_d be the number of the concordant and discordant pairs of the data points, respectively, such that $p = p_c + p_d$. Then the Kendall τ index is defined as [24]

$$\tau = \frac{2(p_c - p_d)}{p(p-1)}. \tag{2.26}$$

The nonparametric correlation between $\Delta\Delta x_i$ and $\Delta IC(i)$ is $\tau = -0.56$, which indicates that both indices rank very differently and almost in a completely un-correlated way. For instance, the ranking of top individuals in terms of $\Delta\Delta x_i$ is as follows: Zakeyo > Chipalo > Adrian > Sign > Enoch > Donald > Meshak > Seans > Kamwefu > Chipata. On the other hand, the ranking in terms of $\Delta IC(i)$ is as follows: Meshak > Adrian > Zakeyo > Chipalo > Chipata > Kamwefu > Ibrahim > Mukubwa > Nkoloya > Enoch. In Fig. 2.6, we show the profiles of the normalised values of $\Delta\Delta x_i$ and $\Delta IC(i)$ for all individuals in this network.

This striking difference between the information centrality and the node displacement can be traced back to (2.25). It tells us that an increase in the information centrality of a node can have two origins: a decrease in the local node displacement $(\Delta x_i)^2$ or a decrease in the global (average) node displacement $\overline{(\Delta x)^2}$ (or both).

More detailed analysis of the two rankings of the nodes tells us that for most nodes, the increase of the information centrality is caused by the decrease of the global node displacement, not by the local one. Many tailors had many social ties and were not very vulnerable in the first place. Their information centrality increased after the seven months mostly because the number of the links generally increased all over the network; on the other hand, their local node displacement (the vulnerability of each tailor) scarcely changed. For tailors such as Zakeyo and Chipalo, however, their local node displacements decreased greatly after the seven months because their own degrees increased dramatically. This demonstrates clearly that the node displacement has a better resolution of the time evolution than the information centrality.

In summary, despite the relation (2.25) between the information centrality and the node displacement, there is a fundamental difference between them. The information centrality can be seen as a composite index containing local information of a node as well as global topological information of the network, whereas with the node displacement we can separate it into the local information as $(\Delta x_i)^2$ and the global one as $\overline{(\Delta x)^2}$. This difference is very relevant when comparing nodes in different networks.

2.10 Outlook

It is a well known fact that there are several common features between very disparate complex systems arising in non-related areas of nature, society or technology. When these systems are represented by complex networks, some of these features are well documented in the scientific literature [1, 27, 30]. In order to discover these universal features, we need to carry out cross-comparative analysis of complex systems and their behaviours by using appropriate mathematical tools and physical concepts. Here we have introduced the concept of the node displacement as a measure of vulnerability of each node in a network. It is defined in terms of the amplitude of vibration caused by thermal fluctuation of a heat bath in which the network is immersed. This physical analogy simulates the situation in which the network in question is under a level of external stress. It is interesting that this fundamental physical concept is related to graph-theoretic invariants previously developed and used in very different scientific disciplines like Chemistry and Social Sciences. In this sense, we have seen in practise the unifying nature of physico-mathematical concepts across the boundaries of many disciplines. Then, we hope that this work contributes to the interdisciplinary search of more universal properties of complex systems that permit a better understanding of their structure and dynamics.

References

1. Albert, R., Barabási, A.L.: Statistical mechanics of complex networks. Rev. Mod. Phys. **74**, 47–97 (2002)

2. Albert, R., Jeong, H., Barabási, A.L.: Error and attack tolerance of complex networks. Nature **406**, 378–382 (2000)
3. Atilgan, A.R., Akan, P., Baysal, C.: Small-world communication of residues and significance for protein dynamics. Biophys. J. **86**, 85–91 (2004)
4. Bahar, I., Atilgan, A.R., Erman, B.: Direct evaluation of thermal fluctuations in proteins using a single-parameter harmonic potential. Fold. Des. **2**, 173–181 (1997)
5. Barthelemy, M., Barrat, A., Vespignani, A.: The role of geography and traffic in the structure of complex networks. Adv. Complex Syst. **10**, 5–28 (2007)
6. Chen, H.Y., Zhang, F.J.: Resistance distance and the normalized Laplacian spectrum. Discrete Appl. Math. **155**, 654–661 (2007)
7. Choi, J., Barnett, G., Chou, B.: Comparing world city networks: a network analysis of Internet backbone and air transport intercity linkages. Glob. Netw. **6**, 81–99 (2006)
8. de Nooy, W., Mrvar, A., Batagelj, V.: Exploratory Social Network Analysis with Pajek. Cambridge University Press, Cambridge (2005)
9. del Rio, G., Koschutzki, D., Coello, G.: How to identify essential genes from molecular networks? BMC Syst. Biol. (2009). doi:10.1186/1752-0509-3-102
10. Dobrynin, A.A., Entringer, R., Gutman, I.: Wiener index of trees: Theory and applications. Acta Appl. Math. **66**, 211–249 (2001)
11. Estrada, E.: Virtual identification of essential proteins within the protein interaction network of yeast. Proteomics **6**, 35–40 (2006)
12. Estrada, E.: Universality in protein residue networks. Biophys. J. **98**, 890–900 (2010)
13. Estrada, E., Bodin, O.: Using network centrality measures to manage landscape connectivity. a short path for assessing habitat patch importance. Ecol. Appl. **18**, 1810–1825 (2008)
14. Estrada, E., Hatano, N.: A vibrational approach to node centrality and vulnerability in complex networks. arXiv:0912.4307
15. Estrada, E., Hatano, N.: Topological atomic displacements, Kirchhoff and Wiener indices of molecules. Chem. Phys. Lett. **486**, 166–170 (2010)
16. Estrada, E., Rodríguez, L., Gutiérrez, A.: Matrix algebraic manipulations of molecular graphs. 1. graph theoretical invariants based on distances and adjacency matrices. MATCH Commun. Math. Comput. Chem. **35**, 145–156 (1997)
17. Fiedler, M.: Algebraic connectivity of graphs. Czechoslov. Math. J. **23**, 298–305 (1973)
18. Freeman, L.C.: A set of measures of centrality based upon betweenness. Sociometry **40**, 35–41 (1977)
19. Freeman, L.C.: The Development of Social Network Analysis. Empirical Press, Vancouver (2004)
20. Harary, F. (ed.): Graph Theory and Theoretical Physics. Academic Press, London (1967)
21. Jeong, H., Mason, S.P., Barabási, A.L., Oltvai, Z.N.: Lethality and centrality in protein networks. Nature **411**(6833), 41–42 (2001)
22. Jordán, F.: Keystone species and food webs. Philos. Trans. R. Soc. Lond. B, Biol. Sci. **364**, 1733–1741 (2009)
23. Kapferer, B.: Strategy and Transaction in an African Factory. Manchester University Press, Manchester (1972)
24. Kendall, M.: A new measure of rank correlation. Biometrika **30**, 81–89 (1938)
25. Klein, D., Randić, M.: Resistance distance. J. Math. Chem. **12**, 81–95 (1993)
26. Lind, P., González, M., Herrmann, H.: Cycles and clustering in bipartite networks. Phys. Rev. E **72**, 056127 (2005)
27. Newman, M.E.J.: The structure and function of complex networks. SIAM Rev. **45**(2), 167–256 (2003)
28. Soheilifard, R., Makarov, D., Rodin, G.: Critical evaluation of simple network models of protein dynamics and their comparison with crystallographic B-factors. Phys. Biol. **5**, 1–13 (2008)
29. Stephenson, K., Zelen, M.: Rethinking centrality: methods and examples. Soc. Netw. **11**, 1–37 (1989)
30. Strogatz, S.H.: Exploring complex networks. Nature **410**, 268–276 (2001)

31. Trinajstić, N.: Chemical Graph Theory. CRC Press, Boca Raton (1992)
32. Wasserman, S., Faust, K.: Social Network Analysis. Cambridge University Press, Cambridge (1994)
33. Watts, D.J., Strogatz, S.H.: Collective dynamics of 'small-world' networks. Nature **393**, 440–442 (1998)
34. Wiener, H.: Structural determination of paraffin boiling points. J. Am. Chem. Soc. **69**, 17–20 (1947)
35. Xiao, W., Gutman, I.: Resistance distance and Laplacian spectrum. Theor. Chem. Acc. **110**, 284–289 (2003)
36. Yang, Y.J., Zhang, H.P.: Some rules on resistance distance with applications. J. Phys. A, Math. Theor. **41**, 445203 (2008)
37. Yuan, Z., Bailey, T., Teasdale, R.: Prediction of protein B-factor profiles. Proteins **58**, 905–912 (2005)
38. Zhou, B., Trinajstić, N.: On resistance distance and Kirchhoff index. J. Math. Chem. **46**, 283–289 (2009)

Chapter 3
From Topology to Phenotype in Protein–Protein Interaction Networks

Nataša Pržulj

Abstract   We have recently witnessed an explosion in biological network data along with the development of computational approaches for their analyses. This new interdisciplinary research area is an integral part of systems biology, promising to provide new insights into organizational principles of life, as well as into evolution and disease. However, there is a danger that the area might become hindered by several emerging issues. In particular, there is typically a weak link between biological and computational scientists, resulting in the use of simple computational techniques of limited potential to explain these complex biological data. Hence, there is a danger that the community might view the topological features of network data as mere statistics, ignoring the value of the information contained in these data. This might result in the imposition of scientific doctrines, such as scale-free-centric (on the modelling side) and genome-centric (on the biological side) opinions onto this nascent research area. In this chapter, we take a network science perspective and present a brief, high-level overview of the area, commenting on possible challenges ahead. We focus on protein–protein interaction networks (PINs) in which nodes correspond to proteins in a cell and edges to physical bindings between the proteins.

3.1 Data Sets

Recent technological advances in experimental biology have been producing large quantities of network data describing gene and protein interactions. These technologies include yeast two-hybrid (Y2H) assays [22, 29, 37, 51, 79, 88, 90, 93], affinity purification coupled to mass spectrometry [27, 28, 36, 45] and synthetic-lethal and suppressor networks [17, 92]. They yield partial networks for many model organisms [28, 29, 34, 37, 45, 51, 71, 92, 93], humans [79, 90], as well as microbial [48,

N. Pržulj (✉)
Department of Computing, Imperial College London, London, UK
e-mail: natasha@imperial.ac.uk

E. Estrada et al. (eds.), *Network Science*,
DOI 10.1007/978-1-84996-396-1_3, © Springer-Verlag London Limited 2010

67, 77] and viral [15, 94, 98] pathogens. Due to their large sizes and systems-level inter-connectedness, these network data sets are offering many important and interesting opportunities for biologists and computational scientists. We are currently at a unique time in the history of science when advances in network analysis and modelling could contribute to biological understanding and therapeutics, thus potentially having huge impacts on public health and well-being.

There are considerable challenges involved with this nascent research area. First, our current observational data are noisy and largely incomplete due to sampling and other biases in data collection, handling and interpretation, as well as to biotechnological limitations [18–20, 32, 33, 91, 99, 103]. An example of a biological network that illustrates sparsity of the data is presented in Fig. 3.1. Despite this, as has been done in physical sciences, we have begun analyzing and modelling them, hoping to obtain concise summaries of the phenomena of interest that might exhibit some unexpected properties that we may experimentally validate. However, the main reason to model network data is to understand laws, since only with the help of such laws we can make predictions and reproduce the phenomena. Finding such models is non-trivial not only due to the low quality of the data, but also due to provable computational intractability of many graph-theoretic problems.

3.2 Network Comparisons

To find similarities and differences between network data sets or between data and models, we need to be able to compare them. However, comparing large real-world networks (also called *graphs*) is computationally intensive. The basis of network comparison lies in finding a graph isomorphism between two networks, which is a node bijection preserving the node adjacency relation [102]. For two networks G and H that are given as input, determining whether G contains a subgraph isomorphic to H is NP-complete, since it includes problems such as Hamiltonian path, Hamiltonian cycle, and the maximum clique as special cases [26]. If graph G on n_G nodes is input and graph H on n_H nodes is fixed, then the subgraph isomorphism can be tested in polynomial time, $O(n_H! \cdot n_H^2 \cdot \binom{n_G}{n_H})$, simply by iterating through all subsets of n_H nodes of G. However, such exhaustive searches are computationally infeasible for large biological (and other real-world) networks and thus approximate, i.e. heuristic, approaches are sought.

Because nature is variable and the data are noisy, traditional graph isomorphism described above is of little use for network comparison and alignment, and more flexible, intentionally approximate approaches are necessary. Thus, easily computable macroscopic statistical *global properties* of large networks have extensively been examined. The most widely used global network properties are the *degree distribution, clustering coefficient, clustering spectra, network diameter* and various forms of network *centralities* [62]. Based on these properties, network models have been proposed for cellular (and other real) networks if their global properties fit the global properties of cellular networks. The *degree* of a node is the number of edges touching the node and the *degree distribution* is the distribution of degrees of all

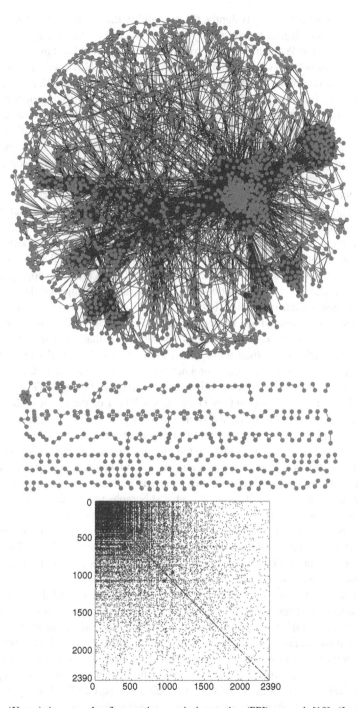

Fig. 3.1 (*Upper*) An example of a protein–protein interaction (PPI) network [18]. (*Lower*) The adjacency matrix of the same network illustrating its sparsity

nodes in the network, or equivalently, the probability that a randomly selected node of a network has degree k (commonly denoted by $P(k)$). Many large real-world networks have non-Poisson degree distributions with a power-law tail, $P(k) \sim k^{-\gamma}$, $\gamma > 0$; all such networks have been termed scale-free [5]. However, networks with exactly the same power-law degree distributions can have vastly different structure affecting their function [50, 73]. For example, a network consisting of four triangles and a network consisting of one 12-node ring (cycle) are of the same size (i.e. have the same number of nodes and edges) and have the same degree distribution (each node has degree two), but their topologies are very different. The same holds for other global network properties [73]. Furthermore, global network properties of largely incomplete cellular networks do not tell us much about the true structure of the real networks; instead, they describe the network structure produced by the sampling techniques used to obtain these networks [20, 33, 91]. Thus, global statistics on such incomplete data may be substantially biased, or even misleading with respect to the currently unknown complete network. Conversely, certain neighborhoods of these networks are well-studied, usually the regions of a network relevant for human disease, so local statistics applied to the well-studied areas are more appropriate.

To overcome the above mentioned problems in modelling cellular networks based on their global properties, bottom-up *local* approaches to studying microscopic network structure have been proposed [57, 73, 86]. Analogous to sequence motifs, *network motifs* have been defined as subgraphs that recur in a network at frequencies much higher than those found in randomized networks [57, 58, 86]. A *subgraph* (or a *partial subgraph*) of a network G with the set of nodes $V(G)$ and the set of edges $E(G)$ is a network whose nodes and edges belong to G. An *induced subgraph H* of G is a subgraph of G on subset $V(H)$ of the set of nodes $V(G)$, such that edges $E(H)$ of H consists of all edges of G that connect nodes of $V(H)$. All approaches based on network motifs ignore subnetworks with "average" frequencies. However, if we are to understand the underlying mechanisms of cellular structure and function, it is as important to understand why certain structures appear at average or low frequencies in the data as it is to understand why some structures are over-represented. Also, it is unclear what subgraphs are more frequent than expected at *random*, since it is not clear what should be expected at random. Thus, approaches based on the frequencies of occurrences of *all* small induced subgraphs in a network, called *graphlets* (Fig. 3.2(A)), have been proposed [72, 73]. These approaches are not based on the assumed correctness of any random graph model (graph models are described below) for the data.

Graphlets do not need to be overrepresented in a network and this, along with being induced, distinguishes them from network motifs [57, 86]. Note that whenever a structure of a graph (or a graph family) is studied, we care about induced rather than partial subgraphs [14]; thus, the definition of graphlets as induced subgraphs, unlike network motifs which are partial. Based on graphlets, systematic measures of a network's local structure have been introduced that impose a large number of local similarity constraints on networks being compared [72, 73]. By counting the frequency of graphlets across a network, we get a statistical characterization of local structure independent of any network null model. Comparing such frequency

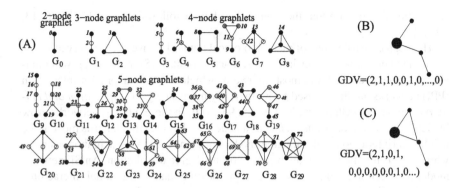

Fig. 3.2 (**A**) All 2-, 3-, 4-, and 5-node graphlets, $G_0, G_1, \ldots, G_{29}$, and the orbits denoted by $0, 1, 2, \ldots, 72$ [72]. In each graphlet, nodes belonging to the same orbit are of the same shade. (**B**) A small 4-node network. The graphlet degree vector of heavy node is $(2, 1, 1, 0, 0, 1, 0, \ldots)$ because it is touched by two edges (orbit 0), the end of one 3-path (orbit 1), the middle of another 3-path (orbit 2), no orbits 3 and 4, the middle of a 4-path (orbit 5), and no other orbits. (**C**) Another small 4-node network. This case is similar to the above but is touched by one triangle (orbit 3), and one orbit 10 from G_6.

distributions gives a new measure of structural similarity between networks [73]. We currently deal only with graphlets with five or fewer nodes, which is enough in practice due to the small-world nature of many real-world networks [101]. There are 30 such graphlets, denoted by $G_0, \ldots, G_{29}$ in Fig. 3.2(A). We may further refine the graphlet idea by noting that in some graphlets, the nodes are distinct from each other. As an example, in a ring (cycle) of five nodes, every node looks the same as every other, but in a chain (path) of five nodes, there are two end nodes, two near-end nodes, and one middle node. We formalize this idea by using graph "automorphism orbits" [72] (described below). In this way, we greatly enhance the sensitivity of using graphlets to compare networks without increasing the computational cost.

3.3 Network Models

There exist many different random graph models that we could compare the data against to find network motifs [3]. The earliest is *Erdős–Rényi* ("ER") random graphs in which the probability that there is an edge between any pair of nodes, p, is distributed uniformly at random [21]. This model is well-studied and many of its properties are well understood [11]. Hence, it is a standard model to compare the data against, even though it is not expected to fit the data well. Since ER graphs, unlike PINs, have Poisson degree distributions and low clustering coefficients, other network models have been sought. In *generalized random graphs* ("ER-DD"), the edges are randomly chosen as in Erdős–Rényi random graphs, but the degree distribution is constrained to match that of the data, which often follows a power-law [1, 59, 60, 65]. *Small-world* ("SW") networks are characterized by small diameters and large clustering coefficients [63, 64, 101]. *Scale-free* ("SF") networks include an additional condition that the degree distribution follows a power-law [5, 6, 13, 50, 87].

The degree distributions of many biological networks have been observed to decay as an approximate power-law. Thus, many variants of SF network growth models have been proposed, the most notable of which for protein–protein interaction (PPI) networks are those based on biologically motivated gene *duplication and mutation* network growth principles [30, 68, 95, 100]. In these models, networks grow by duplication of nodes (genes), and as a node gets duplicated, it inherits most of the neighbors (interactions) of the parent node, but gains some new neighbors as well, while preserving the power-law property of the degree distribution. An SF network model has been used to propose a strategy for time- and cost-optimal interactome detection [49]. Finding cost-effective strategies for completing interaction maps is an active research topic (e.g. see [80]). The dangers of using inadequate network models for such a purpose are at best wasted time and resources and at worst wrong identification of "complete" interactome maps.

The above described new measures of local network structure based on graphlet and orbit frequencies, demonstrated that PPI networks are better modelled by *geometric graphs* (defined below) than by any previous network model [72, 73]. Assume we have a collection of points dispersed in a metric space. Now, pick some constant distance ϵ and say that two points are "related" if they are within ϵ of each other. The relationship can be represented as a graph, where each point in space is a node and two nodes are connected if they are within distance ϵ. This is called a *geometric graph*; if the points are distributed at random, then it is a *geometric random graph*. Illustrations are presented in Fig. 3.3.

Since this insight into the geometric structure of PPI networks, there has been an avalanche of papers questioning scale-freeness of PPI and other biological networks. The geometric model is further corroborated by the demonstration that PPI networks can explicitly be embedded into a low-dimensional geometric space [35]. The geometric graph model can further be refined to fit the data by learning the distribution of proteins in that space [46]. Also, biological reasons why PPI networks are geometric have been argued [76]: it has been noticed that all biological entities, including genes and proteins as gene products, exist in some multidimensional (likely metric) biochemical space. This is an abstract space that does not only include the three-dimensional Euclidean space of protein folds with perhaps time being the additional fourth dimension. It is likely to include as dimensions phenomena such as post-translational modifications, small molecule bindings, etc. Currently, it is hard even to hypothesize about the nature or dimensionality of that space.

Genomes evolve through a series of gene duplication and mutation events [43]. For this reason and also since geometric graphs seem to provide the best fit to the currently available PPI networks, we may bridge the concepts of PPI network geometricity with the evolutionary dynamics [76]. Gene duplications and mutations are naturally modelled in the above mentioned biochemical space: a duplicated gene starts at the same point in biochemical space as its parent, and then natural selection, or "evolutionary optimization", acts either to eliminate one, or cause them to slowly separate in the biochemical space. This means that the child inherits some

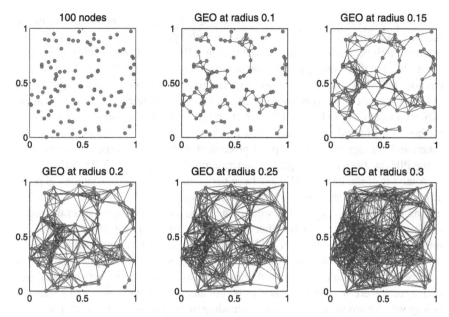

Fig. 3.3 Illustrations of geometric random graphs on 100 nodes when distance (or radius) of 0.1, 0.15, 0.2, 0.25 and 0.3 is chosen for their construction

of the neighbors of its parent, while possibly gaining novel connections as well. The further the "child" is moved away from its "parent", the more different their biochemical properties. Although motivated by biological principles, these current geometric network models are quite crude mathematical approximations of real biology and further refinement is necessary for obtaining well fitting models for PINs.

Another reason for modelling PINs is the development of fast heuristics for data collection and analysis. One property of every heuristic approach is that it performs poorly on some input. Thus, heuristics are designed, with the help of models, to work well for a particular application. As mentioned above, a scale-free network model of PPI networks has been used to propose an algorithmic strategy for optimal interactome detection in humans [49]. However, if the model is not fitting the data well, the heuristics based on it will at best be inefficient in discovering the interactome and at worst misleading and fail to discover parts of the interactome, since the model instructed us not to examine certain interactions. Also, geometric graph models have been used for designing efficient algorithms for graphlet count estimation [74]. For these reasons, it is important to make network models as accurate as possible.

3.4 Network Topology and Biological Function and Disease

The relationship between network topology and biological function has received much attention. Approaches for network-based prediction of protein function have

been proposed; for a review, see [82]. Also, the role of protein networks in disease
has been examined; for a review, see [85]. An early approach was to find correlations
between high protein connectivity (degree) in a PIN and its essentiality in baker's
yeast [38], but this technique failed on some newer PIN data [108] (also see the discussion in [78]). Correlations between connectivity and protein function were used
in [75]. Other methods were based on the premise that proteins that are closer in the
PIN are more likely to have similar function [16, 81], or used some graph theoretic
methods [96] including cut-based and network flow-based approaches [61]. Also,
functional homogeneity of groups of proteins that show some type of "coherence"
in the PIN has been used for protein function prediction [4, 44, 45, 75, 83].

Analyses of the human PIN have been performed in search for topological properties of disease-related genes (and proteins as gene products) with the hope of
getting insights into disease that would lead to better drug design. General conclusions are that these genes have high connectivity, are closer together, and are centrally positioned within the PIN [85]. However, these results might be biased, since
disease-causing proteins may exhibit these properties in a PIN simply because they
have been better studied than non-disease proteins. Furthermore, network analyses
of drug action are starting to be used as part of an emerging field of *systems pharmacology* which aims to develop an understanding of drug action across multiple scales
of organismal complexity, from cellular to tissue to organismal [9]. Multiple studies
have constructed network types that link biochemical interaction networks, such as
PINs, with networks of drug similarities, interactions, or therapeutic indications. For
example, a bipartite network connecting drug targets (proteins affected by a drug)
and drugs was constructed and used to generate two "projections:" (a) a network in
which nodes are drugs and they are connected if they share a common target; and
(b) a network in which nodes are targets and they are connected if they are affected
by the same drugs [107]. By analyzing the former and taking into consideration the
time the drug was introduced, they demonstrated that there are relatively few drugs
acting on novel targets that enter the market. When analyzing the latter by overlay-
ing it with the PIN, they showed that drug targets tend to have higher degrees than
non-targets in the PIN. However, as mentioned above, this observation might be an
artifact of disease-related parts of the PIN receiving more attention. For a survey of
network-based analyses in systems pharmacology, see [9].

Graphlets have also been used to isolate the structural characteristics of individual nodes and relate them to protein function and involvement in disease [54, 55].
Recall that the "degree" of a node is the number of edges it touches. Note that an
edge is the only graphlet on two nodes (graphlet G_0 in Fig. 3.1(A)). Thus, we can
similarly define a "graphlet degree" of a node v with respect to each graphlet G_i
in Fig. 3.1(A), in the sense that the G_i-degree of v counts "how many graphlets of
type G_i touch node v" [72]. Referring to Fig. 3.1(A), note that the traditional degree
is simply the G_0-degree. Since there are 30 graphlets, this would provide a vector
of 30 "graphlet degrees". However, specificity can be increased by noting that not
all nodes in a given graphlet are topologically equivalent. For example, the middle
node in G_1 is topologically distinct from the end nodes of G_1. Figure 3.1(A) shows
the 73 topologically distinct nodes across all 2-, 3-, 4- and 5-node graphlets. Each

is called an *orbit* (an *automorphism orbit*, see [54, 72] for details), and we label them 0, ..., 72. The *graphlet degree vector* (GDV), or *GD-signature* of a node v, thus has 73 elements: element i represents the number of times node v "touches" a graphlet at orbit i, across all the graphlets in its neighborhood. Simple examples of a GD-signatures appear in Figs. 3.1(B) and 3.1(C). As mentioned above, node degree of a protein in a PPI network has previously been used as a predictor of biological function, but the evidence of a link between such a simple measure of topological similarity between proteins in a PPI network and their biological functions has since been questioned. GD-signature is superior to such a simple measure, since it is based on all up to 5-node graphlets. We demonstrated that GD-signatures correspond to similarity in biological function and involvement in disease [54] and our function predictions were phenotypically validated [55]. By observing only the topology around nodes in PPI networks and finding nodes that are topologically similar to nodes that are known regulators of melanogenesis, we successfully identified novel regulators of melanogenesis in human cells and our predictions were validated by systems-level functional genomics siRNA screens [25, 55].

3.5 Network Alignment

A related problem is that of network alignment. Sequence comparison and alignment has had a deep impact on our understanding of evolution, biology, and disease, so it is expected that comparison and alignment of biological networks will have a similar impact. Thus, it has been argued that comparing networks of different organisms in a meaningful manner is one of the most important problems in evolutionary and systems biology [84].

Network alignment is the general problem of finding the best way to "fit" graph G into graph H even if G does not exist as an exact subgraph of H [84]. A simple example illustrating network alignment is presented in Fig. 3.4. Biological networks, such as PINs, may contain noise, e.g. missing edges, false edges, or both [97]. Biological variation makes it further non-obvious how to measure the "goodness" of this fit. Analogous to sequence alignments between genomes, alignments of biological networks are useful for knowledge transfer, since we may know a lot about

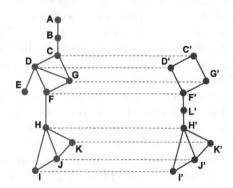

Fig. 3.4 An example of an alignment of two networks

some nodes in one network and almost nothing about topologically similar nodes in the other network. Also, network alignments can be used to measure the global similarity between biological networks of different species and to construct the matrix of pairwise global network similarities that can be used to infer phylogenetic relationships.

Analogous to sequence alignments, there exist *local* and *global* network alignments. With local alignments, mappings are chosen independently for each local region of similarity. Hence, local alignments can be ambiguous, since one node can have different pairings in different local alignments. A global network alignment provides a unique alignment from every node in the smaller network to only one node in the larger network. A disadvantage is that this may lead to suboptimal matchings in some local regions. For biological networks, the majority of methods used for alignment have focused on local alignments [7, 8, 23, 41, 52]. Generally, local network alignments are not able to identify large subgraphs that have been conserved during evolution [7, 41]. Global network alignments have been studied previously in the context of biological networks [24, 89, 110], but existing methods incorporate some *a priori* information about nodes, such as sequence similarities of proteins in PINs [8, 89], or they use some form of learning on a set of "true" alignments [24].

Our new study [47] investigates how much biological information could be obtained from network topology *only*, which makes our method applicable to *any* type of network, not just biological ones. The reason we want to use topology only without integrating it with other types of biological information is two-fold. First, just as genetic sequences describe some part of biological information, so do biological networks. Analogous to sequence alignment algorithms that do not use biological information external to sequences to perform alignments, we do not want to use biological information external to network topology. This is because we believe that it is scientifically interesting to ask how much biological information could be extracted from topology only and that we would only be able to utilize well various sources of biological information after we have reliable topological alignment algorithms for biological network data.

Clearly, if we want to build good alignments based solely upon network topology, we must first have a highly constraining measure of topological similarity. The simplest and weakest description of the topology of a node is its degree. A much more highly constraining measure is the above described generalization of the degree of a node into the vector of "graphlet degrees" [54] that describes the topology of a node's neighborhood and captures the node's interconnectivities out to a distance of four (Fig. 3.1). We argue that reaching out to distance four from a node should be enough to almost uniquely determine the node's position in a network, since many real-world networks have the "small world" property [101] (described in Sect. 3.3).

We define an alignment of two networks G and H to consist of a set of ordered node pairs (u, v), where u is a node in G and v is a node in H. Our algorithm, called GRAAL (GRAph ALigner), incorporates aspects of both local and global alignment. We match pairs of nodes originating in different networks based on their GD-signature similarity [54] described in Sect. 3.4 above, where a higher GD-signature similarity between two nodes corresponds to a higher topological similarity between their extended neighborhoods out to distance four. We align each node in the smaller network to exactly one node in the larger network. Our matching algorithm proceeds using a technique analogous to the "seed and extend" approach of the popular BLAST [2] algorithm for sequence alignment: first, we choose a "seed" pair of nodes, one node from each network, that have high GD-signature similarity. Then, we expand the alignment radially outward around the seed nodes as far as practical using a greedy algorithm.

Although local in nature, GRAAL produces large and dense global alignments in the sense that the aligned subgraphs share many edges. We demonstrate that this would not be the case in a low-quality, or random alignment. We argue that the high quality of our alignments is based less on the details of the extension algorithm, and more on having a good measure of pair-wise topological similarity between nodes [54]. We apply GRAAL to PINs of yeast and human and produce by far the most complete topological alignments of biological networks to date indicating that even distant species share a surprising amount of network topology. This might suggest broad similarities in internal cellular wiring across all life on Earth. We use this alignment for knowledge transfer and demonstrate that detailed biological function of individual proteins can be extracted from our alignments. Notably, when we use GRAAL to align metabolic networks of closely related species and the alignment scores to construct the matrix of pairwise global network similarities to infer phylogenetic relationships, we find that the phylogenetic trees constructed from our purely topological alignments for protists and fungi are very similar to those found by sequence comparison [69]. Thus, topology-based alignments have the potential to provide a completely new, independent source of phylogenetic information; see [47] for details.

In contrast to GRAAL, which is a greedy 'seed-and-extend' approach that relies solely on network topology, Hungarian-algorithm-based GRAAL (H-GRAAL) is an optimal network alignment algorithm also based solely on network topology [56]. As before, we match pairs of nodes originating in different networks based on their GD-signature similarities, with the cost of aligning two nodes being modified to favor alignment of the densest parts of the networks. We use the Hungarian algorithm for minimum-weight bipartite matching to find an optimal matching between the nodes of two networks with the minimum total alignment cost as follows. We construct a complete bipartite graph with $V(G_1)$ and $V(G_2)$ as the bipartition and each edge (u, v) from $V(G_1)$ to $V(G_2)$ is labelled with the node alignment cost between u and v. H-GRAAL then uses the Hungarian algorithm to find an alignment from G_1 to G_2 by minimizing the cost summed over all aligned pairs. Furthermore, we show that a large proportion of the aligned pairs in the optimal alignment returned by H-GRAAL are 'stable' in the sense that they would still be present for a different optimal alignment, so that any one optimal alignment would be highly representative of all optimal alignments. That is, we identify the *core alignment*, which is the subset of all aligned pairs that are present in all optimal alignments, and show that it contains 72.2% of yeast–human protein pairs in the alignment of yeast and human PINs. We apply H-GRAAL to expose large contiguous regions of network similarity between PINs of yeast and human, to transfer function from annotated to unannotated PIN regions, as well as to build phylogenetic trees based on the alignment scores; see [56] for details.

3.6 Data Integration

Molecular networks come in many different types depending on the cellular phenomenon that they model. For example, we have rich datasets of PINs, transcriptional regulation networks, networks of genetic interactions, etc. deposited in databases including DIP [105], MINT [109], and HPRD [70]. They cover different slices of biological information and thus, integrating them would contribute to a comprehensive view of a cellular system. It is currently unclear how to perform such integration in a way that would be biologically informative. However, some approaches have been proposed. They usually integrate diverse networks on the same node sets into a single network with different types of interactions and try to identify functional modules supported by varied interaction types.

For example, we integrated PINs with the information about viable, lethal, and genetic interaction mutants [75]. In *genetic interaction networks* (GINs), nodes correspond to genes and edges between them to changed phenotype (lethal or sick) of cells with simultaneous mutations of the two genes in which a single mutation results in no phenotypic change [12]. We suggested the existence of alternate paths that bypass viable nodes in PPI networks and so offered an explanation why null mutation of these proteins are not lethal. This was later corroborated by a proposition that genetic interactions tend to bridge genes from redundant pathways rather than within a single pathway [42]. Other studies demonstrated that a dense cluster of interactions supported by several network types is more likely to correspond to protein complexes than dense clusters in any one network [31]. Machine learning methods that use graph-theoretic properties of proteins in PINs were also used to predict genetic interactions [66]. Integration of networks with multiple types of edges was also done to predict protein functions and interactions [39, 53, 104]. Also, composite network motifs arising from such combined network data have been studied for the same purposes [106, 111]. For a review on methods for integration of physical and genetic networks, see [10].

3.7 Outlook

The new transdisciplinary field of network biology is still in its infancy, but it is already very fast paced and in a bit of a turmoil. First, currently there is a relatively weak link between biological and computational scientists in the field. Therefore, computational and mathematical analyses performed on these data thus far have been quite simple, even though much stronger mathematical tools have been available. Also, it is necessary to develop new, strong mathematical and algorithmic techniques specifically aimed at solving network biology problems (e.g. see the discussion in Sect. 3.3 above) and this is sometimes frowned upon with claims that such methods are "complicated". This is probably due to the fact that the area gathers researchers from a variety of areas with varied backgrounds in quantitative techniques.

Second, there is a danger of the emergence of scientific doctrines that could further hinder the development of this nascent research area. Early on, one of them involved scale-free-centric modeling of complex biological (and other) networks that Evelyn Fox Keller wrote eloquently about in her 2005 Bioessays article "Revisiting 'scale-free' networks" [40]. Another one involves a genome-centric view of biological systems. While it is certainly true that genetic sequence data has revolutionized our view of biology, we should not let that fact obscure our vision towards new scientific horizons. In particular, even though PPI network data are very new and thus currently noisy and incomplete and even though the mathematical methods applied to them are rather primitive, there is already evidence documenting that these new biological data can reveal biological information that could not have been inferred from sequence alone, at least not by using the currently available sequence analysis tools. Despite, the community has been questioning the value of the network data with unsubstantiated claims, e.g. that PPI network topology and biological function are unrelated. At a recent meeting, this went to the point that a colleague publically asked if the community "should keep analyzing PPI network data at all". Needless to say, such questions could lead to scientific censorship that the area might already be beginning to experience. For example, articles demonstrating that biological information can be obtained from PIN data alone, which cannot be obtained from sequence data, are viewed as "warning signs" that something is wrong with the analysis, rather than as success stories demonstrating that new biology could be learned from these new systems-level biological data. Thus, rather than seeing genome and interactome as complementary data, there is a danger that the community might reject the interactome-based analyses if they cannot be confirmed by the genome-based ones (often despite a provision of biological validation). Conversely, interactome-based studies could be regarded as useless if they are in agreement with genome-based ones. Hence, interactome data are bound to loose in such an unfair game. Furthermore, such opinions might spread, potentially negatively affecting the availability of public resources necessary for continued collection the biological network data towards reliable reference networks for key model organisms, or for the development of reliable computational tools, such as those for computationally challenging problems of foremost scientific interest including network alignment and network data integration.

Finally, amongst computational scientists, there is somewhat of a clash between statistical and descriptive modelling communities. We can all agree that statistical approaches have certainly proved their usefulness. However, they do not describe how things actually work. Thus, while it is fine to look for statistical patterns (e.g. observe power-laws in the degree distributions of PPI networks) and then reason about why they are there, the availability of easy-to-use statistical approaches should not prevent us from searching for descriptive models that could provide us with understanding and enable reproduction of phenomena at study.

References

1. Aiello, W., Chung, F., Lu, L.: A random graph model for power law graphs. Exp. Math. **10**, 53–66 (2001)
2. Altschul, S.F., Gish, W., Miller, W., Lipman, D.J.: Basic local alignment search tool. J. Mol. Biol. **215**, 403–410 (1990)
3. Artzy-Randrup, Y., Fleishman, S.J., Ben-Tal, N., Stone, L.: Comment on "Network motifs: Simple building blocks of complex networks" and "Superfamilies of evolved and designed networks". Science **305**, 1107 (2004)
4. Bader, G.D., Hogue, C.W.V.: An automated method for finding molecular complexes in large protein interaction networks. BMC Bioinform. **4**, 2 (2003)
5. Barabási, A.L., Albert, R.: Emergence of scaling in random networks. Science **286**(5439), 509–512 (1999)
6. Barabási, A.L., Albert, R., Jeong, H.: Mean-field theory for scale-free random networks. Physica A **272**, 173–197 (1999)
7. Berg, J., Lassig, M.: Local graph alignment and motif search in biological networks. Proc. Natl. Acad. Sci. USA **101**, 14689–14694 (2004)
8. Berg, J., Lassig, M.: Cross-species analysis of biological networks by Bayesian alignment. Proc. Natl. Acad. Sci. USA **103**(29), 10967–10972 (2006). doi:10.1073/pnas.0602294103
9. Berger, S.I., Iyengar, R.: Network analyses in systems pharmacology. Bioinformatics **25**, 2466–2472 (2009)
10. Beyer, A., Bandyopadhyay, S., Ideker, T.: Integrating physical and genetic maps: from genomes to interaction networks. Nat. Rev. Genet. **8**, 699–710 (2007)
11. Bollobas, B.: Random Graphs. Academic Press, London (1985)
12. Boone, C., Bussey, H., Andrews, B.J.: Exploring genetic interactions and networks with yeast. Nat. Rev. Genet. **8**, 437–449 (2007)
13. Bornholdt, S., Ebel, H.: World-wide web scaling exponent from Simon's 1955 model. Phys. Rev. E **64**, 046401 (2001)
14. Brandstadt, A., Van Bang, L., Spinrad, J.P.: Graph Classes: A Survey. SIAM Monographs on Discrete Mathematics and Applications. SIAM, Philadelphia (1999)
15. Chatr-aryamontri, A., Ceol, A., Peluso, D., Nardozza, A., Panni, S., Sacco, F., Tinti, M., Smolyar, A., Castagnoli, L., Vidal, M., Cusick, M., Cesareni, G.: VirusMINT: a viral protein interaction database. Nucleic Acids Res. **37**, 669–673 (2009)
16. Chua, H., Sung, W., Wong, L.: Exploiting indirect neighbors and topological weight to predict protein function from protein–protein interactions. Bioinformatics **22**, 1623–1630 (2006)
17. Collins, S., Schuldiner, M., Krogan, N., Weissman, J.: A strategy for extracting and analyzing large-scale quantitative epistatic interaction data. Genome Biol. **7**, R63 (2006)
18. Collins, S., Kemmeren, P., Zhao, X.C., Greenblatt, J., Spencer, F., Holstege, F., Weissman, J., Krogan, N.: Toward a comprehensive atlas of the physical interactome of *Saccharomyces cerevisiae*. Mol. Cell. Proteomics **6**(3), 439–450 (2007)
19. de Silva, E., Stumpf, M.: Complex networks and simple models in biology. J. R. Soc. Interface **2**, 419–430 (2005)
20. de Silva, E., Thorne, T., Ingram, P., Agrafioti, I., Swire, J., Wiuf, C., Stumpf, M.: The effects of incomplete protein interaction data on structural and evolutionary inferences. BMC Biol. (2006). doi:10.1186/1741-7007-4-39
21. Erdős, P., Rényi, A.: On random graphs. Publ. Math. (Debr.) **6**, 290–297 (1959)
22. Fields, S.: High-throughput two-hybrid analysis. the promise and the peril. FEBS J. **272**, 5391–5399 (2005)

23. Flannick, J., Novak, A., Balaji, S., Harley, H., Batzglou, S.: Graemlin general and robust alignment of multiple large interaction networks. Genome Res. **16**(9), 1169–1181 (2006)
24. Flannick, J., Novak, A.F., Do, C.B., Srinivasan, B.S., Batzoglou, S.: Automatic parameter learning for multiple network alignment. In: RECOMB, pp. 214–231 (2008)
25. Ganesan, A., Ho, H., Bodemann, B., Petersen, S., Aruri, J., Koshy, S., Richardson, Z., Le, L., Krasieva, T., Roth, M., Farmer, P., White, M.: Genome-wide siRNA-based functional genomics of pigmentation identifies novel genes and pathways that impact melanogenesis in human cells. PLoS Genet. **4**(12), 1000298 (2008)
26. Garey, M.R., Johnson, D.S.: Computers and Intractability–A Guide to the Theory of NP-Completeness. Freeman, New York (1979)
27. Gavin, A.C., Bosche, M., Krause, R., Grandi, P., Marzioch, M., Bauer, A., Schultz, J., Rick, J.M., Michon, A.M., Cruciat, C.M., Remor, M., Hofert, C., Schelder, M., Brajenovic, M., Ruffner, H., Merino, A., Klein, K., Hudak, M., Dickson, D., Rudi, T., Gnau, V., Bauch, A., Bastuck, S., Huhse, B., Leutwein, C., Heurtier, M.A., Copley, R.R., Edelmann, A., Querfurth, E., Rybin, V., Drewes, G., Raida, M., Bouwmeester, T., Bork, P., Seraphin, B., Kuster, B., Neubauer, G., Superti-Furga, G.: Functional organization of the yeast proteome by systematic analysis of protein complexes. Nature **415**(6868), 141–147 (2002)
28. Gavin, A., Aloy, P., Grandi, P., Krause, R., Boesche, M., Marzioch, M., Rau, C., Jensen, L., Bastuck, S., Dumpelfeld, B., Edelmann, A., Heurtier, M., Hoffman, V., Hoefert, C., Klein, K., Hudak, M., Michon, A., Schelder, M., Schirle, M., Remor, M., Rudi, T., Hooper, S., Bauer, A., Bouwmeester, T., Casari, G., Drewes, G., Neubauer, G., Rick, J., Kuster, B., Bork, P., Russell, R., Superti-Furga, G.: Proteome survey reveals modularity of the yeast cell machinery. Nature **440**(7084), 631–636 (2006)
29. Giot, L., Bader, J., Brouwer, C., Chaudhuri, A., Kuang, B., Li, Y., Hao, Y., Ooi, C., Godwin, B., Vitols, E., Vijayadamodar, G., Pochart, P., Machineni, H., Welsh, M., Kong, Y., Zerhusen, B., Malcolm, R., Varrone, Z., Collis, A., Minto, M., Burgess, S., McDaniel, L., Stimpson, E., Spriggs, F., Williams, J., Neurath, K., Ioime, N., Agee, M., Voss, E., Furtak, K., Renzulli, R., Aanensen, N., Carrolla, S., Bickelhaupt, E., Lazovatsky, Y., DaSilva, A., Zhong, J., Stanyon, C., Finley, R.J., White, K., Braverman, M., Jarvie, T., Gold, S., Leach, M., Knight, J., Shimkets, R., McKenna, M., Chant, J., Rothberg, J.: A protein interaction map of *Drosophila melanogaster*. Science **302**(5651), 1727–1736 (2003)
30. Goh, K.I., Kahng, B., Kim, D.: Hybrid network model: the protein and the protein family interaction networks. arXiv:q-bio.MN/0312009v2 (March 2004)
31. Gunsalus, K.C., et al.: Predictive models of molecular machines involved in *Caenorhabditis elegans* early embryogenesis. Nature **436**, 861–865 (2005)
32. Hakes, L., Pinney, J., Robertson, D.L., Lovell, S.C.: Protein–protein interaction networks and biology—what's the connection? Nat. Biotechnol. **26**(1), 69–72 (2008)
33. Han, J.D.H., Dupuy, D., Bertin, N., Cusick, M.E., Vidal, M.: Effect of sampling on topology predictions of protein–protein interaction networks. Nat. Biotechnol. **23**, 839–844 (2005)
34. Harbison, C.T., Gordon, D.B., Lee, T.I., Rinaldi, N.J., Macisaac, K.D., Danford, T.W., Hannett, N.M., Tagne, J.B., Reynolds, D.B., Yoo, J., Jennings, E.G., Zeitlinger, J., Pokholok, D.K., Kellis, M., Rolfe, P.A., Takusagawa, K.T., Lander, E.S., Gifford, D.K., Fraenkel, E., Young, R.A.: Transcriptional regulatory code of a eukaryotic genome. Nature **431**, 99–104 (2004)
35. Higham, D.J., Rašajski, M., Pržulj, N.: Fitting a geometric graph to a protein–protein interaction network. Bioinformatics **24**(8), 1093–1099 (2008)
36. Ho, Y., Gruhler, A., Heilbut, A., Bader, G.D., Moore, L., Adams, S.L., Millar, A., Taylor, P., Bennett, K., Boutilier, K., Yang, L., Wolting, C., Donaldson, I., Schandorff, S., Shewnarane, J., Vo, M., Taggart, J., Goudreault, M., Muskat, B., Alfarano, C., Dewar, D., Lin, Z., Michalickova, K., Willems, A.R., Sassi, H., Nielsen, P.A., Rasmussen, K.J., Andersen, J.R., Johansen, L.E., Hansen, L.H., Jespersen, H., Podtelejnikov, A., Nielsen, E., Crawford, J., Poulsen, V., Sorensen, B.D., Matthiesen, J., Hendrickson, R.C., Gleeson, F., Pawson, T., Moran, M.F., Durocher, D., Mann, M., Hogue, C.W., Figeys, D., Tyers, M.: Systematic identification of protein complexes in *Saccharomyces cerevisiae* by mass spectrometry. Nature **415**(6868), 180–183 (2002)

37. Ito, T., Tashiro, K., Muta, S., Ozawa, R., Chiba, T., Nishizawa, M., Yamamoto, K., Kuhara, S., Sakaki, Y.: Toward a protein–protein interaction map of the budding yeast: A comprehensive system to examine two-hybrid interactions in all possible combinations between the yeast proteins. Proc. Natl. Acad. Sci. USA **97**(3), 1143–1147 (2000)
38. Jeong, H., Mason, S.P., Barabási, A.L., Oltvai, Z.N.: Lethality and centrality in protein networks. Nature **411**(6833), 41–42 (2001)
39. Kammeren, P., et al.: Protein interaction verification and functional annotation by integrated analysis of genome-scale data. Mol. Cell **9**, 1133–1143 (2002)
40. Keller, E.F.: Revisiting "scale-free" networks. BioEssays **27**, 11060–11068 (2005)
41. Kelley, B.P., Bingbing, Y., Lewitter, F., Sharan, R., Stockwell, B.R., Ideker, T.: PathBLAST: a tool for alignment of protein interaction networks. Nucleic Acids Res. **32**, 83–88 (2004)
42. Kelley, R., Ideker, T.: Systematic interpretation of genetic interactions using protein networks. Nat. Biotechnol. **23**, 561–566 (2005)
43. Kellis, M., Birren, B.W., Lander, E.S.: Proof and evolutionary analysis of the ancient gene duplication in yeast *Saccharomices cerevisiae*. Nature **428**, 617–624 (2004)
44. King, A.D., Pržulj, N., Jurisical.: Protein complex prediction via cost-based clustering. Bioinformatics **20**(17), 3013–3020 (2004)
45. Krogan, N., Cagney, G., Yu, H., Zhong, G., Guo, X., Ignatchenko, A., Li, J., Pu, S., Datta, N., Tikuisis, A., Punna, T., Peregrín-Alvarez, J., Shales, M., Zhang, X., Davey, M., Robinson, M., Paccanaro, A., Bray, J., Sheung, A., Beattie, B., Richards, D., Canadien, V., Lalev, A., Mena, F., Wong, P., Starostine, A., Canete, M., Vlasblom, J., Wu, S., Orsi, C., Collins, S., Chandran, S., Haw, R., Rilstone, J., Gandi, K., Thompson, N., Musso, G., St Onge, P., Ghanny, S., Lam, M., Butland, G., Altaf-Ul, A., Kanaya, S., Shilatifard, A., O'Shea, E., Weissman, J., Ingles, C., Hughes, T., Parkinson, J., Gerstein, M., Wodak, S., Emili, A., Greenblatt, J.: Global landscape of protein complexes in the yeast *Saccharomyces cerevisiae*. Nature **440**, 637–643 (2006)
46. Kuchaiev, O., Pržulj, N.: Learning the structure of protein–protein interaction networks. In: Proc. of 2009 Pacific Symposium on Biocomputing (PSB) (2009)
47. Kuchaiev, O., Milenkovic, T., Memisevic, V., Hayes, W., Pržulj, N.: Topological network alignment uncovers biological function and phylogeny. Journal of the Royal Society Interface (2010). doi:10.1098/rsif.2010.0063
48. LaCount, D.J., Vignali, M., Chettier, R., Phansalkar, A., Bell, R., Hesselberth, J.R., Schoenfeld, L.W., Ota, I., Sahasrabudhe, S., Kurschner, C., Fields, S., Hughes, R.E.: A protein interaction network of the malaria parasite *Plasmodium falciparum*. Nature **438**, 103–107 (2005)
49. Lappe, M., Holm, L.: Unraveling protein interaction networks with near-optimal efficiency. Nat. Biotechnol. **22**(1), 98–103 (2004)
50. Li, L., Alderson, D., Tanaka, R., Doyle, J.C., Willinger, W.: Towards a theory of scale-free graphs: definition, properties, and implications (extended version). arXiv:cond-mat/0501169 (2005)
51. Li, S., Armstrong, C., Bertin, N., Ge, H., Milstein, S., Boxem, M., Vidalain, P.O., Han, J.D., Chesneau, A., Hao, T., Goldberg, D.S., Li, N., Martinez, M., Rual, J.F., Lamesch, P., Xu, L., Tewari, M., Wong, S., Zhang, L., Berriz, G., Jacotot, L., Vaglio, P., Reboul, J., Hirozane-Kishikawa, T., Li, Q., Gabel, H., Elewa, A., Baumgartner, B., Rose, D., Yu, H., Bosak, S., Sequerra, R., Fraser, A., Mango, S., Saxton, W., Strome, S., van den Heuvel, S., Piano, F., Vandenhaute, J., Sardet, C., Gerstein, M., Doucette-Stamm, L., Gunsalus, K., Harper, J., Cusick, M., Roth, F., Hill, D., Vidal, M.: A map of the interactome network of the metazoan *C. elegans*. Science **303**, 540–543 (2004)
52. Liang, Z., Xu, M., Teng, M., Niu, L.: NetAlign: a web-based tool for comparison of protein interaction networks. Bioinformatics **22**(17), 2175–2177 (2006). doi:10.1093/bioinformatics/btl287
53. Lu, L., Xia, Y., Paccanaro, A., Yu, H., Gerstein, M.: Assessing the limits of genomic data integration for predicting protein networks. Genome Res. **15**, 945–953 (2005)
54. Milenković, T., Pržulj, N.: Uncovering biological network function via graphlet degree signatures. Cancer Inform. **6**, 257–273 (2008)

55. Milenković, T., Memisević, V., Ganesan, A.K., Pržulj, N.: Systems-level cancer gene identification from protein interaction network topology applied to melanogenesis-related interaction networks. J. R. Soc. Interface (2009). doi:10.1098/rsif.2009.0192
56. Milenkovic, T., Ng, W.L., Hayes, W., Pržulj, N.: Optimal network alignment with graphlet degree vectors. Cancer Informatics 9, 121–137 (2010)
57. Milo, R., Shen-Orr, S.S., Itzkovitz, S., Kashtan, N., Chklovskii, D., Alon, U.: Network motifs: simple building blocks of complex networks. Science 298, 824–827 (2002)
58. Milo, R., Itzkovitz, S., Kashtan, N., Levitt, R., Shen-Orr, S., Ayzenshtat, I., Sheffer, M., Alon, U.: Superfamilies of evolved and designed networks. Science 303, 1538–1542 (2004)
59. Molloy, M., Reed, B.: A critical point of random graphs with a given degree sequence. Random Struct. Algorithms 6, 161–180 (1995)
60. Molloy, M., Reed, B.: The size of the largest component of a random graph on a fixed degree sequence. Comb. Probab. Comput. 7, 295–306 (1998)
61. Nabieva, E., Jim, K., Agarwal, A., Chazelle, B., Singh, M.: Whole-proteome prediction of protein function via graph-theoretic analysis of interaction maps. Bioinformatics 21, 302–310 (2005)
62. Newman, M.E.J.: The structure and function of complex networks. SIAM Rev. 45(2), 167–256 (2003)
63. Newman, M.E.J., Watts, D.J.: Renormalization group analysis in the small-world network model. Phys. Lett. A 263, 341–346 (1999)
64. Newman, M.E.J., Watts, D.J.: Scaling and percolation in the small-world network model. Phys. Rev. E 60, 7332–7342 (1999)
65. Newman, M.E.J., Strogatz, S.H., Watts, D.J.: Random graphs with arbitrary degree distributions and their applications. Phys. Rev. E 64, 026118 (2001)
66. Paladugu, S., Zhao, S., Ray, A., Raval, A.: Mining protein networks for synthetic genetic interactions. BMC Bioinform. (2008). doi:10.1186/1471-2105-9-426
67. Parrish, J.R., Yu, J., Liu, G., Hines, J.A., Chan, J.E., Mangiola, B.A., Zhang, H., Pacifico, S., Fotouhi, F., DiRita, V.J., Ideker, T., Andrews, P., Finley, R.L. Jr.: A proteome-wide protein interaction map for Campylobacter jejuni. Genome Biol. 8, R130 (2007)
68. Pastor-Satorras, R., Smith, E., Sole, R.V.: Evolving protein interaction networks through gene duplication. J. Theor. Biol. 222, 199–210 (2003)
69. Pennisi, E.: Modernizing the tree of life. Science 300, 1692–1697 (2003)
70. Peri, S., Navarro, J.D., Kristiansen, T.Z., Amanchy, R., Surendranath, V., Muthusamy, B., Gandhi, T.K., Chandrika, K.N., Deshpande, N., Suresh, S., Rashmi, B.P., Shanker, K., Padma, N., Niranjan, V., Harsha, H.C., Talreja, N., Vrushabendra, B.M., Ramya, M.A., Yatish, A.J., Joy, M., Shivashankar, H.N., Kavitha, M.P., Menezes, M., Choudhury, D.R., Ghosh, N., Saravana, R., Chandran, S., Mohan, S., Jonnalagadda, C.K., Prasad, C.K., Kumar-Sinha, C., Deshpande, K.S., Pandey, A.: Human protein reference database as a discovery resource for proteomics. Nucleic Acids Res. 32, 497–501 (2004). 1362-4962 Journal Article
71. Pokholok, D.K., Harbison, C.T., Levine, S., Cole, M., Hannett, N.M., Lee, T.I., Bell, G.W., Walker, K., Rolfe, P.A., Herbolsheimer, E., Zeitlinger, J., Lewitter, F., Gifford, D.K., Young, R.A.: Geome-wide map of nucleosome acetylation and metylation in yeast. Cell 122, 517–527 (2005)
72. Pržulj, N.: Biological network comparison using graphlet degree distribution. Bioinformatics 23, 177–183 (2007)
73. Pržulj, N., Corneil, D.G., Jurisica, I.: Modeling interactome: Scale-free or geometric? Bioinformatics 20(18), 3508–3515 (2004)
74. Pržulj, N., Corneil, D.G., Jurisica, I.: Efficient estimation of graphlet frequency distributions in protein–protein interaction networks. Bioinformatics 22(8), 974–980 (2006). doi:10.1093/bioinformatics/btl030
75. Pržulj, N., Wigle, D., Jurisica, I.: Functional topology in a network of protein interactions. Bioinformatics 20(3), 340–348 (2004)
76. Pržulj, N., Kuchaiev, O., Stevanovic, A., Hayes, W.: Geometric evolutionary dynamics of protein interaction networks. In: 2010 Pacific Symposium on Biocomputing (PSB) (2010)

77. Rain, J.D., Selig, L., De Reuse, H., Battaglia, V., Reverdy, C., Simon, S., Lenzen, G., Petel, F., Wojcik, J., Schachter, V., Chemama, Y., Labigne, A., Legrain, P.: The protein–protein interaction map of *Helicobacter pylori*. Nature **409**, 211–215 (2001)
78. Ratmann, O., Wiuf, C., Pinney, J.W.: From evidence to inference: probing the evolution of protein interaction networks. HFSP J. **3**(5), 290–306 (2009)
79. Rual, J.F., Venkatesan, K., Hao, T., Hirozane-Kishikawa, T., Dricot, A., Li, N., Berriz, G.F., Gibbons, F.D., Dreze, M., Ayivi-Guedehoussou, N., Klitgord, N., Simon, C., Boxem, M., Milstein, S., Rosenberg, J., Goldberg, D.S., Zhang, L.V., Wong, S.L., Franklin, G., Li, S., Albala, J.S., Lim, J., Fraughton, C., Llamosas, E., Cevik, S., Bex, C., Lamesch, P., Sikorski, R.S., Vandenhaute, J., Zoghbi, H.Y., Smolyar, A., Bosak, S., Sequerra, R., Doucette-Stamm, L., Cusick, M.E., Hill, D.E., Roth, F.P., Vidal, M.: Towards a proteome-scale map of the human protein–protein interaction network. Nature **437**, 1173–1178 (2005)
80. Schwartz, A., Yu, J., Gardenour, K.R., Finley, R.L. Jr., Ideker, T.: Cost-effective strategies for completing the interactome. Nat. Methods **6**(1), 55–61 (2009)
81. Schwikowski, B., Uetz, P., Fields, A.: A network of protein–protein interactions in yeast. Nat. Biotechnol. **18**, 1257–1261 (2000)
82. Sharan, R., Ulitsky, I., Shamir, R.: Network-based prediction of protein function. Mol. Syst. Biol. **3**(88), 1–13 (2007)
83. Sharan, R., Ideker, T., Kelley, B.P., Shamir, R., Karp, R.M.: Identification of protein complexes by comparative analysis of yeast and bacterial protein interaction data. In: Proceedings of the Eighth Annual International Conference on Computational Molecular Biology (RE-COMB'04) (2004)
84. Sharan, R., Ideker, T.: Modeling cellular machinery through biological network comparison. Nat. Biotechnol. **24**(4), 427–433 (2006)
85. Sharan, R., Ideker, T.: Protein networks in disease. Genome Res. **18**, 644–652 (2008)
86. Shen-Orr, S.S., Milo, R., Mangan, S., Alon, U.: Network motifs in the transcriptional regulation network of *Escherichia coli*. Nat. Genet. **31**, 64–68 (2002)
87. Simon, H.A.: On a class of skew distribution functions. Biometrika **42**, 425–440 (1955)
88. Simonis, N., Rual, J.F., Carvunis, A.R., Tasan, M., Lemmens, I., Hirozane-Kishikawa, T., Hao, T., Sahalie, J.M., Venkatesan, K., Gebreab, F., Cevik, S., Klitgord, N., Fan, C., Braun, P., Li, N., Ayivi-Guedehoussou, N., Dann, E., Bertin, N., Szeto, D., Dricot, A., Yildirim, M.A., Lin, C., Smet, A.S.D., Kao, H.L., Simon, C., Smolyar, A., Ahn, J.S., Tewari, M., Boxem, M., Milstein, S., Yu, H., Dreze, M., Vandenhaute, J., Gunsalus, K.C., Cusick, M.E., Hill, D.E., Tavernier, J., Roth, F.P., Vidal, M.: Empirically controlled mapping of the *Caenorhabditis elegans* protein–protein interactome network. Nat. Methods **6**(1), 47–54 (2009)
89. Singh, R., Xu, J., Berger, B.: Pairwise global alignment of protein interaction networks by matching neighborhood topology. In: Research in Computational Molecular Biology, pp. 16–31. Springer, Berlin (2007)
90. Stelzl, U., Worm, U., Lalowski, M., Haenig, C., Brembeck, F., Goehler, H., Stroedicke, M., Zenkner, M., Schoenherr, A., Koeppen, S., Timm, J., Mintzlaff, S., Abraham, C., Bock, N., Kietzmann, S., Goedde, A., Toksoz, E., Droege, A., Krobitsch, S., Korn, B., Birchmeier, W., Lehrach, H., Wanker, E.: A human protein–protein interaction network: A resource for annotating the proteome. Cell **122**, 957–968 (2005)
91. Stumpf, M.P.H., Wiuf, C., May, R.M.: Subnets of scale-free networks are not scale-free: Sampling properties of networks. Proc. Natl. Acad. Sci. USA **102**, 4221–4224 (2005)
92. Tong, A.H.Y., Lesage, G., Bader, G.D., Ding, H., Xu, H., Xin, X., Young, J., Berriz, G.F., Brost, R.L., Chang, M., Chen, Y., Cheng, X., Chua, G., Friesen, H., Goldberg, D.S., Haynes, J., Humphries, C., He, G., Hussein, S., Ke, L., Krogan, N., Li, Z., Levinson, J.N., Lu, H., Menard, P., Munyana, C., Parsons, A.B., Ryan, O., Tonikian, R., Roberts, T., Sdicu, A.M., Shapiro, J., Sheikh, B., Suter, B., Wong, S.L., Zhang, L.V., Zhu, H., Burd, C.G., Munro, S., Sander, C., Rine, J., Greenblatt, J., Peter, M., Bretscher, A., Bell, G., Roth, F.P., Brown, G.W., Andrews, B., Bussey, H., Boone, C.: Global mapping of the yeast genetic interaction network. Science **303**, 808–813 (2004)
93. Uetz, P., Giot, L., Cagney, G., Mansfield, T.A., Judson, R.S., Knight, J.R., Lockshon, E., Narayan, V., Srinivasan, M., Pochart, P., Qureshi-Emili, A., Li, Y., Godwin, B., Conover, D.,

Kalbfleish, T., Vijayadamodar, G., Yang, M., Johnston, M., Fields, S., Rothberg, J.M.: A comprehensive analysis of protein–protein interactions in *Saccharomyces cerevisiae*. Nature **403**, 623–627 (2000)

94. Uetz, P., Dong, Y.A., Zeretzke, C., Atzler, C., Baiker, A., Berger, B., Rajagopala, S., Roupelieva, M., Rose, D., Fossum, E., Haas, J.: Herpesviral protein networks and their interaction with the human proteome. Science **311**, 239–242 (2006)

95. Vazquez, A., Flammini, A., Maritan, A., Vespignani, A.: Modeling of protein interaction networks. Complexus **1**, 38–44 (2001)

96. Vazquez, A., Flammini, A., Maritan, A., Vespignani, A.: Global protein function prediction from protein–protein interaction networks. Nat. Biotechnol. **21**, 697–700 (2003)

97. Venkatesan, K., et al.: An empirical framework for binary interactome mapping. Nat. Methods **6**(1), 83–90 (2009)

98. von Brunn, A., Teepe, C., Simpson, J.C., Pepperkok, R., Friedel, C.C., Zimmer, R., Roberts, R., Baric, R., Haas, J.: Analysis of intraviral protein–protein interactions of the SARS coronavirus ORFeome. PLoS ONE **2**, e459 (2007)

99. von Mering, C., Krause, R., Snel, B., Cornell, M., Oliver, S.G., Fields, S., Bork, P.: Comparative assessment of large-scale data sets of protein–protein interactions. Nature **417**(6887), 399–403 (2002)

100. Wagner, A.: How the global structure of protein interaction networks evolves. Proc. R. Soc. Lond. B, Biol. Sci. **270**, 457–466 (2003)

101. Watts, D.J., Strogatz, S.H.: Collective dynamics of 'small-world' networks. Nature **393**, 440–442 (1998)

102. West, D.B.: Introduction to Graph Theory, 2nd edn. Prentice Hall, Upper Saddle River (2001)

103. Wodak, S., Pu, S., Vlasblom, J., Seraphin, B.: Challenges and rewards of interaction proteomics. Mol. Cell. Proteomics **8**(1), 3–18 (2009)

104. Wong, S., et al.: Combining biological networks to predict genetic interactions. Proc. Natl. Acad. Sci. USA **101**, 15682–15687 (2004)

105. Xenarios, I., Rice, D.W., Salwinski, L., Baron, M.K., Marcotte, E.M.., Eisenberg, D: DIP: the Database of Interacting Proteins. Nucleic Acids Res. **28**(1), 289–291 (2000)

106. Yeger-Lotem, E., Sattath, S., Kashtan, N., Itzkovitz, S., Milo, R., Pinter, R., Alon, U., Margalit, H.: Network motifs in integrated cellular networks of transcription-regulation and protein–protein interaction. Proc. Natl. Acad. Sci. USA **101**(16), 5934–5939 (2004)

107. Yildirim, M.A., et al.: Drug-target network. Nat. Biotechnol. **25**, 1119–1126 (2007)

108. Yu, H., et al.: High-quality binary protein interaction map of the yeast interactome networks. Science **322**, 104–110 (2008)

109. Zanzoni, A., Montecchi-Palazzi, L., Quondam, M., Ausiello, G., Helmer-Citterich, M., Cesareni, G.: MINT: A Molecular INTeraction database. FEBS Lett. **513**(1), 135–140 (2002)

110. Zaslavskiy, M., Bach, F., Vert, J.P.: Global alignment of protein–protein interaction networks by graph matching methods. Bioinformatics **25**(12), 259–267 (2009)

111. Zhang, L., et al.: Motifs, themes and thematic maps of an integrated *Saccharomyces cerevisiae* interaction network. J. Biol.. (2005). doi:10.1186/jbiol23

Chapter 4
Networks and Models with Heterogeneous Population Structure in Epidemiology

R.R. Kao

Abstract Heterogeneous population structure can have a profound effect on infectious disease dynamics, and is particularly important when investigating "tactical" disease control questions. At times, the nature of the network involved in the transmission of the pathogen (bacteria, virus, macro-parasite, etc.) appears to be clear; however, the nature of the network involved is dependent on the scale (e.g. within-host, between-host, or between-population), the nature of the contact, which ranges from the highly specific (e.g. sexual acts or needle sharing at the person-to-person level) to almost completely non-specific (e.g. aerosol transmission, often over long distances as can occur with the highly infectious livestock pathogen foot-and-mouth disease virus—FMDv—at the farm-to-farm level, e.g. Schley et al. in J. R. Soc. Interface 6:455–462, 2008), and the timescale of interest (e.g. at the scale of the individual, the typical infectious period of the host). Theoretical approaches to examining the implications of particular network structures on disease transmission have provided critical insight; however, a greater challenge is the integration of network approaches with data on real population structures. In this chapter, some concepts in disease modelling will be introduced, the relevance of selected network phenomena discussed, and then results from real data and their relationship to network analyses summarised. These include examinations of the patterns of air traffic and its relation to the spread of SARS in 2003 (Colizza et al. in BMC Med., 2007; Hufnagel et al. in Proc. Natl. Acad. Sci. USA 101:15124–15129, 2004), the use of the extensively documented Great Britain livestock movements network (Green et al. in J. Theor. Biol. 239:289–297, 2008; Robinson et al. in J. R. Soc. Interface 4:669–674, 2007; Vernon and Keeling in Proc. R. Soc. Lond. B, Biol. Sci. 276:469–476, 2009) and the growing interest in combining contact structure data with phylogenetics to identify real

Elements of Sects. 4.1–4.3 have been adapted from: Kao, R.R., Kiss, I.Z.: Network concepts and epidemiological models. In: Stumpf, M.P.H., Wiuf, C. (eds.) Statistical and Evolutionary Analysis of Biological Networks. Imperial College Press, London (2009).

R.R. Kao (✉)
Faculty of Veterinary Medicine, University of Glasgow, Glasgow, UK
e-mail: r.kao@vet.gla.ac.uk

E. Estrada et al. (eds.), *Network Science*,
DOI 10.1007/978-1-84996-396-1_4, © Springer-Verlag London Limited 2010

contact patterns as they directly relate to diseases of interest (Cottam et al. in PLoS Pathogens 4:1000050, 2007; Hughes et al. in PLoS Pathogens 5:1000590, 2009).

4.1 Simple Mathematical Models

The susceptible/infected/resistant (*SIR*) ordinary differential equation (ODE) model lies at the foundation of modern quantitative epidemiology. Though the original work [46] considered infectious states in greater generality, the most common version of this model makes the simplification of assuming a single exponentially distributed infectious stage, with all infected individuals being equally infectious. With this assumption, the system takes the form of a "compartmental model". Here there are a set of three ordinary differential equations to be integrated over time:

$$\frac{dS}{dt} = -\beta I S,$$

$$\frac{dI}{dt} = \beta I S - \gamma I,$$

$$\frac{dR}{dt} = \gamma I, \tag{4.1}$$

$$S + I + R = N.$$

In the system of equations (4.1), the compartments are: S the number of susceptible individuals, I the number of infected, and R the number of removed (usually considered to be recovered and immune, though other interpretations of this state are possible). The total population size N is fixed. The parameter β is the rate per infected individual at which infections occur, while γ is the rate at which infected individuals are removed. Important principles that have guided mathematical epidemiology over the last century are apparent in this simple formulation. First, interest in the field has concentrated on the nonlinear interactions over time between a host population and a pathogen that exploits it. Second, individuals are treated as indistinguishable except for their disease state. Third, the nonlinear terms incorporate the "mean-field" assumption, where interactions between members of the population are considered to occur at random, with equal probability that any member will interact with any other element of the system. Finally, the model operates in continuous time and population-space.

In contrast, under the network paradigm of disease spread, a population is a network (or "graph") of nodes ("vertices") representing epidemiological units at a relevant scale (e.g. individuals, towns, cities, farms or wildlife communities). Each node i is connected to other nodes by a number k_i links ("edges"), this defining the degree of the node. The links usually represent potentially infectious contacts. For example, for sexually transmitted infections, or STIs, links may be sexual acts or sexual partners [32], while for diseases transmitting within a hospital links may represent contacts occurring through room- and ward-sharing [53]. Multiple, simultaneous exposures to a pathogen are usually assumed to act independently; therefore, if a node is connected to two infected nodes each of which can infect with probability $\bar{p}$, the probability of becoming infected is $(1 - (1 - \bar{p})^2)$, where in this case, all links have the same weight. In directed networks (e.g. where one individual can infect another but not necessarily *vice versa*), links are distinguished as being in- or out-links, with nodes having in- and out-degrees. For infectious diseases, this is more likely to be appropriate for larger scale models, for example, where transmission may be related to the migration of individuals who do not return to their origin. In most epidemiologically relevant examples where network structure is important, $\langle k \rangle \ll N$, where $\langle k \rangle$ is the average node degree, and N the population size. Borrowing the concept from the simple ODE models, nodes typically possess one of a limited number of states (e.g. susceptible, infected or removed as in (4.1)). "Mean-field" models such as described by (4.1) are similar to maximally connected network models—i.e. where every individual in the population is connected to any other individual and $\langle k \rangle = k_i = N - 1$ for all nodes i. Network models can in this sense be considered a generalisation of mean-field models. Both network models and ODE models differ from detailed simulations studies, by being abstractions for gaining insight into how heterogeneity in the contacts amongst individuals can contribute to disease spread and its control. However, mean-field and network models differ in terms of the philosophy behind their representations. Mean-field models often do have population structure, but this structure is imposed on the population, rather than being generated from individual properties. In the network perspective, each node only has information about a limited subset of neighbours. Links are generated from this "local neighbourhood" that defines the social network. Thus the network model displays corresponding "emergent behaviour" in a way that the Kermack–McKendrick model does not. An important question is the extent to which the pattern, or the population structure, and process, or temporally-dependent changes as highlighted in mean-field models, are important in determining how epidemics spread. That most work has previously concentrated on the dynamics amongst simplified compartments is at least partially because observational data on overall disease incidence, and detailed data describing the time course of individual infection states have historically been more available than meaningful population contact structure data, particularly for humans. One of the most detailed and successful models of disease transmission on structured human populations is the description of measles outbreaks in post-WWII Britain (e.g. [7, 28]) which includes comprehensive measles incidence reports, but where location is only specified to the level of city or town. Contact structure is therefore highly abstract (though more recent work in this field has used gravity models to described the underlying demographic contacts between cities [72]). The development of the field has also benefited from the rich literature of dynamical systems, and the development of analogous models in chemical kinetics, reflected in the early appellation of "mass-action" dynamics when referring to what is now commonly known as "density dependent" contact.[1] Nevertheless, many of the ideas explored in social network analyses have been pre-

---

[1]Noting that there has been some confusion on this—see [13].

viously explored using other approaches, though the social network paradigm has often proved to be more natural, and provided new insights.

4.1.1 Introducing R_0

For compartmental models of disease spread, the stability of the disease-free steady state is determined by the basic reproduction number, R_0, which is the central quantity of modern theoretical epidemiology (e.g. [2]). The "simple", commonly accepted biological definition of R_0 is generally stated as "the number of new infections generated by a single infected individual introduced into a wholly susceptible, homogeneously mixed population at equilibrium". For the system of equations (4.1), the definition is equivalent to

$$R_0 = \frac{\beta N}{\gamma}. \tag{4.2}$$

For simple systems, if $R_0 < 1$, then the disease-free state is globally asymptotically stable (but see the section below). Each infected person will typically infect fewer than one person before dying or recovering, so the outbreak itself will die out (i.e. $\frac{dI}{dt}\big|_{t=0^+} < 0$). When $R_0 > 1$, each person who becomes infected will infect on average more than one person, so the epidemic will spread (i.e. $\frac{dI}{dt}\big|_{t=0^+} > 0$). While this definition is intuitive, conceptual problems immediately arise. For example, can one define a "typical" infected individual? At what stage of the infection process is the infected individual introduced? What if there are distinct subpopulations or population structures? Is R_0 then a meaningful concept? Considerable attention has been devoted to these questions (e.g. [31, 60, 66]), in particular due to the generalisation to more complex population and infection structures via the next generation matrix formalism [15]. However, these definitions are meaningful only if meaningful sub-populations can be defined, allowing for an exponential growth phase in an epidemic. Thus most network models with their complex structure do not lend themselves to such simple definitions, and the relationship between R_0 and the network representation is further discussed below.

4.1.2 Density vs. Frequency Dependent Contact

A connection from (4.1) to network models can be established by a closer examination of the contact structure implicit in the nonlinear term βSI, which can be understood if this expression is replaced with a term

$$\tau C(N) I \frac{S}{N}$$

(see, for example, [59]). Here, each individual has $C(N)$ potential infectious contacts (infectious with probability τ), and this is dependent on the total population N.[2] The region in the parameter space where $R_0 < 1$ then defines a globally stable disease-free state if $dC/dN \geq 0$ (usually, $d^2C/dN^2 \leq 0$ but this is not required), and none of $C(N)$, β or γ are functions of I. In particular, if $dC/dI > 0$, $d\beta/dI > 0$, or $d\gamma/dI > 0$, global stability is lost. This can occur if, for example, removal of infected individuals requires the availability of limited resources, so that $d\gamma/dI > 0$ (e.g. foot-and-mouth disease in the UK in 2001, see [30]) or one may have $dC/dI > 0$ if, for example, contacts are increased by otherwise sedentary individuals attempting to flee an epidemic, as may have occurred during the Black Death in the fourteenth century Europe. Each infected individual has a probability S/N per contact of interacting with a susceptible individual. For density dependent contact, $C(N) = N$ and the form of system (4.1) is obtained. For "frequency dependent" contact, $C(N) = \kappa$, a constant. In this case, the rate that new infections appear is $\tau SI\kappa/N$, and $R_0 = \tau\kappa/\gamma$. A critical difference between the two cases is that, with density dependence, thinning of the total population reduces N and therefore the value of R_0, while with frequency dependence the reduction in population density or size has no effect on R_0.

In frequency dependent models, the number of contacts (links) is independent of population size. However, they differ from network models in that the contact is made with a random individual in the population. Thus the two are only equivalent in the case of a dynamic network with links that switch to new partners at an infinite rate [57]. An important consequence of this is that any infected individual still has κ outward potentially infectious contacts in a frequency dependent model, while in static network models with bi-directional links, at least one of them is "used up" because the node was infected along one of its existing links (see, for example, [14]).

As previously noted, in network models individuals can no longer be assumed to be in potentially infectious contact with all members of the population. If the degree distribution $p(k)$ gives the probability that a randomly selected node has exactly k links, then the average number of connections per node is given by $\langle k \rangle = \sum_l lp(l)$. Epidemiologically, the degree of a node gives the maximum number of nodes that a node could infect. Of course, as $\langle k \rangle \ll N$, only a few nodes are likely to be directly infected by any given node. In a Poisson random network (originally studied by Erdős and Rényi [19]), nodes are connected by links, these chosen randomly from the $N(N-1)/2$ possible links. A Poisson network can be constructed via a binomial model where, rather than fixing the number of links and choosing partners at random, every possible pair out of the nodes is connected with probability $\widetilde{p}$. The average number of connections per node is $\langle k \rangle = \widetilde{p}(N-1)$ and the degree distribution is given by

$$P(k) = \binom{N-1}{k} \widetilde{p}^k (1-\widetilde{p})^{(N-1)-k} \cong \frac{\langle k \rangle^k e^{-\langle k \rangle}}{k!}. \tag{4.3}$$

Here, exact equivalence is achieved when $N \to \infty$. When $\widetilde{p}$ is sufficiently large, random networks tend to have relatively small diameters (maximum shortest path

---

[2] We note that this it is sometimes more important to consider population density rather than total population; however, throughout will consider dynamics that depend on the population size.

length considering all possible node pairs). The number of nodes at a distance l from a given node is well approximated by $\langle k \rangle^l$ for the Poisson network [20]. When the whole network is captured starting from a given node, $\langle k \rangle^l \cong N$, and l approaches the network diameter d. Hence, d depends only logarithmically on the number of nodes, and the average path length is also expected to scale only slowly with increasing population size, i.e. $\langle l_{\text{rand}} \rangle \propto \ln(N)/\ln(\langle k \rangle)$, with correspondingly small diameter. In this case, there is a direct relationship to the "simple" SIR model, as $R_0 = \tau \langle k \rangle$. For more complex network structures, the correspondence to R_0 is less clear.

4.2 Networks with Localisation of Contacts: Small Worlds, Clustering, Pairwise Approximations and Moment Closure

4.2.1 Small Worlds

A contact network with a small diameter such as found in Poisson networks supports epidemics that can spread broadly throughout the network in a few generations. Thus even for a disease with low probability of transmission and where the disease has been identified within a few generations of infection after its introduction, it would be difficult to identify and isolate subgroups of individuals who are at higher risk of becoming infected. Localisation is exemplified by spatial spread, such as found in lattice models, where nodes are positioned on a regular grid of locations, and neighbouring individuals are connected. Such lattice models/networks exhibit homogeneous contact but have much longer average path lengths and diameters than Poisson networks. Empirical measurements confirm that many real-world networks are characterised by greater localisation of connections—i.e. the tendency for links to occur with greater probability than average amongst subgroups of nodes, but have small average path lengths very similar to that of Poisson random networks. Motivated by social structures where most individuals belong to localised communities composed of work colleagues, neighbours or people sharing similar interests, but some individuals also have connections with individuals that belong to other localised communities (e.g. relatives living considerable distances away and thus likely to belong to distant social communities as well) and old acquaintances, Watts and Strogatz [71] proposed the famous "small-world network" (SWN) model, which uses a one-parameter model to interpolate between a regular lattice model and a Poisson network. Their model starts with a ring lattice with N nodes where each node is connected to an arbitrary fixed number K of its closest neighbours. Two types of SWNs have commonly been studied. In the original version, a random rewiring of all links is carried out with probability q. A variant with similar properties does not rewire, but adds long range links randomly, with probability q to generate the same number of long range links as in the original model (Fig. 4.1).

Both approaches produce on average $qKN/2$ "long-range" links (or more correctly, they connect nodes at random). As the latter approach simplifies some calculations but has the same key properties as the original model, it will be referred to

Fig. 4.1 An example
small-world network, with
each node connected locally
to its four nearest neighbours

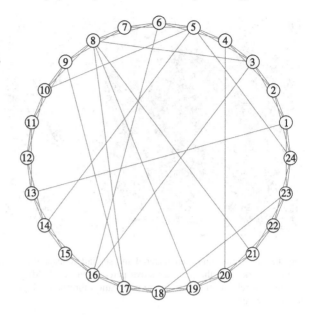

later in the chapter. For a broad range of q, the SWN generates average path lengths
approaching those observed in Poisson random graphs, yet with much greater localisation. The smaller average path length driven by the limited number of long-
range connections (shortcuts) makes the network more connected, with fewer edges
needed to connect any two nodes. A smaller average path length also means a
smaller number of infectious generations with a shorter epidemic time scale, and
a lower threshold for a large epidemic. The critical idea put forward by this model
is that a relatively few "long-distance" connections are important for the transmission and persistence of disease. This has long been established, for example, within
the metapopulation paradigm developed in the 1960s [50] where occasional migration between habitat patches was invoked to explain the persistence of species that
would otherwise go extinct—in the case of epidemiology, the metapopulation is the
pathogen operating on the host (or communities of hosts), which represent the habitat patches, such as the cities and towns in the previously mentioned measles models
[7, 28]. Where the model of Watts and Strogatz' differed, however, was showing in
an elegantly simple model, and in a quantifiable way, how simple couplings defined
only as a property of individuals could be weak, yet produce dramatic effects in
communities.

4.2.2 Clustering on Networks and Moment Closure

The SWN model is a very specific, illustrative example of a highly clustered network. More generally, there are often subgroups or communities of individuals that

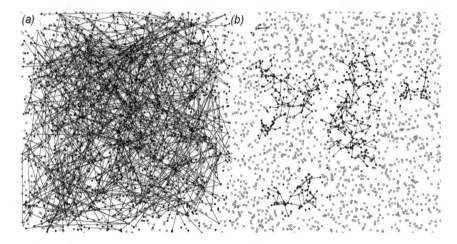

Fig. 4.2 Transmission on unclustered and spatially clustered networks. Transmission on unclustered networks fills the picture (above percolation threshold) while on clustered networks, the epidemic is self-limiting (below the percolation threshold). Figure courtesy of Dr. D.M. Green, Stirling University

are more likely to be associated with each other, and there is an extensive literature devoted to identifying network-based measures of community (for a review, see [12]). One measure of localisation is the clustering coefficient which can be quantified as $c = \frac{3 \cdot triangles}{triples}$, where a triangle is defined by a set of three nodes X, Y and Z in a triplet, where X is connected to Y which is connected to Z, and X is also connected to Z. Clustering can be viewed as expressing the probability of two friends of any one individual being themselves friends of each other, and this is illustrated in the classic signature of the small world effect, which is the rapid decline in the average path length between nodes, when the clustering coefficient remains high [71]. This definition is not unique; for example, clustering can also be computed by averaging the clustering coefficients of individual nodes $c_i = \frac{E_i}{k_i(k_i-1)/2}$, which represents the ratio between the number of links E_i present amongst the neighbours of node and the possible maximum number of such links. For any meaningful definition, in networks approximating the structure of Poisson random networks have small inherent clustering, and in the limit of infinite populations, zero. Clustered networks can be generated by randomly distributing individuals/nodes in a given n-dimensional space (e.g. a specified two-dimensional surface) and assuming that the probability of a connection between two individuals is a function of their distance. By choosing an appropriate function, the average degree and clustering can be varied. Of course, clustering alone does not uniquely define a network; for example, an infinite number of networks can be generated with zero clustering.

While the definition of clustering and its extensions to higher order loops including four or more nodes allows for the description of heterogeneous structures in networks, it does not create an analytical tool for describing the effect on disease transmission (Fig. 4.2). One approach to this is "moment closure" [42, 44].

A population can be described in terms of the frequency of clusters of individuals of various types (e.g. S, I, and R) and of various sizes (singlets, doublets, triplets and so on; i.e. the 'moments' of the distribution). By including the frequency of moments of increasingly higher order, the population can be described with increasing accuracy, but at the cost of increasing complexity. Disease transmission is dependent on whether one of the pairs is connected to an infectious individual, i.e. if $[SS]$ is the number of $S + S$ pairs, and $[SSI]$ the number of $S + S + I$ triplets then $\frac{d[SS]}{dt} \propto [SSI]$. Similarly, $\frac{d[SSS]}{dt} \propto [SSSI]$, etc. For the simple SIR model, the number of $[SI]$ pairs is determined by the equation

$$\frac{d[SI]}{dt} = \tau[SSI] - \tau[SI] - \tau[ISI] - g[SI],$$

where $\tau[SSI]$ denotes the creation of an SI pair through the infection of S in the central position of the triple. In a similar fashion, the number of triplets requires knowledge about the number of quadruplets, and so on, and the system soon becomes completely intractable. Analytical tractability is achieved by "closing" the system at the level of pairs and approximating triplets as a function of pairs and individual classes [44]. In clustered networks there will be some heterogeneity in the probability of association between two nodes (in social networks, for example, the probability that two people will be friends will increase if they have a friend in common, or for spatially clustered populations, that the Voronoi tessellation for three nodes produces a common boundary point [45]). To account for the correlation between the node in state X and node in state Z, a closure relation is considered [42], where if N is the total population size, and Φ the expected proportion of triplets that are triangles, then

$$[XYZ] \approx \frac{\langle k \rangle - 1}{\langle k \rangle} \frac{[XY][YZ]}{[Y]} \left((1 - \Phi) + \frac{\Phi N}{\langle k \rangle} \frac{[XZ]}{[X][Z]} \right).$$

This approach has the attractive feature that is transparent, easy to parameterise and builds on understanding global properties of the system based on local/neighbourhood interactions. The closure at the triplet level (i.e. ignoring loops incorporating four or more nodes) is a compromise between incorporating contact heterogeneity and retaining analytical tractability, and it has been successful in accounting for correlations that form due to diseases spreading amongst clusters of connected individuals. An important feature of even moderate levels of clustering is the rapid decrease in the average number of new infections produced by each infectious individual. Largely due to the depletion of the susceptible neighbourhood; past the first generation, infected nodes often have at least one neighbour that is already infected. In networks clustered in two dimensions, there is a corresponding spatial localisation of epidemics (Fig. 4.2). While moment closure can provide a good approximation to the time course of stochastic simulations on clustered networks [42], as always such good agreement depends on the underlying model being considered. Based on a model using Poisson-random networks with contact tracing and a delay before infectiousness [47], Fig. 4.2 shows how, even with no "forced" clustering (i.e. clustering only occurs due to population size effects), there is poor agreement between simulations and the analytic approximation, and this difference quickly becomes pronounced as clustering increases. While the sources of the discrepancy are not entirely clear, the delay in the onset of infectiousness and the addition of contact tracing add considerably to the complexity of the system being studied, highlighting the need for further research into analytical models of this type of contact heterogeneity.

Despite these difficulties, as a strategic tool, moment closure equations allow us to explore the relationship between clustering and epidemic spread [42], showing how clustering can lead to a dramatic reduction in the value of R_0 if generations of infection overlap with equivalent effects on the probability of successful disease invasion. Using additional equations incorporating links between nodes along which tracing takes place, the moment closure approach can also be used to explore the effect of network dependent disease control, such as contact tracing, i.e. identifying potentially infectious connections from infected individuals (e.g. [17, 34, 47]). On a practical level, moment closure approaches have been used to explore the consequences of exploiting spatial proximity in the case of the Great Britain 2001 foot-and-mouth disease epidemic [21].

4.3 Heterogeneity in Contacts per Individual

4.3.1 Models for Sexually Transmitted Diseases and HIV

While moment closure approaches can be used in systems with both clustering and heterogeneity in contact frequency [18], it is not a natural tool for exploring heterogeneity in the number of contacts. For models where contact heterogeneity is important, such as is found for sexually transmitted infections, or STIs, the starting assumption is often that the population is homogeneously mixed. For STIs, the nature of the potentially infectious contact is well-defined, and it has long been understood that modelling their transmission and control must account for heterogeneities in sexual activity [2, 32]. Assume that the probability of transmission of an STI to an individual depends only on the number of potentially infectious contacts per individual and the probability of transmission per contact. Then the population can be divided into distinct groups, with each group defined solely by the number of contacts. The number of individuals with k contacts is N_k ($k = 1, \ldots, n$). For simplicity, only the case of an *SIR* model in an infinite closed population is considered. Following [2], (4.1) can then be extended to

$$
\begin{aligned}
\frac{dS_k}{dt} &= -\beta k S_k(t) \sum_l p(l|k) \frac{I_l(t)}{N_l}, \\
\frac{dI_k}{dt} &= \beta k S_k(t) \sum_l p(l|k) \frac{I_l(t)}{N_l} - \gamma I_k(t),
\end{aligned}
\qquad k = 1, \ldots, n. \qquad (4.4)
$$

Here S_k and I_k represent the number of susceptible and infectious individuals with k contacts, and (frequency dependent) per contact transmission rate β between an infected and a susceptible individual. The rate at which new infections are produced is proportional to β, the degree k of the susceptible nodes being considered, the number of susceptible nodes with k connections, and the probability that any given neighbour of a susceptible node with k connections is infectious. When proportionate random mixing is assumed, the probability that a node with k contacts is connected to a node with l contacts is given by $P(l|k) = lp(l)/\langle k \rangle$, where $p(l) = N_l/N$, and $\langle k \rangle = \sum_l lp(l)$ is the average number of connections in the population.

The basic reproduction number R_0 can be calculated for this system, which has no higher order structure, using the more general definition

$$R_0 = \lim_{N,n\to\infty} \left(\sqrt[n]{\prod_{m=1}^{n} \frac{I_{m+1}}{I_m}} \right), \tag{4.5}$$

where N is the population size, n is the generation number, and I_m is the number of infected individuals in all classes in generation m [15]. In this abstract model, heterosexual transmission, which requires cycles of length two, is not considered. This reduces (4.5) to $R_0 = \lim_{N,n\to\infty}(I_{n+1}/I_n)$. A simple approach to calculating R_0 in this latter case follows [40]. Consider the introduction of infection into an arbitrary node in a network. This node will be of degree k with probability $p(k)$. Then for a given probability of transmission per link $\bar{p}$, the number of infected elements of an arbitrary degree l following the first generation of transmission is

$$I_{l,1} = \bar{p} \sum_k P(l|k)kp(k)$$
$$= \frac{\bar{p}lp(l) \sum_k kp(k)}{\langle k \rangle}$$
$$= \bar{p}lp(l) \tag{4.6}$$

since $\langle k \rangle = \langle l \rangle$. In the following generation,

$$I_{m,2} = \bar{p} \sum_l P(m|l)I_{l,1}. \tag{4.7}$$

It is easy to show using (4.6) and (4.7) and summing over all node degrees, that $I_2/I_1 = I_{n+1}/I_n$ for all subsequent successive generations n and $n+1$, and therefore

$$R_0 = \bar{p}\frac{\langle k^2 \rangle}{\langle k \rangle}, \tag{4.8}$$

i.e. R_0 is proportional to the variance-to-mean ratio of the contact degree distribution in the population, where $\langle k^2 \rangle = \sum_l l^2 p(l)$ is the second moment of the contact distribution. In a directed network, with unbalanced in- and out-degrees, this can easily be generalised to

$$R_0 = \bar{p}\frac{\langle k_{in}k_{out}\rangle}{\langle \sqrt{k_{in}k_{out}}\rangle}. \tag{4.9}$$

Equations (4.8) and (4.9) illustrate the disproportionate role played by highly connected individuals or 'super-spreaders'. Such models can be further extended to account for additional properties of the population contact structure or disease characteristics, though at the cost of losing analytical tractability and model generality.

4.3.2 Disease Transmission on Scale-Free Networks

These investigations have been mirrored by equivalent investigations of social networks with high variance in the degree distribution. Although random graphs have been extensively used as models of real-world networks, particularly in epidemiology, they can have serious shortcomings when compared to empirical data characterising social structures such as networks of friendship within various communities, as well as structures in physical and biological systems, including food webs, neural networks and metabolic pathways. With surprising frequency, the empirically measured degree distribution has significantly higher variance-to-mean ratio compared to a Poisson distribution. Examples include the World Wide Web, the Internet, ecological food webs, protein–protein interactions at the cellular level (e.g. [25]), and most relevant for this discussion, human sexual networks, all with degree distributions reasonably approximated as scale-free, i.e. $p(k) \approx k^{-\gamma}$ with $2 < \gamma \leq 3$, over several orders of magnitude (but see also [38]). As noted above, to account for the fact that each infected node past the first generation must have at least one link that ends in another infected node, the value of R_0 differs slightly from (4.8):

$$R_0 = \bar{p}\langle k\rangle\left(\frac{\langle k^2\rangle}{\langle k\rangle^2} - \frac{1}{\langle k\rangle}\right). \tag{4.10}$$

The translation in terms of the epidemiological parameters β and γ is slightly more difficult as the depletion of links from an infected node means that the transmission rate must be increased to maintain the same R_0 [43] and this, in turn, changes the infection rate [26]. While the empirically determined distribution of sexual contacts is more precisely fit with a truncated scale-free distribution [38], in the limiting approximation of a scale-free infinite population with no truncation, $R_0 \to \infty$ since $\langle k^2\rangle/\langle k\rangle \to \infty$ even though $\langle k\rangle$ is finite. It follows that even an arbitrarily small transmission rate β can sustain an epidemic [58]. As implied by the name "scale-free", random removal of nodes does not reduce the variance. Therefore, no amount of randomly applied, incomplete control (i.e. vaccination, quarantine) can prevent an epidemic. However, this is not the case for finite populations where the threshold behaviour is recovered [52], and targeting the small pool of highly connected nodes is sufficient to prevent an epidemic, so long as these individuals can be identified

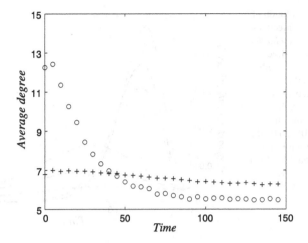

Fig. 4.3 Average degree of new infectious nodes for random (+) and truncated scale-free networks ($p(k) = Ck^{-\gamma}e^{-k/L}$ with $\gamma = 2.5$, $L = 100$ and $k \geq 3$) (o). Both networks with $N = 2000$, $\langle k \rangle = 6$. The model includes four classes (susceptible—S, exposed—E, infectious—I, results in tracing—T, and removed—R) with rate of susceptible becoming infected ($S \rightarrow E$) $0.15d^{-1}$, and, tracing occurring at rate $0.5d^{-1}$ (for all of $S \rightarrow R$, $E \rightarrow R$, $I \rightarrow R$), latent period $10d$, infectious period $3.5d$, nodes trigger tracing for $2.0d$. Figure courtesy of Dr. I.Z. Kiss, University of Sussex

and treated or removed. Further, even in the absence of control, the supply of highly connected nodes is quickly depleted, resulting in rapid disease extinction.

Barthélemy et al. [6] showed that a further consequence of high variance distributions is the non-uniform spread of the epidemic. The higher probability that any node will be connected to a highly connected node means that disease spread follows a hierarchical order, with the highly connected nodes becoming infected first, and the epidemic thereafter cascading towards groups of nodes with smaller degree (Fig. 4.3 and [48]).

The initial exponential growth in the time-scale of epidemics is inversely proportional to the network degree fluctuations, $\langle k^2 \rangle / \langle k \rangle$. Thus the high variance in heterogeneous networks also implies an extremely small time-scale for the outbreak and a very rapid spread of the epidemic, implying that in populations with these characteristics there is a window of opportunity, in which diseases can be controlled with relatively little impact on the majority of individuals (Fig. 4.4 and [48]), though this window becomes small with increasing degree fluctuations.

May and Lloyd [52] defined $\rho_0 = \beta \langle k \rangle / \gamma$ to be the transmission potential, equal to R_0 in homogeneously mixing (i.e. random) networks. For $\rho_0 < 1$, $R_0 < 1$ on a random network, but for networks with higher variance-to-mean ratio, we can have $R_0 > 1$. For $\rho_0 > 1$, because scale-free networks lose high-degree nodes more rapidly than low-degree nodes, the variance in the degree of the remaining susceptible nodes is quickly reduced, and thus the low-degree nodes are effectively protected. Thus for sufficiently high ρ_0, epidemics on random networks last longer, and also are able to reach more nodes. Above a value ρ_{crit}, the final epidemic size

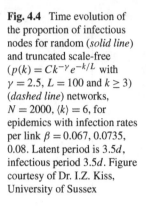

Fig. 4.4 Time evolution of the proportion of infectious nodes for random (*solid line*) and truncated scale-free ($p(k) = Ck^{-\gamma}e^{-k/L}$ with $\gamma = 2.5$, $L = 100$ and $k \geq 3$) (*dashed line*) networks, $N = 2000$, $\langle k \rangle = 6$, for epidemics with infection rates per link $\beta = 0.067, 0.0735, 0.08$. Latent period is $3.5d$, infectious period $3.5d$. Figure courtesy of Dr. I.Z. Kiss, University of Sussex

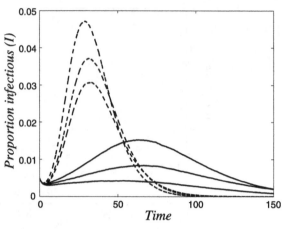

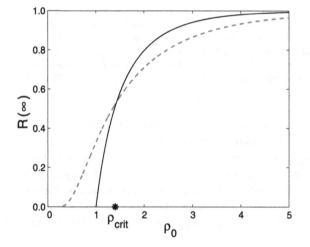

Fig. 4.5 Final epidemic size $R(\infty)$ as a function of the transmission potential ρ_0 computed analytically for the mean-field SIR model (*solid line*) and semi-analytically for Barabasi–Albert or BA networks (*dashed line*). For the BA networks R_∞ increases from close to zero; however, for the mean-field case it only increases from $\rho_0 = 1$. The value of $R(\infty)$ for the scale-free network increases more slowly, however, due to the depletion of highly connected nodes. Figure courtesy of Dr. I.Z. Kiss, University of Sussex

on random networks is larger [49, 52] and as $\rho_0 \rightarrow \infty$, approaches its asymptote (the total population size) more rapidly than for scale-free networks (Fig. 4.5).

4.3.3 Link Dynamics and STI Partnership Models

In the simplest network models, the connections of the population are fixed with no switching of links; in contrast, models of the Kermack–McKendrick type can be viewed as populations where the links switch at an infinitely rapid rate [57]. Of interest is the interaction between the two extremes, i.e. when do the dynamics of the network change the dynamics of disease? The concurrency of links is well-studied [16, 18, 23, 55, 70] in the modelling of STIs, where the nature of the partnerships between individuals is emphasised, rather than the individuals themselves. This dyad-based approach often assumes that epidemic dynamics are driven by serially monogamous relationships [16, 55]. Despite this abstraction, they are of interest because of the emphasis on the dynamics of the network itself—in the simplest case, no epidemic can occur if all partnerships are sufficiently long. The networks generated from partnership models illustrate the importance of both "traditional" static network properties, for example, number of partners and the network structures such as the centrality of an individual in a network, as well as dynamic properties such as the concurrency of partnerships.

The effect of link dynamics are seen in a simple SWN example [62]. In this variant of the SWN, all local links are fixed (for all nodes, $k_{\text{local}} = n$, where n is an even constant) but a fixed number of random links are "lifted" and "dropped" randomly on the network at a fixed rate σ, so that, if all nodes are labelled $0, \ldots, n_{\text{pop}} - 1$, then nodes are joined by random links where the nodes are more than $n/2$ locations apart (i.e. all random links are longer than local links). It has previously been suggested that if link dynamics evolve ergodically, then an appropriate static representation of the network will have the same characteristics as the original, dynamic network [41]. An example of an ergodic, dynamic network is one where the network evolution is a Markov chain, and all states are accessible from the initial state. This is considerably less restrictive than other explorations of network dynamics, where the number of links for each node is assumed fixed (e.g. [57, 68]). Here, the static network is generated by assigning to each node an infectious period drawn from an exponential distribution with mean period τ_{inc}. Then a number v_{rand} of random links are generated and placed on the SWN with the restriction that the distance between the two connected nodes is greater than $n/2$.

Identification of the static network immediately identifies one consequence of link dynamics. Because the removal and replacement of a link "frees" up the link from already connecting two infected nodes, epidemic dynamics would be expected to be different on the static and dynamic networks (Fig. 4.6). Early on, it is more likely that a "used" up link will be replaced by a "free" link, whereas the opposite would become true later in the epidemic, as more nodes are infected. Here, link dynamics are represented by a switching rate that defines an effective infectious period over a given link. Construction of a transmission network where every node has the same infectious period distribution is equivalent to a bond percolation model [65]. The static representation allows us to quantify these differences, by considering the effective infectious period of a node, with respect to a dynamic random link. Assuming SIR infection dynamics with exponentially distributed periods, the average infectious period is $\tau_{\text{inc}} = 1/r_{\text{inc}}$ and for transmission over the random links, the average effective infectious period must be modified by the switching rate, and therefore $\tau_{\text{eff}} = 1/(r_{\text{inc}} + r_{\text{switch}})$. The relative probability of infection over random links is given by $e^{-\beta \tau_{\text{eff}}}/e^{-\beta \tau_{\text{fixed}}}$. To correct an effective transmission rate τ_{eff} must

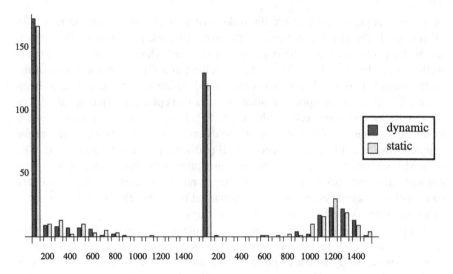

Fig. 4.6 Comparison of final epidemic size for different switching rates σ, showing the equivalence between the dynamic networks and a static representation. Epidemic simulations are run on a dynamic small world network (size $n = 2000$), with switching rate to infectivity removal rate ratio $\sigma/\gamma = 0.1$ (*left*) and $\sigma/\gamma = 10.0$ (*right*), and transmission rate per link $\tau = 1.0$. Simulations run using the Gillespie algorithm

be defined by

$$\frac{1 - \exp(-\beta_{\mathrm{eff}}\tau_{\mathrm{eff}})}{1 - \exp(-\beta\tau_{\mathrm{fixed}})} = \frac{\tau_{\mathrm{eff}}}{\tau_{\mathrm{inc}}}, \tag{4.11}$$

that is,

$$\beta_{\mathrm{eff}} = -\ln\left(\frac{\tau_{\mathrm{eff}}}{\tau_{\mathrm{inc}}}\exp(-\beta\tau_{\mathrm{fixed}})\right)\Big/\tau_{\mathrm{eff}}$$

$$= -\ln\left(1 - \frac{\tau_e}{\tau_f}(1 - \exp(-\beta_f\tau_f))\right)\Big/\tau_e. \tag{4.12}$$

The mean probability of transmission per link is therefore given by

$$p_{\mathrm{dyn}} = \int_0^\infty p(t)P(t)\,dt$$

$$= \int_0^\infty (1 - \exp(-\beta t))(\gamma + \sigma)\exp\big(-(\gamma + \sigma)t\big)\,dt$$

$$= \frac{\beta(\gamma + \sigma)}{(\beta + \gamma + \sigma)}, \tag{4.13}$$

similar to the link saturation result relating static networks to mean-field models [43]. An immediate consequence of this is that epidemics are made larger by link

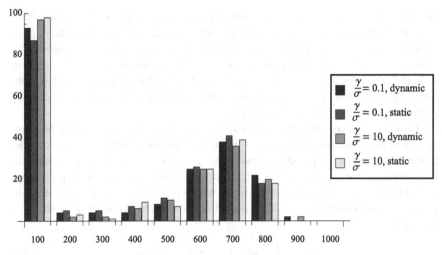

Fig. 4.7 Comparison of adjusted networks, $\gamma/\sigma = 0.1$ and $\gamma/\sigma = 1.0$, showing correction for link switching using (4.14). Simulations and parameters otherwise as in Fig. 4.6

switching. To conserve the total epidemic size, this requires that the overall probability of transmission be the same, i.e. $\frac{p_2}{p_1} = \frac{\tau_2}{\tau_1}$, which results in a corrected value of β:

$$\beta_{\text{dyn}} = \frac{(\beta_{\text{stat}}\gamma + \sigma)\beta_{\text{stat}}\gamma}{\beta_{\text{stat}}\sigma + \gamma(\gamma + \sigma)}. \tag{4.14}$$

This correction in (4.14) results in final epidemics that have the same distribution under stochastic simulation for different switching rates, and both for static and dynamic representations (Fig. 4.7). Of course, while the epidemic size is the same, the adjustment in β results in substantially different epidemic dynamics [26].

4.3.4 Integrating Networks and Epidemiology: Transmission Networks

Thus far, only the properties of the social network of potentially infectious contacts, i.e. which nodes could a node infect, if it were infectious, have been considered. This is often the only logical approach if, for instance, no disease data are available, or if the properties of the underlying social network are being exploited for disease control. For example, for the purposes of analysing the efficacy of tracing of potentially infectious contacts for disease control, understanding the social network is vital [17, 34, 47]. However, in the absence of control, or when control is not based on exploiting social network structure, given a contact network and the characteristics of a disease that can spread on the network, one can thin links to generate the network of truly infectious links (as disease will not necessarily spread across all available links), referred to as the "transmission" network. Such a network is inherently directed (since one must consider separately the probability of infection in each direction) even when the social network is undirected; however, the thinned network is usually significantly more sparse. Further, while the social network may have weights attached to links and nodes, the transmission network is unweighted so long as the infectious state of any node is not dependent on any network parameters (e.g. one cannot have a node that is more infectious if it has been infected by exposure to multiple infected neighbours).

It is also often the case that networks generated with different disease assumptions will have different properties to the underlying social network. For example, following Trapman [65], consider two systems in which both have a constant infectiousness per link per unit time $\tau(t)$, but with either fixed infectious periods θ_A (system A), or bimodal infectious periods, with a proportion $1 - X$ with a zero infectious period, and proportion X with an infectious period of length θ_B (system B), such that

$$\bar{p}_{av} = \int_0^{\theta_A} \tau(t)\,dt = X \int_0^{\theta_B} \tau(t)\,dt, \qquad (4.15)$$

i.e. for the two systems the average probability of infection per link $\bar{p}_{av}$ is the same. This latter system B can be thought of as a population where only some individuals are susceptible to disease. In system A, there is a fixed probability of transmission per link—in this case, the epidemic threshold $R_0 = 1$ corresponds to the "bond percolation" threshold (i.e. all sites occupied, but links present only with the probability $\bar{p}_{av}$). In system B, consider the limit where $\theta_B \to \infty$. Then the individuals in the proportion X are able to transmit with 100% probability, while the remainder never do. As $\bar{p}_{av}$ increases, X increases and $R_0 = 1$ corresponds to the "site percolation" threshold. Similarly, perfect vaccination could be viewed as having an effect on the site percolation of the "original" transmission network, removing whole nodes from the network, and thus the most relevant question is the coverage required, i.e. how many individuals must be vaccinated? Imperfect vaccination, however, is more closely related to bond percolation, if it is assumed that there is perfect coverage but imperfect protection.

4.3.5 The Basic Reproduction Number on Transmission Networks and Network Percolation Thresholds

In a transmission network, any disease starting in a strong component or at a source node will infect all elements of the strong component, and will infect all sink nodes as well, but not necessarily all sources. Thus, the largest or giant strongly connected component (GSCC), in the absence of any interventions or control measures, is an estimate of the lower bound of the maximum epidemic size, while the giant weakly connected component is an estimate of its upper bound (e.g. [41]). The transmission network construction allows us to establish a connection between the network percolation threshold and R_0. In a randomly mixed transmission network, R_0 is the network percolation threshold [64], loosely defined as the point at which the final epidemic size is expected to scale with the size of the population (discussed in [41]).

The result of (4.8) can be easily extended to consider weighted, directed links and with variable susceptibility of nodes. In this case, it can be shown that

$$R_0 = \bar{p} \frac{\langle \tau k_{\text{out}} \sigma k_{\text{in}} w \rangle}{\langle \sqrt{\tau k_{\text{out}} \sigma k_{\text{in}} w} \rangle}, \tag{4.16}$$

where τ and σ are the weights of the out- and in-links, w the weight associated with each node, k_{in} is the number of inward links, and k_{out} the number of outward links [41, 64], and the form of the denominator is to account for the fact that in- and out-links may not balance. Note that in (4.10), the node at the end of one of the links after the initial generation is already infected, while in (4.16), because the in-links and out-links are distinct, this does not occur. In this case, the equation for R_0 reduces to $R_0 = \frac{\langle l_{\text{in}} l_{\text{out}} \rangle}{\langle l_{\text{out}} \rangle}$ in the transmission network generated from a directed network where nodes have uncorrelated in- and out-links or a network with dynamic links, or $R_0 = \frac{\langle l_{\text{in}} l_{\text{out}} \rangle}{\langle l_{\text{out}} \rangle} - \frac{\bar{p}^2}{\langle l_{\text{out}} \rangle}$ when generated from static networks, where l_{in} and l_{out} are the number of inward and outward "truly infectious" links per node and $\bar{p}^2$ arises as the probability that an undirected potentially infectious link generates transmission links in both directions.

While this approach is only valid for randomly connected networks, it can be more broadly useful, provided a network can be transformed into a randomly-connected structure. This is illustrated in the case of the small-world network for which both the bond and site percolation threshold problems have been solved [54]. In the absence of long range connections, increases in the transmission probability per link will result in the growth of local clusters in the transmission network that would correspond to the local epidemic size, should an element in that cluster become infected. In the simplest case of a one-dimensional small-world lattice (i.e. with all nodes having local connections to exactly two neighbours), the probability $\widehat{p}_C$ that a local cluster of infected individuals will be of size C depends in a straightforward fashion on the probability $\bar{p}$ that a given link is infectious, if one assumes that, during the initial spread of the disease, the probability of a long range link returning to an already infected cluster is small. Then in this case, $\widehat{p}_C = (1 - \bar{p})^2 \bar{p}^{C-1}$, since the two end links must be non-infectious and all others $C - 1$ links in the cluster must be infectious. Moore and Newman [54] use the expression for the local cluster size to determine the percolation threshold via a direct calculation based on the number and size of clusters connected together by long range shortcuts. Another, related approach is to construct a directed transmission network and contract all nodes in connected components joined by only local links into a single "supernode". The probability that there will be a supernode of size C in the (now directed) transmission network is $p_C = C(1 - \bar{p})^2 \bar{p}^{C-1}$; e.g. for a cluster of size $C = 3$, with three consecutive nodes X, Y and Z, one could have a cluster of size C with $X \rightarrow Y \rightarrow Z$, $X \leftarrow Y \rightarrow Z$ or $X \leftarrow Y \leftarrow Z$. Each supernode will have an average of $\bar{p}qC$ infectious long range connections if the probability of a node having a long range connection in the original network was q. For a sufficiently

large population, with all clusters contracted into supernodes, the resultant network
of supernodes is randomly connected, and so (4.16), while not equal to R_0, is the
epidemic percolation threshold of the network, and therefore what one might call
R_0^{SN} (i.e. for the system of supernodes) reduces to

$$R_0^{SN} = \bar{p}q \sum_{C=1}^{\infty} Cp_C$$

$$= (1 - \bar{p})^2 q \sum_{C=1}^{\infty} C^2 \bar{p}^C$$

$$= q\bar{p}\frac{(1 + \bar{p})}{(1 - \bar{p})}. \tag{4.17}$$

The expression for the distribution of local cluster sizes becomes significantly more
complicated for higher-dimensional small world networks; however, the principle
remains the same. The interpretation of local clusters linked by long range connections is closely related to a household model of disease transmission [4], in which
the distribution of epidemic sizes within households is used to generate the value of
the between-household value of R_0. Multi-scale percolation as described here has
also been analysed in several real networks [39, 41].

4.4 Use of Social Networks with Real Epidemic Data

The previous section was largely concerned with the identification of phenomena that can influence the transmission of disease over a heterogeneous network.
Whether or not such phenomena have a bearing on the transmission of real diseases
over real networks is dependent on the interaction between the disease transmission characteristics and the underlying pattern of contact. A rule of thumb for the
appropriateness of social network approaches is through a comparison of the relative timescale and distance of the activity of the host, compared to the transmission
range and duration of infectiousness of the pathogen, which defines the scale over
which social network-based approaches are useful. In the case of sexually transmitted diseases, transmission occurs over a very short range, specific action. In the
case of SARS, at the worldwide scale, the airline transport network occurs over a
much greater range than person-to-person disease transmission—equivalently, the
action of the person has longer range than the action of the virus, and this is a similar case to the spread of pandemic influenza. In the case of livestock infectious
diseases, the long range movement of livestock is greater than the local airborne
spread of the pathogen. Here, examples related to all three of these cases are examined.

4.4.1 The Global Airline Network and SARS

Severe Acute Respiratory Syndrome or SARS is a respiratory disease caused by the SARS coronavirus. The index case was identified in Hong Kong in 2002, and over the course of the epidemic there were 8,096 known infected human cases, including 774 deaths worldwide, as listed by the World Health Organisation. While the SARS virus may persist in a wildlife host reservoir, it has been fully eradicated in the human population, with the last infected human case seen in June 2003 (disregarding a laboratory induced infection case in 2004). While the local spread is difficult to typify in terms of contact heterogeneity, the situation at the global level is much clearer. Within a matter of weeks in early 2003, SARS spread from the index case, believed to have been in Guangdong province of China, to rapidly infect individuals in some 37 countries around the world, mainly via the airline network. The airline interaction network in SARS has been extensively studied [9, 35] and some key elements are described here.

The model formulation is similar to that of the measles metapopulation models [7]; however, the SARS/airline network models are able to utilise the extensive data regarding the potentially infectious social contacts, rather than inferring them from the disease reporting numbers. The populations are reported as $V = 3,880$ vertices (major airports) joined by $E = 18,810$ weighted edges. These data are supplemented by the urban population data associated with these nodes (the human populations serviced by them) and, in the case of the later paper, the full disease outbreak data by reporting location. This does not consider the country of origin of the cases. In this example, "multi-scale" modelling abstracts the dynamics at the metropolitan level to stochastic homogeneous mixing models—no attempt is made to integrate more complex dynamics at this level, as is found in other studies.

Hufnagel et al. [35] considered the effect of stochasticity at the local level on global disease dynamics. Here, the more recent results of Colizza et al. [8] are discussed, which extend this using a Langevin equation formulation (originally to describe Brownian motion), based on stochastic *SIR* models with density dependence, discretized for numerical simulation. The approach results in a system of almost 10,000 differential equations where there are variables associated with 3,100 major centres with large airports, and three differential equations per centre. Demographic parameters are well-described by the airline network data, allowing for an analysis of the effects of well-described demographic stochasticity on epidemic occurrence. Of interest is the issue of repeatability—how often is a single set of events replicated, given an initial starting point for disease introduction? This has several implications: first, it impinges upon the usefulness of modelling exercises to predict, at a tactical level, how to target epidemic control. Second, comparison of simulation repeatability to a single simulation output (where the model structure is identical to that of the data) to repeatability in replicating a real epidemic is an indicator that, even if a model is a "poor" fit, it may, nevertheless, be a "good" model from the model selection point-of-view. Colizza et al. identify the "Hellinger" affinity $sim(\overrightarrow{\pi}^{\mathrm{I}}, \overrightarrow{\pi}^{\mathrm{II}}) = \sum_j \sqrt{\pi_j^{\mathrm{I}} \pi_j^{\mathrm{II}}}$ measure of repeatability, where $\overrightarrow{\pi}^{I}(t)$ is the vector

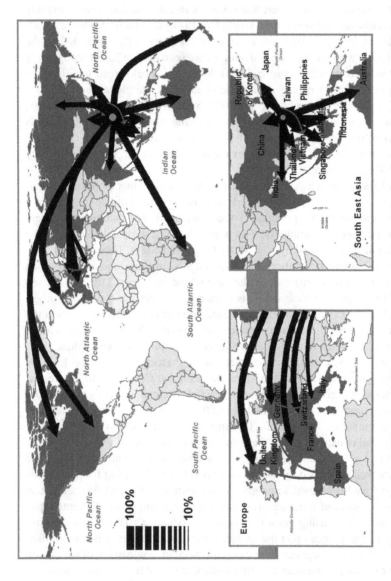

Fig. 4.8 Epidemic pathways on the global airline network. The *arrows* show the transmission pathways of greater probability than 10%, assuming Hong Kong is the source. The thickness of the arrows represents the probability associated to a given path. Paths that transmit the virus directly from Hong Kong are in *black*; paths that start from the first level of infected countries are in *grey*. The *shading* of countries represent the relative risk of infection, darker representing higher risk. From Colizza et al., BMC Medicine 5:34 (2007), doi:10.1186/1741-7015-5-34. Figure reproduced with permission of corresponding author, Dr. V. Colizza, Institute for Scientific Exchange, Turin

whose jth component represents the probability that an active individual (i.e. carrying infection) is in city j at time t. As the measure is scale invariant, it is only a measure of the epidemic pattern; therefore, a comparison of the overall prevalence between any two iterations I and II must also be included as an additional term, $sim(\vec{d}^{\,\mathrm{I}}, \vec{d}^{\,\mathrm{II}}) = \sum_j \sqrt{a_j^{\mathrm{I}}(1 - a_j^{\mathrm{I}})}$, resulting in an overall measure

$$\Theta(t) = sim\left(\vec{d}^{\,\mathrm{I}}(t), \vec{d}^{\,\mathrm{II}}(t)\right) \cdot sim\left(\vec{\pi}^{\,\mathrm{I}}(t), \vec{\pi}^{\,\mathrm{II}}(t)\right), \qquad (4.18)$$

which takes a value from zero to one, zero indicating no cities with infected individuals in both realisations, and one indicating identical realisations. The measure does not apportion the relative contribution of overall prevalence and pattern; however, this is easily extracted from the individual terms in (4.18).

However, there remain questions regarding the relative importance of the stochastic mechanisms identified here and other unexplored factors. Within-region modelling is defined by a compartmental model with homogenised mixing and density dependent contact, implemented with discrete probabilities of transition between states, and discrete time steps. An underlying assumption is that the pattern of air travel reflects the mean characteristics of the population—whether or not some individuals are more likely to travel than others, and whether or not that is correlated with within-region behaviour, susceptibility or transmissibility, is not considered. Compartments are also treated generically, with the same structure and parameters for all regions despite the likelihood of epidemiologically important differences in the way people behave around the world. Thus the within-centre model remains highly abstract, and there is no consideration of the balance in detail accorded the disease model and the network model complexity. Is the detail of the transport network necessary for understanding the level of stochasticity and outputs generated? These simplifications imply that direct interpretation of model parameters must be treated with caution; scientifically this relatively parsimonious approach is appropriate if the intention is to concentrate on the relationship between air transport contact heterogeneity and disease transmission. The availability of epidemiological data is critical for getting this balance right. Optimisation is relatively unsophisticated, using a least squares approach to optimise the Hong Kong data (in the paper, they do not seek to optimise the Hellinger measure of (4.18)). Despite these issues, the integration of more explicit disease dynamics at a lower population scale, with the explicit demographic interaction is a welcome consideration, and the approaches used in this analysis have the potential to be broadly applicable across other disease systems, and would provide useful insights. Here, the critical result of the model is that it is a good predictor of regions that did have meaningful numbers of cases, with the majority of these being directly related to the activity originating from Hong Kong. The most telling indicator of the role of network heterogeneity and the interaction between the network model and within-node dynamics is the risk to Spain, which is mainly due to secondary connections from other European countries (UK, France, and Germany) rather than direct links from Hong Kong.

4.4.2 Bovine Tuberculosis and the Network of Livestock Movements in GB

The movement of livestock in Great Britain is exceptionally well recorded, with detailed informing concerning the movement of large livestock between agricultural premises in Great Britain. Such data, recorded on a day-to-day basis, is an exceptional record of a dynamic disease-relevant network for which there exists disease data on which to test our concepts of social networks in epidemiology. These livestock networks have been extensively analysed, and have been shown to exhibit both small world and scale-free properties [41, 48]. Particularly well described is the movement of cattle, as individual animal movements are recorded, largely due to concerns over the spread of bovine spongiform encephalopathy in the 1990s. Bovine Tuberculosis (BTB) is a zoonotic disease of cattle caused by *Mycobacterium bovis*, a member of the tuberculosis clonal complex and an important cause of tuberculosis in humans, though less importantly in developed countries due to milk pasteurisation. It has been an endemic disease in British cattle for centuries which, however, was largely eliminated from most herds with the introduction of a widespread test-and-slaughter programme in the first half of the twentieth century. However, BTB incidence in cattle has been steadily on the rise for the last four decades, with the estimated cost of control reaching £90 million in 2005 and including £35 million in compensation to farmers. Disease spread at the national level is likely due to both cattle movements [24] and other factors, most controversially transmission from infected badgers in high-risk areas. As BTB in cattle is a notifiable disease, all cattle testing positive for BTB are recorded centrally, with regular tests of all herds occurring every one, two, three or four years, depending on the perceived risk of transmission to cattle. This combination of long term disease plus demographic data allows for an exceptional opportunity to identify the role of detailed network structure in the transmission of disease.

In Green et al. [27], a livestock network is constructed probabilistically so that each premises i maintains a probability of infection through the simulation, P_i, updated using one-day time-steps. Each potential infection event causes infection with probability p. This causes an increase in P_i, conditional on the probability of i already being infected, such that $P_i \mapsto P_i + \Delta P$, where $\Delta P = (1 - P_i)p$. The summation of ΔP across all infection events gives the expectation of the total number of infections produced during the simulation, I, and it may be partitioned into the causes of infection listed below: total infections due to livestock movements (M), infections within high-risk areas (G) and background rate, countrywide (B). The expected prevalence at a given time is given by $\sum_i P_i$, according to the following criteria:

- Livestock movement: A livestock movement from premises j to premises i is considered potentially infectious where j has a high probability of infection and where the number of animals moved is large:

$$p = \left(1 - (1 - \mu)^c\right)P_j, \tag{4.19}$$

where c is the batch size and μ is a model parameter denoting probability of infection of a single animal moved off infected premises. Risk of infection is therefore positively correlated with numbers of cattle moved onto a premises, but is not affected by herd size.

- High risk area: Each premises has a variable ϱ_i, set at 0 for premises not considered in 'high-risk' areas, and 1 for those that are. There are thus $n = \sum_i \varrho_i$ premises in high-risk areas. A fixed probability of infection per day χ is applied to premises in high-risk areas, which is normalised according to the number of premises n in these areas; χ / n is thus the mean daily rate of production of infected premises through this mechanism in a susceptible population. High-risk areas were defined as either (a) all premises in one- or two-year testing areas, or (b) all premises within a radius r of an index case, defined here as a breakdown in a previous, fixed period. No higher risk was assigned to premises in overlapping radii.

- Background rate: Each premises is exposed to infection on a daily basis with a fixed probability ω, independently of location or movement; the model considers an infection event $p = \omega$ once per day for each premises. This simulates infection due to unknown causes such as unknown long-distance animal movements or fomite transmission.

Model predictions for 2004 were tested against the data. The variable Y_i represented an estimate from the breakdowns data of the premises status, assigned in a manner analogous to P. Y_i was set as $Y_i = 1$ between times $t - w$ and t, where t is the time of a breakdown occurring in 2004–2005, and $Y_i = 0$ otherwise. Additionally for these events, P was set to 0 on day $t + 1$ to account for culling and movement restriction. With $\mathcal{Y}$ being the set of all premises not assigned as index cases on any day in 2004, model likelihood was calculated as

$$L = \prod_{i \in \mathcal{Y}} P_i^{Y_i} (1 - P_i)^{(1 - Y_i)}. \tag{4.20}$$

The goodness of fit of the model was expressed in terms of log-likelihood, and the best model selected using the Akaike Information Criterion (AIC) [1]: $AIC = 2k - 2\ln L$, where k is the number of parameters fitted—this is equivalent to a likelihood ratio test (and thus statistical significance can be attached to differences in AIC score) where models are nested, as is the case when comparing models without background-rate spread to those with background-rate spread, and models with low cattle-to-cattle transmission (where only cattle with a life history that include residence in high risk areas are considered a risk of onward infection) nested within those with high cattle-to-cattle transmission (where all cattle are potentially a risk). Maximum likelihood estimates were initially determined using the Nelder–Mead algorithm [56], and the Metropolis–Hastings algorithm [29] was then used to explore parameter space around the best-fit parameters through a Markov chain Monte Carlo simulation (MCMC). The model showed that the outbreak data are best explained by a model attributing roughly 16% of observed breakdowns to recorded cattle movements, and with only low levels of cattle-to-cattle transmission. High

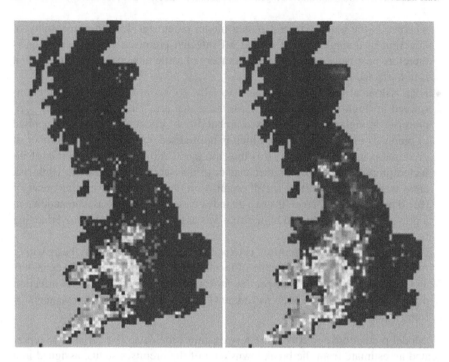

Fig. 4.9 Observed (*left*) and predicted (*right*) distribution of cattle herd breakdowns due to Bovine Tuberculosis in 2004. The best fit model attributes roughly 16% of spread to the movement of cattle, 9% of spread to unknown causes, and 75% of BTB spread to being present in high risk areas, where these areas are defined as 6 km radial disks surrounding breakdowns in the previous year. The movement of cattle that have previously passed through high risk areas is a better predictor than the full network of movements (i.e. allowing for secondary infection outside of high risk areas), indicating that networks must be carefully chosen. From Green et al., Proc. Biol. Sci. 275:1001–1005 (2008), doi:10.1098/rspb.2007.1601

risk areas by circles surrounding BTB breakdowns were found to be better predictors of future risk of BTB breakdowns than officially designated high risk parishes, with predictions based on these unidentified high-risk herds being also responsible for an estimated 47 breakdowns through movements of infected cattle. The results also suggest that eliminating transmission associated with high-risk areas would reduce the number of BTB breakdowns by 75% in the first year alone. Of particular relevance here is the identification of cattle life histories as a better indicator of the role of network spread, than simply the connections between premises, emphasising the importance of accurate definition of the appropriate network structure. Here, because BTB appears to be of relatively low infectiousness via cattle-to-cattle transmission, transient residence of cattle on premises is insufficient to seed infection in many cases, and thus outward links from premises only exposed to BTB via cattle movements are unlikely to be a risk themselves. This result is similar to a more detailed comparison between static and dynamic representations of the cattle network [67].

4.5   Integrating Networks and Epidemiology—Phylodynamics and the Identification of Transmission Networks

The ability to rapidly and inexpensively sequence large proportions of the genetic code of pathogens has resulted in the development of approaches to incorporate phylogenetic information in the reconstruction of transmission pathways. This provides a direct insight into the likely underlying network of transmission contacts. If the pathogen mutation rate per replication per base pair analysed is sufficiently high, then the genetic sequences from samples taken from infected individuals provides a signature indicating how closely related the virus population from different individuals are. Bayesian MCMC approaches are used to obtain the best fit transmission tree, using a measure such as the Hamming distance from information theory to identify the relatedness between individuals (i.e. how many genetic substitutions must be made to create identical sequences?). Standard phylogenetic fitting models assume that the rate of replication is not affected by density dependence considerations; however, the integration of epidemiological models can be used to correct this. While most current approaches are bespoke and require generalisation to be broadly applicable, theoretical foundations are being built to support the general development of these "phylodynamic" models [69]. Two excellent examples of the use of phylogenetics as tracers of the transmission network are the documentation of the clusters within the HIV/AIDS epidemic, and the transmission of foot-and-mouth disease in GB in 2001. In both cases, a connection to network models is shown, and these data represent an exciting opportunity to validate the importance of putative social network connections for the transmission of infectious diseases, and an opportunity for social network analyses to inform our understanding of phylogenetic models.

4.5.1   Models of HIV Infection

Acquired immune deficiency syndrome (AIDS) is a (primarily) sexually transmitted disease caused by the human immunodeficiency virus (HIV). AIDS progressively compromises the immune system and leaves individuals vulnerable to opportunistic infections and tumors. Despite the development of increasingly effective drug therapies, in 2007, it was estimated that 33.2 million people lived with the disease worldwide, with AIDS and AIDS-related complications having killed an estimated 2.1 million people, including 330,000 children. Over three-quarters of all these deaths occurred in sub-Saharan Africa.

The high rate of HIV evolution, combined with the availability of a very high density sample of viral sequences from routine clinical care in GB creates a system highly amenable to using phylodynamic approaches. Hughes et al. [36] studied extensive viral sequences from 11,071 heterosexual patients infected with HIV. Of these, 2774 were closely linked to at least one other sequence by nucleotide distance. Including the closest sequences, 296 individuals were identified to be in

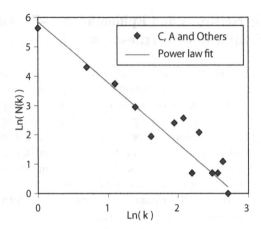

Fig. 4.10 Log–log plot of numbers of individuals with k contacts ($N(k)$) vs. the number of contacts (k), based on an analysis of sequence data. Individuals are assumed to be in contact within the clusters only if the time to the most recent common ancestor of their virus sequences is less than or equal to five years. The best fit to a power law (straight line in log–log space) has $R^2 = 0.95$ (95% CI: 0.84–0.99), $p < 10^{-6}$, and shape parameter (negative gradient) = 2.1. From Hughes et al., PLoS Pathog 5(9):e1000590 (2009), doi:10.1371/journal.ppat.1000590. Figure reproduced with permission of the corresponding author, Prof. A. Leigh-Brown, University of Edinburgh

groups of three or more individuals in the UK. The analysis revealed that heterosexual HIV transmission in the UK is clustered, but compared to transmission amongst MSM (men who have sex with men) groups, are on average in smaller groups and with slower transmission dynamics. Despite the reduced clustering compared to MSM, highly heterogeneous contact rates were indicated, consistent with heavy-tailed distributions indicated in previous studies [37, 51]. Using molecular clock estimates, temporal patterns could also be analysed, rather than just social ones, which is crucial when relationship concurrency (i.e. network dynamics) is important [70]. The analysis of these data revealed extremely long intergenerational periods (27 months), almost twice as long as for MSM. This long generational time makes contact tracing (and thus direct identification of the social contact network) difficult. However, the relationship between the identified clusters and the known heavy-tailed distributions from epidemiological studies (Fig. 4.10) would suggest that, while a snapshot of the direct contact network would not identify truly at risk individuals, the overall pattern is consistent with the dynamic, evolving network over which HIV is transmitted.

One problem with such data is that sampling is always only partial, both in terms of its reflection of pathogen genetic diversity, and in its sampling of the population. Random sampling is unlikely to identify directly critical links if these are few in number. However, if the sample is random at the population level, differences in the relatedness between individuals measured directly by epidemiological contact tracing, and via genetic relatedness should show the existence of these missing links. However, this does not allow for direct inference into the nature of such missing links. Indeed, such approaches on their own, cannot distinguish between sequential events that occur at different scales. For example, if a sequence AAA is taken from individual X, a sequence ABA from individual Y and ABC from individual Z, this implies that X and Y are more closely related by the Hamming distance measure, but it is not known, for example, if all the mutations occurred in X and therefore whether or not Z is a descendant of Y, or they are "siblings". For better estimates of this, more detailed demographic data is required, which are not usually available for human sexual contacts.

4.5.2 Foot-and-Mouth Disease in Great Britain

FMD is the most infectious disease of livestock in the world, with implications for animal health and productivity, and is particularly harmful to young livestock. Endemic in large parts of Africa, South America and Asia, both Western Europe and North America are FMD free, and derive considerable economic benefit from this status. FMD was introduced into GB in 2001, and the resulting epidemic cost well over £5 billion to control, with the loss of over 3 million livestock [30]. In 2007, FMD was again introduced into GB, this time via an escaped strain derived from virus held either the World Reference Laboratory in Pirbright, or the adjacent Meriel vaccine production facility; while considerably less extensive, nevertheless, the epidemic caused widespread disruption of the livestock industry at the national level, and cost almost £100 million to control [11]. Both the 2001 and 2007 foot-and-mouth disease epidemics are exceptionally well described, with detailed demographic and epidemiological information, including virus samples from across the entire epidemic. It is therefore an exceptional model system for understanding and developing phylodynamic principles [33]. FMD virus is an RNA virus with an exceptionally high mutation rate, sufficient so that discrimination of mutations down to the individual-to-individual level is possible. Preliminary studies into the phylodynamics of the 2001 epidemic have used a combined likelihood function that incorporates both Hamming distance measures and the spatio-temporal dynamics models used in previous studies. In this case, the likelihood function is fixed by epidemiological parameters. The most likely date of infection for each farm was estimated to be the date on which disease was reported on the farm, minus the age of the oldest lesion on the farm as estimated by veterinary investigation, less five days for the maximum within-host incubation period. There is uncertainty around the most likely date of infection, due to errors in the lesion dating, and possible variation in the incubation period by $I_i(t)$, and the possibility of missed, infected livestock. Given the estimated most likely date of infection of farm i, the most likely infection date of the first on-farm infection, and the examination date of the farm, allowing for a two day incubation period, determined the very latest possible infection time. The probability that a farm i was infectious at time $F_i(t)$ is then given in terms of $I_i(t)$ and the incubation period distribution $L(k)$ (where k is the incubation period

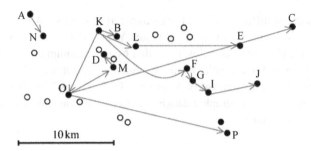

Fig. 4.11 The spatial relationship of 15 agricultural premises where infection was confirmed by laboratory testing (*filled circles*) and 12 infected premises (determined by clinical observations) that were subsequently found to be negative for virus by laboratory testing (*open circles*). A–P indicate the infected premises from which virus has been sequenced. The direction of most likely transmission events as determined by Cottam et al. is shown by the *grey arrows*. Figure from Cottam et al., Proc. B. 275:887–895 (2008). Figure reproduced with permission of the corresponding author, Prof. D.T. Haydon, University of Glasgow

in days) as

$$
F_i(t) = \begin{cases} \sum_{\tau=0}^{t}\big(I_i(\tau) \cdot \big(\sum_{k=1}^{t-\tau} L(k)\big)\big), & \text{if } t \le C_i, \\ 0, & \text{if } t > C_i. \end{cases} \tag{4.21}
$$

If one then considers the probability λ_{ij} that each infected premises i infects susceptible premises j then

$$
\lambda_{ij} = \frac{\sum_{t=0}^{\min(C_i,C_j)}(I_i(\tau) \cdot F_j(t))}{\sum_{k \neq i}\big(\sum_{t=0}^{\min(C_j,C_k)}(I_i(\tau) \cdot F_k(t))\big)}, \tag{4.22}
$$

where n is the number of infected premises in the population. Summed over all possible pairs, this represents the likelihood function for a particular epidemiological transmission tree. It is implicitly assumed that each premises is infected by only one other, and that all infected premises are known. A direct comparison to the set of transmission trees to the phylogenetic trees allows for the identification of the joint most-likely trees, which are significantly different from those identified by epidemiological considerations alone, and shows marked asymmetry in the infection direction, even when considering the underlying distribution of the susceptible population (Fig. 4.11).

This analysis shows the striking role that molecular sequencing can play in providing deeper insight into the underlying contact processes that drive observed epidemics. In this analysis, in (4.21) and (4.22) only the infected premises are considered, and not the underlying uninfected population, though detailed models of the epidemiology exist [21, 45].

4.5.3 Conclusions

There is a rich interplay between two recent, but now mature, subject areas: disease dynamics and social network analysis. While the history of mathematical epidemiology contains many of the ideas that have since been replicated in social network theory, nevertheless, the study of social networks has generated both new ideas and new impetus to understanding the role that contact heterogeneity can play in the spread, persistence and control of infectious diseases. This interplay offers new ideas that are applicable to many other fields where heterogeneous structure is important. Apologies are offered to the authors of many valuable and interesting papers originating from both traditions that have been omitted. Of particular note amongst the omissions are the numerous recent epidemiological analyses that consider complex population structure and its impact on the H1N1 influenza pandemic starting in 2009 (e.g. [3, 10, 22]). While many of these analyses are of epidemiological interest, the models are fundamentally similar to those discussed here in the context of SARS. In general, rather than presenting an exhaustive study of the results from either, illustrations have been presented of how it is only by considering a combination of both pattern and process can disease dynamics be properly understood. Critical to this is the interplay of individuals from both traditions, who will bring together the analytical strengths and insights they both have to offer (e.g. [5]). Of growing interest is the increasing use of molecular epidemiology as a tracing tool, which brings both new opportunities and new challenges, as a coherent, rigorous framework for dealing with phylogenetics, disease dynamics, high dimensional statistical inference and network structure is yet to be established. This will undoubtedly be a major subject of interest over the next decade, and this is the central problem in the growing field of phylodynamics [33].

References

1. Akaike, H.: Information theory and an extension of the maximum likelihood principle. In: Petrov, B.N., Csaki, F. (eds.) Proc. of 2nd International Symposium on Information Theory. Akad. Kiadó, Budapest (1973)
2. Anderson, R.M., May, R.M., Anderson, B.: Infectious Diseases of Humans: Dynamics and Control. Oxford University Press, Oxford (1992)
3. Balcan, D., Hu, H., Goncalves, B., Bajardi, P., Poletto, C., Ramasco, J.J., Paolotti, D., Perra, N., Tizzoni, M., den Broeck, W.V., Colizza, V., Vespignani, A.: Seasonal transmission potential and activity peaks of the new influenza A(H1N1): a Monte Carlo likelihood analysis based on human mobility. BMC Med. (2009). doi:10.1186/1741-7015-7-45
4. Ball, F., Mollison, D., Scalia-Tomba, G.: Epidemics with two levels of mixing. Ann. Appl. Probab. 7, 46–89 (1997)
5. Bansal, S., Grenfell, B.T., Meyers, L.A.: When individual behaviour matters: homogeneous and network models in epidemiology. J. R. Soc. Interface 4, 879–891 (2007)
6. Barthelemy, M., Barrat, A., Pastor-Satorras, R., Vespignani, A.: Velocity and hierarchical spread of epidemic outbreaks in scale-free networks. Phys. Rev. Lett. 92, 178701 (2004)
7. Bolker, B., Grenfell, B.T.: Space, persistence and dynamics of measles epidemics. Philos. Trans. R. Soc. Lond. B, Biol. Sci. 348, 309–320 (1995)

8. Colizza, V., Barrat, A., Barthelemy, M., Vesipignani, A.: The role of the airline transportation network in the prediction and predictability of global epidemics. Proc. Natl. Acad. Sci. USA **103**, 2015–2020 (2006)
9. Colizza, V., Barrat, A., Barthelemy, M., Vesipignani, A.: Predictability and epidemic pathways in global outbreaks of infectious diseases: the SARS case study. BMC Med. (2007). doi:10.1186/1741-7015-5-34
10. Colizza, V., Vespignani, A., Perra, N., Poletto, C., Goncalves, B., Hu, H., Balcan, D., Paolotti, D., den Broeck, W.V., Tizzoni, M., Bajardi, P., Ramasco, J.J.: Estimate of novel influenza A/H1N1 cases in Mexico at the early stage of the pandemic with a spatially structured epidemic model. PLoS Curr Influenza, RRN1129 (2009)
11. Cottam, E.M., Wadsworth, J., Shaw, A.E., Rowlands, R.J., Goatley, L., Maan, S., Maan, N.S., Mertens, P.P.C., Ebert, K., Li, Y., Ryan, E.D., Juleff, N., Ferris, N.P., Wilesmith, J.W., Haydon, D.T., King, D.P., Paton, D.J., Knowles, N.J.: Transmission pathways of foot-and-mouth disease virus in the United Kingdom. PLoS Pathogens **4**, 1000050 (2007)
12. Danon, L., Díaz-Guilera, A., Duch, J., Arenas, A.: Comparing community structure identification. J. Stat. Mech. Theory Exp. (2005). doi:10.1088/1742-5468/2005/09/P09008
13. De Jong, M.C.M., Bouma, A., Diekmann, O., Heesterbeek, H.: Modelling transmission: mass action and beyond. Trends Ecol. Evol. **17**, 64 (2002)
14. Diekmann, O., Heesterbeek, J.A.P.: Mathematical Epidemiology of Infectious Diseases: Model Building, Analysis and Interpretation, Mathematical and Computational Biology. Wiley, New York (2000)
15. Diekmann, O., Heesterbeek, J.A.P., Metz, J.A.J.: On the definition and the computation of the basic reproduction ratio R0 in models for infectious diseases in heterogeneous populations. J. Math. Biol., **28**, 365–382 (1990)
16. Dietz, K., Hadeler, K.P.: Epidemiological models for sexually transmitted diseases. J. Math. Biol. **26**, 1–25 (1988)
17. Eames, K.T., Keeling, M.J.: Contact tracing and disease control. Proc. R. Soc. Lond. B, Biol. Sci. **270**, 2565–2571 (2003)
18. Eames, K.T., Keeling, M.J.: Monogamous networks and the spread of sexually transmitted diseases. Math. Biosci. **189**, 115–130 (2004)
19. Erdös, P., Rényi, A.: On random graphs. Publ. Math. (Debr.) **6**, 290–297 (1959)
20. Chung, F., Lu, L.: The diameter of sparse random graphs Adv. Appl. Math. **26**, 257–279 (2001)
21. Ferguson, N.M., Donnelly, C.A., Anderson, R.M.: The foot-and-mouth epidemic in Great Britain: pattern of spread and impact of interventions. Science **292**, 1155–1160 (2001)
22. Fraser, C., Donnelly, C.A., Cauchemez, S., Hanage, W.P., Kerkhove, M.D.V., Hollingsworth, T.D., Griffin, J., Baggaley, R.F., Jenkins, H.E., Lyons, E.J., Jombart, T., Hinsley, W.R., Grassly, N.C., Balloux, F., Ghani, A.C., Ferguson, N.M., Rambaut, A., Pybus, O.G., Lopez-Gatell, H., Alpuche-Aranda, C.M., Chapela, I.B., Zavala, E.P., Guevara, D.M.E., Checchi, F., Garcia, E., Hugonnet, S., Roth, C.: Pandemic potential of a strain of influenza A (H1N1): early findings. Science **324**, 1557–1561 (2009)
23. Ghani, A.C., Swinton, J., Garnett, G.P.: The role of sexual partnership networks in the epidemiology of gonorrhea. Sex. Transm. Dis. **24**, 45–56 (1997)
24. Gilbert, M., Mitchell, A., Bourn, D., Mawdsley, J., Clifton-Hadley, R., Wint, W.: Cattle movements and bovine tuberculosis in Great Britain. Nature **435**, 491–496 (2005)
25. Goh, K.-I., Oh, E., Jeong, H., Kahng, B., Kim, D.: Classification of scale-free networks. Proc. Natl. Acad. Sci. USA **99**, 12583–12588 (2002)
26. Green, D.M., Kiss, I.Z., Kao, R.R.: Parameterisation of individual-based models: comparisons with deterministic mean-field models. J. Theor. Biol. **239**, 289–297 (2006)
27. Green, D.M., Kiss, I.Z., Mitchell, A.P., Kao, R.R.: Estimates for local and movement-based transmission of bovine tuberculosis in British cattle. Proc. R. Soc. Lond. B, Biol. Sci. **275**, 1001–1005 (2008)
28. Grenfell, B.T., Bjornstad, O.N., Kappey, J.: Travelling waves and spatial hierarchies in measles epidemics. Nature **414**, 716–723 (2001)

29. Hastings, W.K.: Monte Carlo sampling methods using Markov chains and their applications. Biometrika **57**, 97–109 (1970)
30. Haydon, D., Kao, R.R., Kitching, P.: On the aftermath of the UK foot-and-mouth disease outbreak. Nat. Rev., Microbiol. **2**, 675–681 (2004)
31. Heesterbeek, J.A.P., Roberts, M.G.: The type-reproduction number T in models for infectious disease control. Math. Biosci. **206**, 3–10 (2007)
32. Hethcote, H.W., Yorke, J.A., Nold, A.: Gonorrhea modeling: a comparison of control methods. Math. Biosci. **58**, 93–109 (1982)
33. Holmes, E.C., Grenfell, B.T.: Discovering the phylodynamics of RNA viruses. PLoS Comput. Biol. **5**, 1000505 (2009)
34. Huerta, R., Tsimring, L.S.: Contact tracing and epidemic control on social networks. Phys. Rev. E **66**, 056115 (2002)
35. Hufnagel, L., Brockmann, D., Geisel, T.: Forecast and control of epidemics in a globalized world. Proc. Natl. Acad. Sci. USA **101**, 15124–15129 (2004)
36. Hughes, G.J., Fearnhill, E., Dunn, D., Lycett, S.J., Rambaut, A., Brown, A.J.L.: Molecular phylodynamics of the heterosexual HIV epidemic in the United Kingdom. PLoS Pathogens **5**, 1000590 (2009)
37. Jones, H.J., Handcock, M.S.: An assessment of preferential attachment as a mechanism for human sexual network formation. Proc. R. Soc. Lond. B, Biol. Sci. **270**, 1123–1128 (2003)
38. Jones, H.J., Handcock, M.S.: Social networks: sexual contacts and epidemic thresholds. Nature **423**, 605–606 (2003)
39. Jonkers, A.R., Sharkey, K.J., Christley, R.M.: Preventable H5N1 avian influenza epidemics in the British poultry industry network exhibit characteristic scales. J. R. Soc. Interface **7**, 695–701 (2010)
40. Kao, R.R.: Evolution of pathogens towards low R0. J. Theor. Biol. **242**, 634–642 (2006)
41. Kao, R.R., Danon, L., Green, D.M., Kiss, I.Z.: Demographic structure and pathogen dynamics on the network of livestock movements in Great Britain. Proc. R. Soc. Lond. B, Biol. Sci. **273**, 1999–2007 (2006)
42. Keeling, J.J.: The effects of local spatial structure on epidemiological invasions. Proc. R. Soc. Lond. B, Biol. Sci. **266**, 859–867 (1999)
43. Keeling, M.J., Grenfell, B.T.: Individual-based perspectives on R0. J. Theor. Biol. **203**, 51–61 (2000)
44. Keeling, M.J., Rand, D.A., Morris, A.J.: Correlation models for childhood epidemics. Proc. R. Soc. Lond. B, Biol. Sci. **264**, 1149–1156 (1997)
45. Keeling, M.J., Woolhouse, M.E.J., Shaw, D.J., Matthews, L., Chase-Topping, M., Haydon, D.T., Cornell, S.J., Kappey, J., Wilesmith, K., Grenfell, B.T.: Dynamics of the 2001 UK foot and mouth epidemic, stochastic dispersal in a heterogeneous landscape. Science **294**, 813–817 (2001)
46. Kermack, W.O., McKendrick, A.G.: A contribution to the mathematical study of epidemics. Proc. R. Soc. Lond. Ser. A, Math. Phys. Sci. **115**, 700–721 (1927)
47. Kiss, I.Z., Green, D.M., Kao, R.R.: Disease contact tracing in random and clustered networks. Proc. R. Soc. Lond. B, Biol. Sci. **272**, 1407–1414 (2005)
48. Kiss, I.Z., Green, D.M., Kao, R.R.: Disease contact tracing in random and scale-free networks. J. R. Soc. Interface **3**, 55–62 (2006)
49. Kiss, I.Z., Green, D.M., Kao, R.R.: The effect of contact heterogeneity and multiple routes of transmission on final epidemic size. Math. Biosci. **203**, 124–136 (2006)
50. Levins, R.: Some demographic and genetic consequences of environmental heterogeneity for biological control. Bull. Entomol. Soc. Am. **15**, 237–240 (1969)
51. Liljeros, F., Edling, C.R., Amaral, L.A., Stanley, H.E., Aberg, Y.: The web of human sexual contacts. Nature **411**, 907–908 (2001)
52. May, R.M., Lloyd, A.L.: Infection dynamics on scale-free networks. Phys. Rev. E, Stat. Nonlinear Soft Matter Phys. **64**, 066112 (2001)
53. Meyers, L., Newman, M., Martin, M., Schrag, S.: Applying network theory to epidemics: control measures for mycoplasma pneumoniae outbreaks. Emerg. Infect. Dis. **9**, 204–210 (2003)

84 R.R. Kao

54. Moore, C., Newman, M.E.: Exact solution of site and bond percolation on small-world networks. Phys. Rev. E **62**, 7059–7064 (2000)
55. Morris, M., Kretzschmar, M.: Concurrent partnerships and the spread of HIV. AIDS **11**, 641–648 (1997)
56. Nelder, J.A., Mead, R.A.: Simplex method for function minimization. Comput. J. **7**, 308–313 (1965)
57. Parham, P.E., Ferguson, N.M.: Space and contact networks: capturing the locality of disease transmission. J. R. Soc. Interface **3**, 483–493 (2006)
58. Pastor-Satorras, R., Vespignani, A.: Epidemic spreading in scale-free networks. Phys. Rev. Lett. **86**, 3200–3203 (2001)
59. Roberts, M.G., Heesterbeek, H.: Bluff your way in epidemic models. Trends Microbiol. **1**, 343–348 (1993)
60. Roberts, M.G., Heesterbeek, J.A.P.: A new method for estimating the effort required to control an infectious disease. Proc. R. Soc. Lond. B, Biol. Sci. **270**, 1359–1364 (2003)
61. Robinson, S.E., Everett, M.G., Christley, R.M.: Recent network evolution increases the potential for large epidemics in the British cattle population. J. R. Soc. Interface **4**, 669–674 (2007)
62. Saramäki, J., Kaski, K.: Modelling development of epidemics with dynamic small-world networks. J. Theor. Biol. **234**, 413–421 (2005)
63. Schley, D., Burgin, L., Gloster, J.: Predicting infection risk of airborne foot-and-mouth disease. J. R. Soc. Interface **6**, 455–462 (2008)
64. Schwartz, N., Cohen, R., ben Avraham, D., Barabási, A.L., Havlin, S.: Percolation in directed scale-free networks. Phys. Rev. E **66**, 015104 (2002)
65. Trapman, P.: On analytical approaches to epidemics on networks. Theor. Popul. Biol. **71**, 160–173 (2007)
66. van den Driessche, P., Watmough, J.: Reproduction numbers and sub-threshold endemic equilibria for compartmental models of disease transmission. Math. Biosci. **180**, 29–48 (2002)
67. Vernon, M.C., Keeling, M.J.: Representing the UK's cattle herd as static and dynamic networks. Proc. R. Soc. Lond. B, Biol. Sci. **276**, 469–476 (2009)
68. Volz, E., Meyers, L.A.: Epidemic thresholds in dynamic contact networks. J. R. Soc. Interface **6**, 233–241 (2009)
69. Volz, E.M., Kosakovsky Pond, S.L., Ward, M.J., Leigh Brown, A.J., Frost, S.D.W.: Phylodynamics of infectious disease epidemics. Genetics **183**, 1421–1430 (2009)
70. Watts, C.H., May, R.M.: The influence of concurrent partnerships on the dynamics of HIV/AIDS. Math. Biosci. **108**, 89–104 (1992)
71. Watts, D.J., Strogatz, S.H.: Collective dynamics of 'small-world' networks. Nature **393**, 440–442 (1998)
72. Xia, Y., Bjørnstad, O.N., Grenfell, B.T.: Measles metapopulation dynamics: a gravity model for epidemiological coupling and dynamics. Am. Nat. **164**, 267–281 (2004)

Chapter 5
NESSIE: Network Example Source Supporting Innovative Experimentation

Alan Taylor and Desmond J. Higham

Abstract We describe a new web-based facility that makes available some realistic examples of complex networks. NESSIE (Network Example Source Supporting Innovative Experimentation) currently contains 12 specific networks from a diverse range of application areas, with a Scottish emphasis. This collection of data sets is designed to be useful for researchers in network science who wish to evaluate new algorithms, concepts and models. The data sets are available to download in two formats (MATLAB's .mat format and .txt files readable by packages such as Pajek), and some basic MATLAB tools for computing summary statistics are also provided.

5.1 Motivation

Network science has developed rapidly over the last decade. The dramatic increase in activity may be attributed in large part to

- progress in science and technology making it possible, and desirable, to generate large networks (for example, in telecommunications, in internet applications and in high-throughput genomics), and simultaneously,
- increased computing power making it feasible to store and compute with these large data sets.

Analysing, summarising, comparing and modelling such large networks presents fascinating challenges to computational scientists, and new algorithms are being developed and tested across a range of disciplines. The motivation for this work is to provide a test set of example networks, drawn from a diverse range of application areas, that forms a useful resource for prototyping, benchmarking and comparing

A. Taylor (✉) · D.J. Higham
Department of Mathematics and Statistics, University of Strathclyde, Glasgow, UK
e-mail: a.taylor@strath.ac.uk

D.J. Higham
e-mail: d.j.higham@strath.ac.uk

E. Estrada et al. (eds.), *Network Science*,
DOI 10.1007/978-1-84996-396-1_5, © Springer-Verlag London Limited 2010

algorithms in network science. The networks are provided as matrices, that is, two-dimensional arrays. In most cases, the networks are unweighted and undirected, corresponding to binary, symmetric adjacency matrices, but in some cases we have directed or weighted edges.

The URL address for NESSIE is www.mathstat.strath.ac.uk/nessie.

Although we are not aware of any directly comparable resource, it is appropriate to mention some related projects here.

- CONTEST [27] is a MATLAB-based package that makes available networks as instances drawn from classes of random graphs. Since these random graph classes have been shown to reproduce key properties of real networks, they may be regarded as realistic examples on which to test software, especially with regard to linear system and eigenvalue routines. The random graph classes implemented in CONTEST are Erdős–Rényi/Gilbert [6, 9], Barabási–Albert type scale-free [1], Watts–Strogatz small-world [16, 22, 31], range-dependent [11, 14, 15], Kleinberg [18], geometric [13, 23, 25], stickiness [24] and lock-and-key [21, 28], along with some simple post-processing utilities. A major design principle behind CONTEST is that all random graph classes can be accessed with a single input argument—the number of nodes, but more input parameters can be specified if desired. So, for example, A = geo(n,r,m,per,pnorm) returns an instance of a geometric random graph (placing nodes uniformly at random in $\mathbb{R}^m$ and connecting those within a target distance), where
  - r specifies the target distance, defaulting to 0.1,
  - m specifies the dimension of Euclidean space, defaulting to 2,
  - per is a logical variable specifying whether periodic distance is to be used, defaulting to per = 0; not periodic,
  - pnorm specifies the L_p-norm to be used, defaulting to 2,
  but with the call A = geo(n) the default values r = 0.1, m = 2, per = 0 and pnorm = 2 are used.
- GraphCrunch [20] is a tool for comparing networks. For a given input network, it will compute **global properties**: degree distribution, clustering coefficient, clustering spectrum, diameter, shortest path lengths spectrum; and **local properties**: relative graphlet frequency distance, graphlet degree distribution agreement. GraphCrunch will compare these statistics with those of random network models (including Erdős–Rényi/Gilbert [6, 9], Barabási–Albert type scale-free [1], geometric [13, 25] and stickiness [24]). All generated model networks are calibrated to have a number of nodes and edges within 1% of those in the target network.
- The University of Florida Sparse Matrix Collection [5] is a collection of specific instances of sparse matrices from a wide spectrum of domains. Like CONTEST [27], the collection is designed to provide test data for development and performance evaluation in the field of sparse matrix algorithms. The emphasis is on large matrices arising in science and engineering, for example, from the discretisation of problems in computational fluid dynamics, electromagnetics, semiconductor devices, thermodynamics, computer graphics/vision and robotics/kinematics, and directly from mathematical models in circuit simulation,

economic and financial modelling and quantum chemistry. Although it is not the main focus of this set, some of these matrices represent network connectivity patterns. CONTEST differs in that it is tightly focused on matrices in network science, and that it offers parameterised matrices, allowing control over dimension, and features such as sparsity, and degree distribution. The University of Florida collection can be accessed in MATLAB, Fortran, or C, using software provided. Matrix Market [2] with website URL http://math.nist.gov/MatrixMarket/ is a similar facility, with an interactive, web-based feel and indeed there is overlap between the test sets.

- UCINET IV Datasets at http://vlado.fmf.uni-lj.si/pub/networks/data/Ucinet/ UciData.htm provides small (between 10 and 58 nodes) networks collected by social scientists that describe interactions between individuals.
- Pajek (a Slovene word meaning "spider") is a tool for analysis and visualisation of large networks. Although not the main feature, it provides about 40 examples of networks or collections of networks, with a bias towards text mining applications, at http://vlado.fmf.uni-lj.si/pub/networks/data/.

5.2 Philosophy

In creating NESSIE, we aimed for an uncluttered, accessible and informative repository. To this end,

- Networks can be downloaded in two formats: .mat files directly readable into MATLAB and .txt files with the data taking the form of a list of node pairs. The .txt files can easily be read into network tools such as Pajek. In the case of MATLAB, the arrays have the `sparse` attribute [10, 16].
- A small number of useful utility tools have been added including a code for Estrada's classification system [7], a function to compute the matrix of Pearson correlation coefficients for a dataset and produce a "similarity" network consisting of pairs of nodes with correlation coefficient above a certain threshold, and some simple plotting tools.
- For each network, basic information about the meaning of a node and edge is provided, and references are given for further information.

5.3 The Networks

In this section, we describe the 12 networks making up the example set. In each case, we illustrate the adjacency matrix in a MATLAB `spy` plot, and show some basic network properties: degree distribution (as both a log–log plot and a histogram), clustering coefficients, eigenvalue distribution, normalised Fiedler vector and a `spy` plot of the adjacency matrix reordered by the normalised Fiedler vector. Following the classification system in [7], we also show the spectral scaling property of the network; here we plot $\log_{10} {}^S C_{\text{odd}}(i)$ against $\log_{10} \gamma_1(i)$, where

- γ_1 is a dominant eigenvector of the adjacency matrix, and
- $^S C_{odd}(i)$ is the *odd subgraph centrality* of node i, which may be defined by summing over all possible walk lengths k, the number of odd-length closed walks starting and finishing at node i, scaled by $1/(k!)$. On the same axes, we also plot the straight line defined by $y = 0.5x - 0.5 \log_{10} \lambda_1$, where λ_1 is the eigenvalue corresponding to γ_1.

Estrada [7] distinguishes four topological classes.

Class I: the points $(\log_{10} {}^S C_{odd}(i), \log_{10} \gamma_1(i))$ lie **close to** the straight line.
Class II: the points $(\log_{10} {}^S C_{odd}(i), \log_{10} \gamma_1(i))$ lie **below** the straight line.
Class III: the points $(\log_{10} {}^S C_{odd}(i), \log_{10} \gamma_1(i))$ lie **above** the straight line.
Class IV: the points $(\log_{10} {}^S C_{odd}(i), \log_{10} \gamma_1(i))$ are scattered **above and below** the straight line.

Estrada further argues that Class II is typified by networks with central 'holes' and Class III is typified by networks with central 'cores'.

5.3.1 Network 1: European Economic Regions

European countries may be broken down into smaller territories [8]. An undirected network consisting of 255 nodes and 580 undirected edges is established by connecting territories that are physically contiguous, i.e. they share a border, therefore a node in the network represents a territory and an edge between two nodes means that they are physically adjacent. For such a network, it may be useful to establish optimal paths between two territories, e.g. routes that pass through a minimal number of foreign countries. Similarly, measures of centrality may be of interest to establish which territories are best connected in some sense. Figures 5.1 and 5.2 show plots of some simple measures on the network of contiguous European economic regions.

5.3.2 Network 2: Guppy Social Interactions

This dataset consists of social interactions in a population of guppies [4]. Each node represents a free-ranging guppy and each edge an observed social interaction. The network consists of 99 nodes and 726 undirected edges. Recurring social interactions result in weighted edges and these may be of interest in identifying close-knit communities within the population. Figures 5.3 and 5.4 show plots of some simple measures on the binarised network of guppy social interactions.

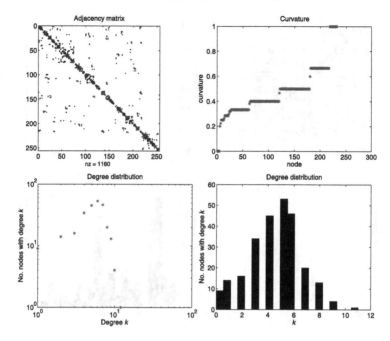

Fig. 5.1 Spyplot, curvature and degree distributions for the network of European economic regions

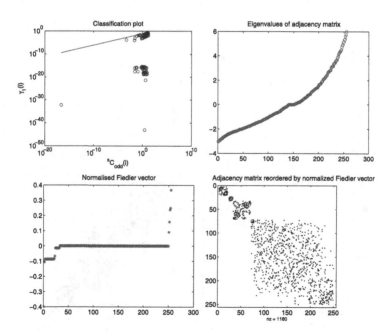

Fig. 5.2 Network classification, eigenvalue distribution, normalised Fiedler vector and reordered adjacency matrix for the network of European economic regions

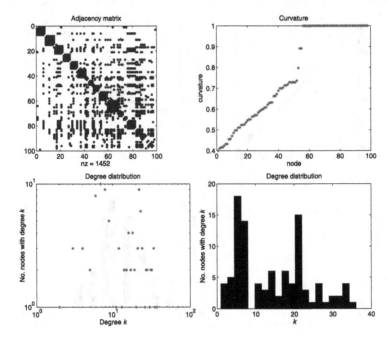

Fig. 5.3 Spyplot, curvature and degree distributions for the network of guppy social interactions

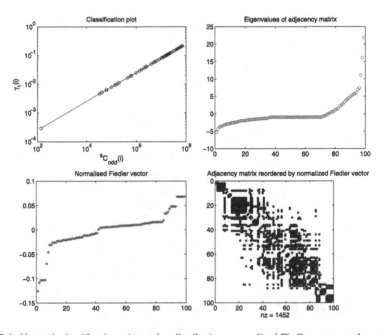

Fig. 5.4 Network classification, eigenvalue distribution, normalised Fiedler vector and reordered adjacency matrix for the network of guppy social interactions

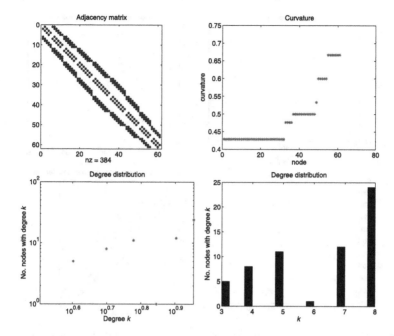

Fig. 5.5 Spyplot, curvature and degree distributions for the network of reactor components

5.3.3 Network 3: Reactor Core Modelling

The function hexgrid.m generates a graph representing the connections between graphite blocks used to encase fuel rods in nuclear reactors. The blocks are modelled as a set of hexagonal tiles arranged in concentric rings, with each node in the network representing a hexagonal block and each edge representing a "keyed connection" between two blocks. The primary aim is to discover how removal of keyed connections influences the modes of movement available to the blocks. Another question is that of symmetry in the network: is it possible, given a pattern of keyed connections to be removed, to eliminate all the analogous cases (i.e. sets of connections whose removal will result in the same modes of movement)? Figures 5.5 and 5.6 show plots of some simple measures on a network obtained by running the program hexgrid.m with input argument 5 (meaning five layers of hexagonal tiles). This results in a network comprising 61 nodes and 192 undirected edges.

5.3.4 Network 4: Classification of Whiskies

In [32], 86 malt whiskies are scored between 0–4 for 12 different taste categories including sweetness, smokiness and nuttiness. Additionally, geographical coordinates

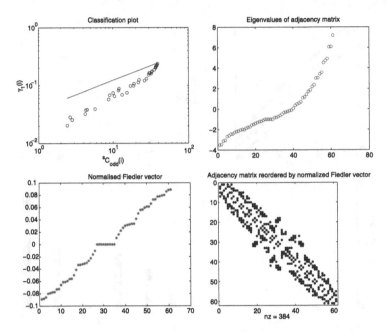

Fig. 5.6 Network classification, eigenvalue distribution, normalised Fiedler vector and reordered adjacency matrix for the network of reactor components

of distilleries allow us to obtain pairwise distance information. Using a combination of these datasets it is possible to look for correlations between particular attributes of taste and physical location, for example, does a shared local resource have a significant effect on nearby whiskies? By using correlation data, it may be possible to provide whisky recommendations based upon an individual's particular preferences. By computing the Pearson correlation coefficient and specifying a threshold value between 0 and 1, we can establish an adjacency matrix where each node is a malt whisky and an edge represents a level of similarity above the threshold. By varying the threshold value, the density of nonzeros in the adjacency matrix will change. A high threshold will result in a more sparse adjacency matrix since a higher level of similarity between two whiskies is required to "earn" a nonzero. Figures 5.7 and 5.8 show plots of some simple measures on the network obtained by computing the Pearson correlation coefficient of pairs of whiskies and taking a threshold level of 0.7. This particular network contains 493 undirected connections between 86 nodes.

5.3.5 Network 5: Scottish Football Transfers

Twice annually, Scottish football clubs have an opportunity to transfer players. A list of these transfers is available from http://en.wikipedia.org/wiki/Seasons_in_Scottish_football. The movement of players between clubs forms a directed graph

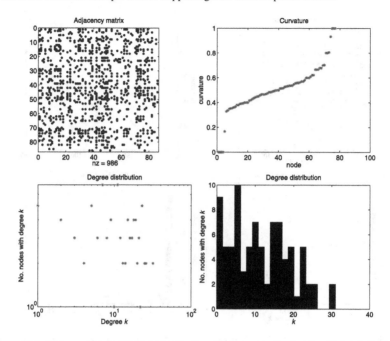

Fig. 5.7 Spyplot, curvature and degree distributions for the network of malt whisky similarity

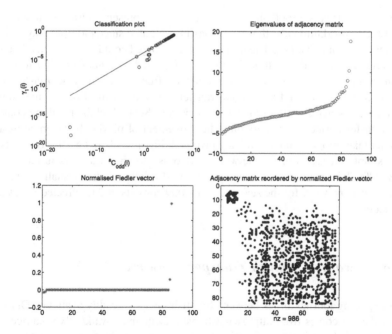

Fig. 5.8 Network classification, eigenvalue distribution, normalised Fiedler vector and reordered adjacency matrix for the network of malt whisky similarity

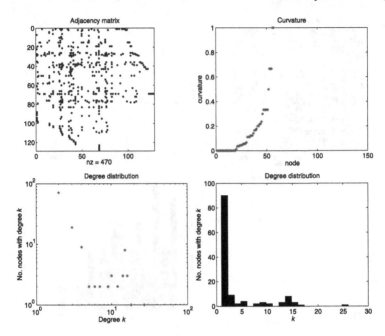

Fig. 5.9 Spyplot, curvature and degree distributions for the undirected network of Scottish football transfers in the season 2008–2009

where each vertex is a football club and each edge represents a transfer in a particular direction. Additionally, this graph may be weighted since multiple players may transfer between two clubs. The transfer fee exchanged could be also considered as the weight on each edge, although this is complicated by a number of factors. Out of contract players may move between clubs for free, players may be transfered on short-term loan deals and very often transfer fees are not disclosed to the public. Our dataset, which lists the transfers to and from Scottish clubs for three consecutive transfer periods, considers only the movement of players between clubs and does not take into account any money involved. Figures 5.9 and 5.10 show plots of some simple measures on the network of Scottish football transfers in the season 2008–2009. The network has been symmetrised to allow better visualisation. The unsymmetric network for the season 2008–2009 consists of 242 directed edges and 128 nodes.

5.3.6 Network 6: Scottish Transport Networks

Data regarding journey times between Scottish towns is readily available. Our particular dataset comes from http://www.transportscotland.gov.uk/. Two matrices list typical travel times between Scottish towns, by train or by car. The matrices are non-square, that is to say, the data is incomplete. For instance, the travel times from

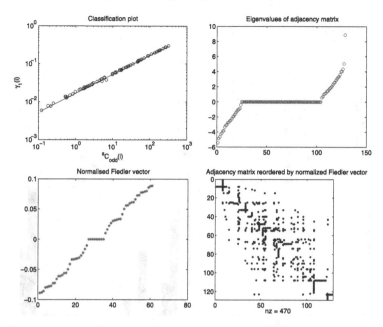

Fig. 5.10 Network classification, eigenvalue distribution, normalised Fiedler vector and reordered adjacency matrix for the undirected network of Scottish football transfers in the season 2008–2009

Wick and Tain to Stirling are included, but the travel time from Wick to Tain is not. The dataset lends itself to graph-layout problems. Given this limited data, can we find a two dimensional distribution of the towns in question such that the distance between them respects the average travel times? By following the same procedure outlined in Sect. 5.3.4, we may obtain an undirected adjacency matrix for a given threshold level of "similarity". In this case, a node represents a town or city and an edge represents a given level of similarity (or inverse-distance) between two towns. Figures 5.11 and 5.12 show plots of some simple measures on the network obtained by computing the Pearson coefficient of pairs of car journey times and taking a threshold level of 0.9. This value yields a network of 25 nodes and 77 undirected edges.

5.3.7 Network 7: Metabolite Network

Here the nodes are potential chemical formulas obtained by searching databases for formulas with mass with 10 ppm of peaks measured in a sample derived from the Trypanosome parasite [26]. Connections are made between two formulas if they differ by one of 80 known transforms. For example, a difference of two hydrogen atoms suggests the possibility of (de-)hydrogenisation $\pm H_2$. Figures 5.13 and 5.14 show plots of some simple measures on the metabolite network which consists of 376 nodes and 343 edges.

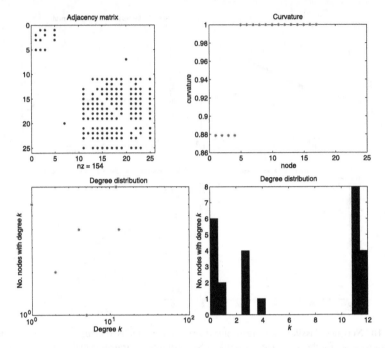

Fig. 5.11 Spyplot, curvature and degree distributions for the transportation network derived from journey times by car

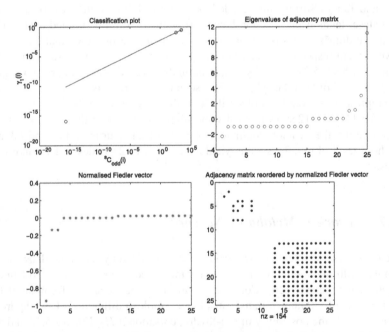

Fig. 5.12 Network classification, eigenvalue distribution, normalised Fiedler vector and reordered adjacency matrix for the transportation network derived from journey times by car

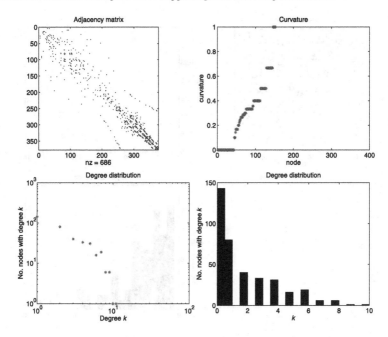

Fig. 5.13 Spyplot, curvature and degree distributions for metabolite network

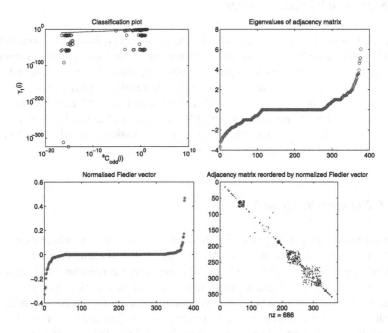

Fig. 5.14 Network classification, eigenvalue distribution, normalised Fiedler vector and reordered adjacency matrix for the metabolite network

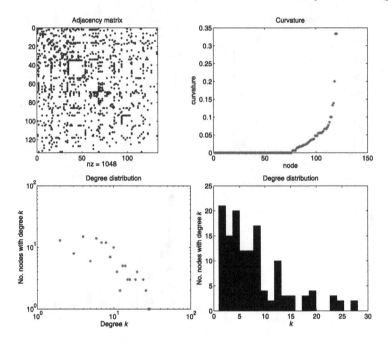

Fig. 5.15 Spyplot, curvature and degree distributions for the p53 network

5.3.8 Network 8: p53 Network

A directed network of genes related to the oncogene p53 is obtained by considering
pairwise expression levels measured by microarray technology. An edge is inserted
from gene i to j if i tends to express significantly above its usual level when j
expresses significantly below its usual level. The resulting 'plus–minus' network
is a directed network consisting of 133 nodes (genes) and 558 edges (changes in
expression level with opposite polarity) [30]. Figures 5.15 and 5.16 show plots of
some simple measures on the directed gene co-expression network. The data has
been symmetrised for presentation purposes.

5.3.9 Network 9: Gene Network

Gene expression is typically recorded in a matrix of size $N \times M$ where expression
levels of N genes are recorded over M samples. This leukaemia data set has been
used in many studies, including [3, 12]. By computing correlation coefficients on
such a matrix, we can obtain a square matrix of samples (patients) or genes. For
the gene network presented here, we have computed a matrix where each node is a
patient and an edge exists between two patients if their gene expression levels yield
a correlation coefficient above a threshold value of 0.65. This results in a network
of 38 nodes and 180 undirected edges. Applying clustering to such a dataset may

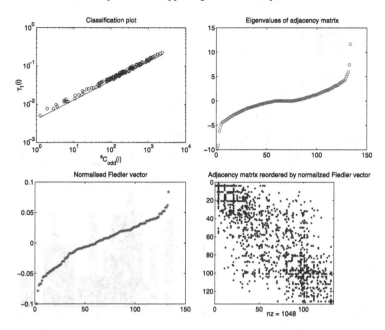

Fig. 5.16 Network classification, eigenvalue distribution, normalised Fiedler vector and reordered adjacency matrix for the p53 network

allow classification of a new sample into an existing group of patients. In Figs. 5.17 and 5.18, we show plots of measures on the gene network.

5.3.10 Network 10: Protein–Protein Interaction Network

Protein–protein interaction networks consist of observed physical interactions between proteins [17, 29]. Each edge represents a protein and an edge exists between two proteins if they have been observed to interact. Interactions between proteins are bidirectional so the set of interactions between proteins in an organism forms an undirected unweighted network. Protein–protein interaction networks are widely available from repositories such as http://www.thebiogrid.org, and we include here an example of a network for yeast consisting of 4388 nodes and 38102 edges (915 of which are self-links). Plots of measures on this network are shown in Figs. 5.19 and 5.20.

5.3.11 Network 11: Benguela Marine Ecosystem

A network can be obtained by observing trophic interactions between species. One such network is that of the Benguela ecosystem consisting of species found off

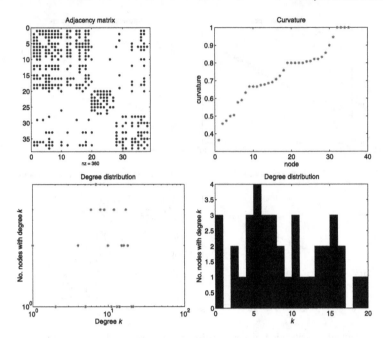

Fig. 5.17 Spyplot, curvature and degree distributions for the gene network

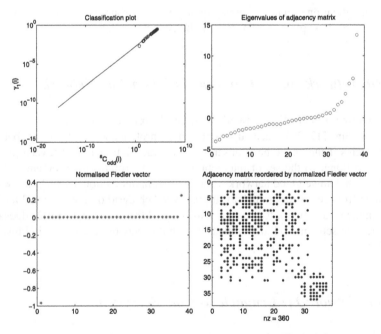

Fig. 5.18 Network classification, eigenvalue distribution, normalised Fiedler vector and reordered adjacency matrix for the gene network

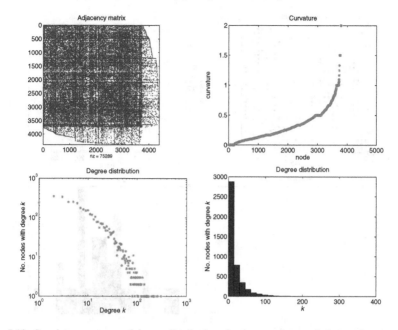

Fig. 5.19 Spyplot, curvature and degree distributions for the protein–protein interaction network

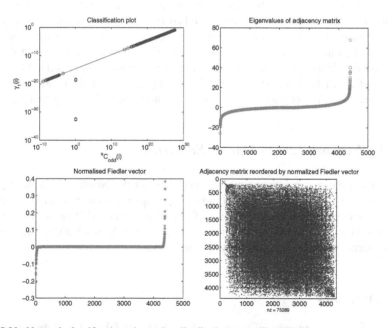

Fig. 5.20 Network classification, eigenvalue distribution, normalised Fiedler vector and reordered adjacency matrix for the protein–protein interaction network

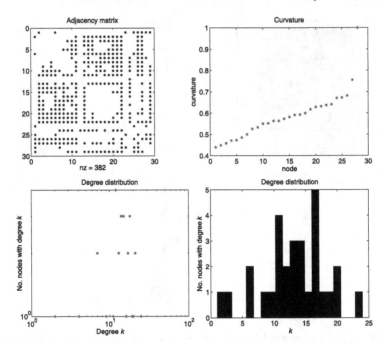

Fig. 5.21 Spyplot, curvature and degree distributions for the Benguela marine ecosystem network

the southwest coast of South Africa [33]. In this instance, each node represents a particular species, and two species are linked if they interact at the trophic level, i.e. one population impacts upon the size of another. The network considered here consists of 29 nodes and 191 undirected edges. Such networks may be useful if we wish to assess the importance of longer paths in a food-web, i.e. to find out how two species affect each other despite a lack of a direct path between them. We show plots of measures on the Benguela marine ecosystem network in Figs. 5.21 and 5.22.

5.3.12 Network 12: US Marine Ecosystem

Similarly, we can consider the marine ecosystem of the Northeast US shelf [19]. Once again, nodes represent species and an edge represents an interaction at the approximate trophic level of each species. The network obtained from this ecosystem contains 81 nodes and 1451 undirected edges. In Figs. 5.23 and 5.24, we show plots of measures on the US marine ecosystem network.

5.4 Summary

Table 5.1 gives a summary of the networks included in NESSIE; for each network the number of nodes and percentage of nonzeros in the adjacency matrix is given, as

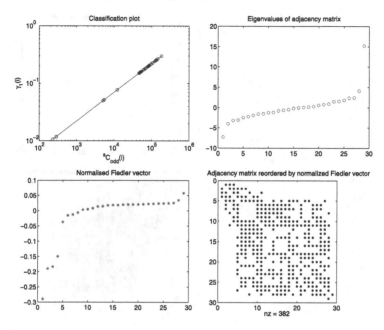

Fig. 5.22 Network classification, eigenvalue distribution, normalised Fiedler vector and reordered adjacency matrix for the Benguela marine ecosystem network

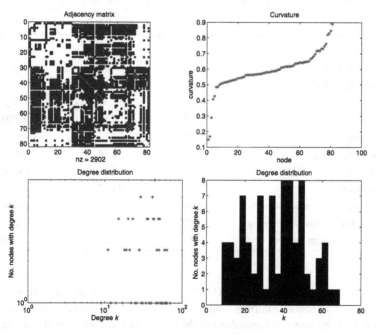

Fig. 5.23 Spyplot, curvature and degree distributions for the US marine ecosystem network

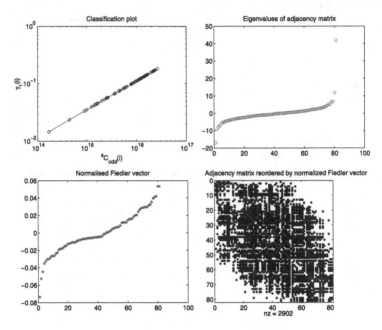

Fig. 5.24 Network classification, eigenvalue distribution, normalised Fiedler vector and reordered adjacency matrix for the US marine ecosystem network

Table 5.1 Number of nodes and percentage of nonzeros in NESSIE networks described here

Network	No. nodes	% nonzeros	MATLAB file
European economic regions	255	1.78	eer.mat
Guppy social interactions	99	14.81	guppy.mat
Reactor core modelling	61	3.92	hex5.mat
Whisky classifications	86	13.33	whisky.mat
Football transfers	128	2.87	spl0809.mat
Transport network	25	24.64	transport.mat
Metabolite network	376	0.49	Tr.mat
p53 network	133	3.15	p53.mat
Gene network	38	24.93	gene.mat
Protein–protein interaction network	4388	0.39	ppi.mat
Benguela marine ecosystem network	29	45.42	benguela.mat
US marine ecosystem network	81	44.23	shelf.mat

well as the name of the relevant MATLAB file available from the NESSIE webpage. In the case of adjacency matrices computed using correlation coefficients, the values listed are for the network created using the threshold value given in the appropriate section of this chapter.

Acknowledgements   These networks are available from the NESSIE website, www.mathstat. strath.ac.uk/nessie. This work was supported by grants from the Medical Research Council (project grant G0601353), and the Engineering and Physical Sciences Research Council (project grant GR/S62383/01 and "Bridging the Gap"). The authors would like to thank the following colleagues for their contributions to NESSIE: Darren Croft, Ernesto Estrada, Bernard Fingleton, Nataša Pržulj, Simon Rogers and Marcus Wheel.

References

1. Barabási, A.L., Albert, R.: Emergence of scaling in random networks. Science **286**(5439), 509–512 (1999)
2. Boisvert, R., Pozo, R., Remington, K., Barrett, R., Dongarra, J.: Matrix market: a web resource for test matrix collections. In: Boisvert, R. (ed.) The Quality of Numerical Software: Assessment and Enhancement, pp. 125–137. Chapman and Hall, London (1997)
3. Brunet, J.P., Tamayo, P., Golub, T.R., Mesirov, J.P.: Metagenes and molecular pattern discovery using matrix factorization. Proc. Natl. Acad. Sci. USA **101**, 4164–4169 (2004)
4. Croft, D.P., Krause, J., James, R.: Social networks in the guppy (*Poecilia reticulata*). Proc. R. Soc. Lond. B, Biol. Sci. **271**, 516–519 (2004)
5. Davis, T.: The University of Florida sparse matrix collection. Technical Report, University of Florida, USA (2007)
6. Erdös, P., Rényi, A.: On random graphs. Publ. Math. (Debr.) **6**, 290–297 (1959)
7. Estrada, E.: Topological structural classes of complex networks. Phys. Rev. E **75**, 016103 (2007)
8. Fingleton, B., Fischer, M.: Neoclassical theory versus new economic geography: competing explanations of cross-regional variation in economic development. Ann. Reg. Sci. **44**, 467–491 (2010)
9. Gilbert, E.N.: Random graphs. Ann. Math. Stat. **30**, 1141–1144 (1959)
10. Gilbert, J.R., Moler, C., Schreiber, R.: Sparse matrices in MATLAB: design and implementation. SIAM J. Matrix Anal. Appl. **13**, 333–356 (1992)
11. Grindrod, P.: Range-dependent random graphs and their application to modeling large small-world proteome datasets. Phys. Rev. E **66**, 066702 (2002)
12. Higham, D.J., Kalna, G., Kibble, M.: Spectral clustering and its use in bioinformatics. J. Computational and Applied Math. **204**, 25–37 (2007)
13. Higham, D.J., Pržulj, N., Rašajski, M.: Fitting a geometric graph to a protein–protein interaction network. Bioinformatics **24**, 1093–1099 (2008)
14. Higham, D.J.: Unravelling small world networks. J. Comput. Appl. Math. **158**, 61–74 (2003)
15. Higham, D.J.: Spectral reordering of a range-dependent weighted random graph. IMA J. Numer. Anal. **25**, 443–457 (2005)
16. Higham, D.J., Higham, N.J.: MATLAB Guide. SIAM, Philadelphia (2000), 283 pp.
17. Ito, T., Chiba, T., Ozawa, R., Yoshida, M., Hattori, M., Sakaki, Y.: A comprehensive two-hybrid analysis to explore the yeast protein interaction interactome. Proc. Natl. Acad. Sci. USA **98**(8), 4569–4574 (2001)
18. Kleinberg, J.M.: Navigation in a small world. Nature **406**, 845 (2000)
19. Link, J.: Does food web theory work for marine ecosystems? Mar. Ecol. Prog. Ser. **230**, 1–9 (2002)
20. Milenkovic, T., Lai, J., Przulj, N.: GraphCrunch: A tool for large network analyses. BMC Bioinform. **9**, 70 (2008)
21. Morrison, J.L., Breitling, R., Higham, D.J., Gilbert, D.R.: A lock-and-key model for protein–protein interactions. Bioinformatics **2**, 2012–2019 (2006)
22. Newman, M.E.J., Moore, C., Watts, D.J.: Mean-field solution of the small-world network model. Phys. Rev. Lett. **84**, 3201–3204 (2000)
23. Penrose, M.: Geometric Random Graphs. Oxford University Press, Oxford (2003)

24. Pržulj, N., Higham, D.J.: Modelling protein–protein interaction networks via a stickiness index. J. R. Soc. Interface **3**, 711–716 (2006)
25. Pržulj, N., Corneil, D.G., Jurisica, I.: Modeling interactome: Scale-free or geometric? Bioinformatics **20**(18), 3508–3515 (2004)
26. Rogers, S., Sceltema, R.E., Girolami, M., Breitling, R.: Probabilistic assignment of formulas to mass peaks in metabolomics experiments. Bioinformatics **25**(4), 512–518 (2009)
27. Taylor, A., Higham, D.J.: CONTEST: A controllable test matrix toolbox for MATLAB. ACM Trans. Math. Softw. **35**, 1–17 (2009)
28. Thomas, A., Cannings, R., Monk, N.A.M., Cannings, C.: On the structure of protein–protein interaction networks. Biochem. Soc. Trans. **31**, 1491–1496 (2003)
29. Uetz, P., Giot, L., Cagney, G., Mansfield, T.A., Judson, R.S., Knight, J.R., Lockshon, E., Narayan, V., Srinivasan, M., Pochart, P., Qureshi-Emili, A., Li, Y., Godwin, B., Conover, D., Kalbfleish, T., Vijayadamodar, G., Yang, M., Johnston, M., Fields, S., Rothberg, J.M.: A comprehensive analysis of protein–protein interactions in *Saccharomyces cerevisiae*. Nature **403**, 623–627 (2000)
30. Vass, J.K., Higham, D.J., Mao, X., Crowther, D.: New controls of TCA-cycle genes revealed in networks built by discretization or correlation. Technical Report No. 10, Department of Mathematics (2009)
31. Watts, D.J., Strogatz, S.H.: Collective dynamics of 'small-world' networks. Nature **393**, 440–442 (1998)
32. Wishart, D.: Whisky Classified: Choosing Single Malts by Flavour, 2nd edn. Pavilion Books, London (2006)
33. Yodzis, P.: Diffuse effects in food webs. Ecology **81**, 261–266 (2000)

Chapter 6
Networks in Urban Design. Six Years of Research in Multiple Centrality Assessment

Sergio Porta, Vito Latora, and Emanuele Strano

Abstract Multiple Centrality Assessment (MCA) is a methodology of mapping centrality in cities that applies knowledge of complex network analysis to networks of urban streets and intersections. This methodology emerged from research initiated some six years ago at Polytechnic of Milan, Italy, and now continuing at University of Strathclyde, Glasgow, through a close partnership and collaboration between scholars in urban planning and design and in the physics of complex networks. After six years and many publications, it is probably time for us to **make a point on** what has been achieved and what remains to be achieved in the future. As most of the whole research has already been published, we forward the reader to those publications for more detailed information. The scope of this paper is to provide the overall sense of this experience so far and a road-map to its main results.

6.1 Introduction

A central place has one special feature to offer to those who live or work in a city: easy accessibility from immediate surroundings and more distant places. Accessibility may be transformed to visibility and popularity. Therefore, a central place tends to attract more customers and has a greater potential to develop into a social catalyst. Important landmarks (i.e. "primary functions") such as museums, the-

S. Porta (✉) · E. Strano
Urban Design Studies Unit, Department of Architecture, University of Strathclyde, Glasgow, UK
e-mail: sergio.porta@strath.ac.uk

E. Strano
e-mail: emanuele.strano@gmail.com

V. Latora
Dipartimento di Fisica ed Astronomia, Universitá di Catania and INFN Sezione di Catania, Catania, Italy
e-mail: latora@ct.infn.it

E. Estrada et al. (eds.), *Network Science*,
DOI 10.1007/978-1-84996-396-1_6, © Springer-Verlag London Limited 2010

atres, or office headquarters as well as service and retail at the community level (i.e. "secondary locations") are preferentially attracted by central locations. A more central location commands a higher real estate value and is occupied by a more intensive land use. Central locations in an urban area have the potential to sustain higher densities of retail and services, and are a key factor for supporting the formation and vitality of urban 'nodes' [22]. Thus, centrality emerges as one of the most powerful determinants for urban planners and designers to understand how a city works and to decide where renovation and redevelopment need to be placed.

Centrality not only affects how a city works today, but also plays an important role in shaping its growth. If one looks at where a city centre is located, it is most likely to sprout from the intersection of main routes, where some special configuration of the terrain or some particular layout of the river system (or water bodies in general) makes the place compulsory to pass through [6, 21]. Then, departing from such central locations, the city grows up over time with gradual additions of dwellings, residents, and activities: first along the main routes, then filling the in-between areas, and then developing streets that realise loops and points of return. As the structure becomes more complex, new central streets and places are formed and stimulate a growth in the number of residents and activities around them. As a result, centrality appears to be somehow at the heart of that marvellous hidden order that supports the formation of 'spontaneous' and organic cities [15, 16]. It is also a crucial issue in the contemporary debate on searching for more bottom-up and 'natural' strategies of urban planning beyond the modernistic heritage. This is strictly related to the capacity of street centrality to act as a driver in the location of economic activity during one city's process of formation.

Urban researchers including geographers have always been interested in understanding how economic activities are distributed in a city, what factors influence their spatial pattern, and how the urban structure and functions are formed [37]. On the one hand, that question has to do with methods to assess how economic activities cluster, diffuse or correlate with each other as well as with other land uses and collective behaviours; on the other hand, it has to do with how centrality is conceived, depicted and measured in space. In this view, accessibility to centres and orders of economic activities should be related to each other. Based on the same ground, planners envision the structure of primary functions relying on the primary street network at a larger scale such as citywide, and the structure of secondary functions served by the secondary street network at the neighbourhood level. As the theoretical debate continues, little empirical evidence is reported to support or reject the relation between different categories of economic activities and spatial centrality.

A substantial amount of research in Space Syntax analysis has been devoted to establishing the correlation between centrality of urban spaces and economic or social dynamics [12, 32]. The self-organised evolutions of a city's topological and functional structures are driven by how the "natural movement" of people finds its way throughout, and in turn contributes to the formation of, the street network and urban spaces [14]. This "natural movement" turns out to be a product of both the "architecture" of the street network (macro-scale factor) and the level of "constitutedness" of the streets themselves (micro-scale factor). The interplay between macro- and micro-scale spatial factors is regarded as the sign of a traditional self-organised way of building cities since ancient times [20].

A more complex definition of centrality came from a non-spatial discipline like structural sociology (for an overview, see [36]). Due to the non-spatial nature of social links, structural sociologists designed several sets of centrality indices, each capturing a different way of being central [11]. For instance, "degree" and "closeness" centrality examine one being near the others, and "betweenness" focuses on one being between the others. More recently, the characteristics of networked structures *in space* have been recognised as an emerging field of study in the physics of complex networks [4] and their mechanisms of formation investigated and modelled [3].

This paper offers an overview of the authors' research on the application of the sciences of complex networks to spatial networks of streets and intersections in cities. In particular, this research is the result of six years of collaboration between scholars in urban design and the physics of complex networks: as such, and because of the importance of centrality in urban sciences, this research has initially focused on the many ways of understanding and measuring centrality in spatial networks, ultimately defining a Multi Centrality Assessment (MCA) set of tools and concepts. The Postscript from the first author illustrates the deep motivations that fuelled the emerging of this experience as an interdisciplinary research effort with roots in city planning and design: with the crisis of the rational–comprehensive model in city planning, the "organic" analogy is now quickly gaining empirical support and the debate about the optimum location of economic activities and their relationship with street centrality is part of a larger effort to elucidate the dynamics of self-organisation and evolution in urban structures [2, 30]. The overall MCA research has to be intended as a contribution to this wider effort.

6.2 Multiple Centrality Assessment

Starting in 2003, the MCA research has been proceeding in three phases. At first, we got engaged in developing the methodological structure of our approach, achieving and testing the tools and understanding the meaning of the results. Another activity that deeply engaged us in this first phase was to achieve the acknowledgement of the scientific communities both in the physics of complex networks and in city planning. During a second phase, we expanded the scope of our research by experimenting with measures of city form that go beyond the analysis of centrality to enter the field of the characterisation of the network's structure. More recently, we have lifted the scale of our analysis up to entire cities and regions and turned our attention to understanding how centrality actually works in space by mapping *density* of centrality instead of centrality on links.

6.2.1 The One-Square-Mile Study: Establishing Centrality
Analysis for Cities

The two fundamental papers [23, 24] that introduced the concept and the methodology of Multiple Centrality Assessment were both published in 2006. These papers where initially written as a single article and then were split into two separate ones during the process of peer review. Thus, they together constitute a very consistent and coherent whole. Our effort was primarily oriented to develop an in-depth understanding of how to analyse street networks in metrical terms. Space Syntax [12, 13], the model for "configurational" analysis of space developed by Bill Hillier since the mid-1980s and well known in urban planning, is, in fact, inherently non-metrical: what appeared to us a geographical analysis of networks, at a deeper insight turned out to be not geographic at all and, by the way, even not primarily based on networks. The "axial" representation of street patterns is not properly a network as the axis represents one linear street and does not break at intersections with other streets as long as it does not present a curve. Axes are then turned into nodes and intersections into links, so no matter how long an axis is it gets collapsed into a node and loses every geographical content. As a result, a proper network is actually created in Space Syntax, but it stays "behind" the stage: calculations are operated on this "dual" network and then, in a final elaboration, values are reported on the axial map which is the one we see at the end of the process. This passage is clearly not easy to capture for the wider audience, but it deeply informs about the model. We wanted something different, especially we wanted to operate all calculations on the same graph that represents what is openly mapped. So we very plainly represented streets as links and intersections as nodes, the good-old traffic engineering way. The advantages of that are so evident that it is even hardly worth telling: first, the metric information stays embedded in the graph; second, because this is the absolute standard way of representing street networks worldwide, virtually all cities in the advanced world already have all the information that is needed to run our model, and they constantly keep that information updated for their ordinary tasks of city planning and management. It is an enormous amount of information that does not need to be replicated at every application of the model.

Box n.1: Indices of centrality. *Closeness centrality* C^C measures to what extent a node is close to all the other nodes along the shortest paths of the network. C^C for a node i is defined as:

$$C_i^C = \frac{N-1}{\sum_{j=1; j \neq i}^{N} d_{ij}}$$

where N is the total number of nodes in the network, and d_{ij} is the shortest distance between nodes i and j. In other words, the closeness centrality for a node is the inverse of the average distance from this node to all other nodes.

Betweenness centrality C^B is based on the idea that a node is more central when it is traversed by a larger number of the shortest paths connecting all couples of nodes in the network. C^B is defined as:

$$C_i^B = \frac{1}{(N-1)(N-2)} \sum_{j=1;k=1;j\neq k\neq i}^{N} \frac{n_{jk}(i)}{n_{jk}}$$

where n_{jk} is the number of shortest paths between nodes j and k, and $n_{jk}(i)$ is the number of these shortest paths that contain node i.

Straightness centrality C^S originates from the idea that efficiency of communication between two nodes increases when there is less deviation of their shortest path from the virtual straight line connecting them, i.e. more "straightness" of the shortest path. C^S is defined as:

$$C_i^S \frac{1}{N-1} \sum_{j=1;j\neq i}^{N} \frac{d_{ij}^{\text{Eucl}}}{d_{ij}}$$

where d_{ij}^{Eucl} is the Euclidean distance between nodes i and j, or the distance with the virtual straight connection.

Information Centrality C^I measures the importance of a node from the ability of the network to respond to the deactivation of the node itself. The delta-centrality of node i is defined as:

$$C_i^I = \frac{\Delta E_{\text{glob},2}}{E_{\text{glob},2}} = \frac{E_{\text{glob},2}(G) - E_{\text{glob},2}(G')}{E_{\text{glob},2}(G)}$$

where G indicates the original graph, G' is the graph with N nodes and $K - k_i$ edges obtained by removing from G the k_i edges incident in node i, and the efficiency $E(G)$, defined as:

$$E = \frac{1}{N(N-1)} \sum_{i,j,i\neq j} \frac{d_{ij}^{\text{Eucl}}}{d_{ij}}$$

measures the mean flow-rate of information over a graph and has the nice property of being finite even for unconnected graphs.

Notice that all four centrality measures are normalised, by definition, to take values in the interval [0, 1].

But the metric issue was really fundamental. Waldo Tobler's "first law of geography", which states that "everything is related to everything else, but near things are more related than distant things", is reflected in countless very ordinary real-life dynamics. Mostly important, all dynamics related with the collective uses of space, including pedestrian flows, visibility, navigation and access, are very strictly related with distance. The "first law" is also reflected in models that economic geographers and regional planners have always been developing on the basis of a *gravitational*

Fig. 6.1 Venice, Italy.
Grey-scaled maps
representing the spatial
distributions of node
centrality. The four indices
(*1*) closeness C^C,
(*2*) betweenness C^B,
(*3*) straightness C^S, and
(*4*) information C^I, are
visually compared over the
spatial graph. Different scales
of grey represent classes of
nodes with different values of
centrality

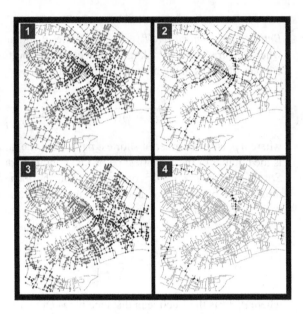

analogy. So we decided to weight our networks by using the most obvious and straightforward way that we knew for accounting distance—by metric length.

Moreover, we decided to experiment with different indices of centrality, not just the closeness/integration index. Some of them, like Closeness and Betweenness, where taken directly from classics of structural sociology, others, like the Efficiency and Information indices, were introduced by Vito [18, 19], and others again, like the Straightness index, had been already conceived for a different use [33] and were then adapted by Vito to our spatial case.

With these two inaugural works, we showed that our primal approach resulted in a very consistent geographical image: the distribution of centrality was not only visually catching but also internally coherent in that it did not exhibit "jumps" or scattered peaks. All indices resulted in beautiful lines and hubs of higher centralities that, in addition, turned out to make a lot of sense when compared with real-life cities. For example, the hierarchy of the most popular streets in Venice, Italy, which are those where shops and service also are located, was nicely highlighted in different grades of centrality (Fig. 6.1). That was extremely important especially for the urban design side of our teamwork: after all, understanding what makes a place popular and doing it quickly and effectively does mean to understand one of the most fundamental aspects of city life and evolution in time. Understanding that as the outcome of a completely self-organised dynamic appeared to us like the sign of relevance for all our efforts. Of course, the correlation between centrality and land uses, for example, the location of shops, was at this stage just *visual* and *experiential*. We felt the need to add a much more formal analysis of correlation in order to strengthen this fundamental achievement, but we did not exactly know how to do that, yet. Moreover, two problems of a conceptual nature appeared: maps of centrality were very different depending on the index of centrality that they represented, while land uses are roughly stable in space and so is the popularity of streets. So how could those highly different geographies equally support highly localised and stable phenomena like land uses? Or, put the other way around, how could different ways of being central "work together" in the urban space, as they evidently do in real life? This problem, as illustrated below in Sect. 6.2.3, was to inform the third and latest phase of this research by taking advantage of a reflection on another fundamental of urban phenomenon: *density*.

But this first phase of research also led to another very important result: centrality values are statistically distributed across street patterns of different cases in a fairly consistent manner. Moreover, and most important, *self-organised* patterns are characterised by a distribution that is different from that of *planned* patterns. Finally, the distribution of one index, the Information centrality, exhibits in self-organised patterns—and just in that case—a clear scaling behaviour. We expanded this topic in two further publications that involved a wider set of one square mile cases [8, 9], which fully confirmed the achievement.

Parallel to this work of research, we began experimenting its achievements as urban design tools in the professional practise. The occasion for that emerged in late 2005, when the University of Parma, a city in northern Italy, decided to commission a project for the regeneration of its external Campus denominated "Area of the Sciences", one of the largest in Europe with some 8,600 students and 980 staff working in it on a daily basis. The Campus had been developing since its foundation in the 1980s under an early plan that devised separated spaces for every department thus resulting in a collage of patches that had never really worked together. That in time generated two problems: on the one side, a problem of traffic, with parking lots everywhere, on-street irregular parking, congestion at peak hours and an abandonment during the rest of the day; on the other side, a problem of public space and liveability, with scattered open spaces separated by traffic arterials and large parking lots. Despite the abundance of open areas, even on sunny mild days students and staff did not really use open spaces and retreated to the covered areas of departmental buildings. That was a typical loop of complex problems that merge the technical, environmental and social dimensions of public life in a built environment. The office in charge, Rivi Engineering, asked for our help to develop a scientifically grounded understanding of the problem and an evaluation of alternative scenarios of development. The project is illustrated in a paper that got published only in 2008 but was actually written and submitted two years earlier [25]. The experience was quite encouraging: the project took advantage of the study of centrality in the Campus spaces by modelling not just the internal streets and paths, but also the open areas. As a result, two graphs were constructed representing the two systems, and two different sets of maps were produced that were eventually compared. What emerged was a clear asynchronicity, or better inconsistency, of centrality in the two domains: central open spaces were served by marginal paths and vice-versa. The project addressed this issue by reframing the connectivity of paths through the addition of several short new strategic links. That set up a new long central spine that ensured an effective re-tuning of the two systems into a unique whole. The study of centrality showed a stunning capacity to penetrate the complexity of a real-world multifaceted problem, unfold drivers and unexpected factors, provide interpretive scenarios, assess practical solutions and deliver decisions in a process of urban design.

That was really exciting: we had found the long-sought connection of spatial systems with the last decade advancements in the analysis of complex systems in other fields and positively tested it in practise. There was definitely scope for renovating our investment and going ahead with a further effort.

6.2.2 Expanding the Scope: From Centrality to Network Analysis and from One-Square-Mile Samples to Entire Cities

Fundamental as it is, centrality is not all in networks. Since the beginning we felt the need to expand the study of centrality with a wider set of indices that characterise the networks themselves. This came from a reflection on the comparability of centrality across cases. So far, we had focused on cases and found internal structures of relationships that turned out to be recurrent across cases. But we had never compared cases in terms of the actual values that centrality indices take on them. In short, we could not say that a street with a certain value of centrality is more or less central than one *in another graph*. Centrality values were strictly case-relative and posed a problem of *normalisation*. But at a deeper insight, it appeared that the same could be said for measures of the structural properties of graphs that are widely used in graph analysis, such as the characteristic path length L, the clustering coefficient C, or the number of short cycles or specific motifs. All these indices are used to evaluate the local and the global efficiency of a system so that, by comparing these properties in the original graph and in a randomised version of it, we can understand its fundamental character, for instance, if it has a small-world structure. The randomised graph, i.e. a graph with the same number of nodes and links as the original but where the links are distributed at random, acts here as the normalising element of the original graph. But in our cases, because street networks are embedded in space and are planar in nature, the randomised version of a graph is simply useless because it is almost surely a non-planar graph due to the edge crossings induced by the random rewiring of the edges. Moreover, because of the presence of long-range edges, a random graph corresponds—in a spatial context—to an extremely costly street pattern configuration. So the problem of normalisation was clearly assuming a specific consistency due to the spatial nature of our field of investigation.

We dealt with these problems in two subsequent papers [7, 28]. The only possible solution was to find a better graph than the randomised one, to be used as normalisation term for the original graph. This was done by actually defining two such comparison graphs, the Minimum Spanning Tree (MST) and the Greedy Triangulation (GT). Given a real graph, and the positions of its nodes in a two-dimensional plane, the Minimum Spanning Tree is the planar graph with the minimum number of edges in order to ensure connectedness, while the GT is the graph with the maximum number of edges compatible with the condition of planarity. In short, MST and GT represent the planar graphs with respectively the lowest and the highest possible cost, with the cost being defined as the total length of links (streets) in the network. The study was developed again on the one square mile maps, but this time over a good 20 cases. The reason behind this was our desire to understand whether the structural properties of street patterns, once made comparable through our normalisation procedure, were specific of particular *types* of cities. City types, in this case, were defined according to the *form* of the street network. As a result, looking at all the one square mile samples that we had, we identified six such types, namely medieval, grid-iron, modernist, baroque, mixed and "lollipop" (the typical configuration of low-density, post-war, "sprawled" suburbs). For example, samples from Ahmedabad and Bologna were classified "medieval", while those from Richmond and San Francisco were "grid-iron".

Box n.2: Minimum Spanning Tree (MST) and Greedy Triangulation (GT).

Spanning trees are connected planar graphs with the minimum number of edges, while greedy triangulations are graphs with the maximum number of edges compatible with the planarity. Spanning trees and greedy triangulations will serve as the two extreme cases to normalise the values of the structural measures we are going to compute, namely efficiency and cost. The cost W is defined as the sum of the length of edges in the network:

$$W = \sum_{i,j} a_{ij} l_{ij}.$$

As a measure of the efficiency in the communication between the nodes of a spatial graph, we use the global efficiency E, defined as in box 1 [18]. The two quantities are evaluated for each city and for the MST and the GT with the same set of nodes as in the original graph of the city. The values of CMST, CGT, EMST and EGT serve to normalise the results, being respectively the minimum and maximum cost, and the minimum and the maximum value of efficiency that can be obtained in a planar graph having the same number of nodes as the graph of the city. Finally, the normalised cost and efficiency are defined as:

$$W_{\text{rel}} = \frac{w - W^{\text{MST}}}{W^{\text{GT}} - W^{\text{MST}}},$$

$$E_{\text{rel}} = \frac{E - E^{\text{MST}}}{E^{\text{GT}} - E^{\text{MST}}}.$$

By definition, the MST has a relative cost $W_{\text{rel}} = 0$ and $E_{\text{rel}} = 0$, while GT has $W_{\text{rel}} = 1$ and $E_{\text{rel}} = 1$. In general, the counterpart of an increase in efficiency is an increase in the cost of construction, i.e. an increase in the number and length of the edges.

Results of this second phase are twofold. On the one hand, after local and global properties of the graphs had been calculated, we understood that, differently from non-spatial graphs, in our case the efficiency of networks at the *global* level increases with the increase of their efficiency at the *local* level. This means that a street pattern that exhibits strong local efficiency is more likely to also present strong global efficiency. The reason behind that is the network cost being measured as the simple total length of streets: that makes a denser and highly interconnected street network which, of course, exhibits higher clustering, also more efficient as a whole in the sense that it is more straightforwardly traversable. This achievement confirms that small-world behaviours are not compatible with the spatial case, at least when metric distance is used to compute the cost of the system. It is reasonable, however, to expect a different result if distance is measured in terms of trip duration. In this latter case, the effect of long, wide and straight channels of movements like boulevards, motorways or subways, which had typically been superimposed on the former dense pre-modern systems in all major western cities (as well as in colonial capitals) after the Haussmanian renovation of Paris in the nineteenth century, would be a significant drop in the duration of *long-range* trips and therefore an increase in global efficiency. But this is grist for the mill of further research.

On the other hand, the normalisation of structural properties measures of one spatial graph against its MST and GT, and in particular of *Efficiency* and *Cost*, made it possible for us to characterise street networks in a very synthetic and comparable way in terms of the relationship between the two variables of *Relative Efficiency* (E_{rel}) and *Relative Cost* (W_{rel}). What came out of that is a very significant clustering of cities of the same type so that, for example, most medieval patterns are characterised by the best combination of high efficiency and low cost, where *Efficiency* measures to which extent on average the connecting route between two nodes approximates the virtual straight line, and *Cost* represents the overall length of all streets in the network. "Lollipop" and modernist patterns show the worst combination of low efficiency and relatively high cost (Fig. 6.2). Grid-iron patterns, finally, do exhibit a high efficiency but at high overall cost. General as it is, this result was completely satisfying to us: we had now a quantitative and comparable measure of the form of street networks in cities at the level of their inner structure that showed a high capacity to discriminate between *historically characterised types*.

This achievement put us in a condition to experiment more widely. The occasion for this came with the invitation to participate to a large effort aimed at understanding the relationship between urban form and sustainability, the "City Form" project [31]. The structure of the project was very simple: the form of urban fabric would have been measured and these measures would have been correlated with the performances that it offered on a number of key-aspects of sustainability, as for social, demographic, economic and environmental aspects. Our work was to substantially contribute to the measurement of urban form. Cases were individuated in five UK cities in central, peripheral and in-between locations. Both the vehicular and pedestrian networks were successfully analysed and the overall results of this study are reported in [17].

Our effort within the City Form project was a considerable challenge for us in many respects. One of the challenges was something we had long been looking at: expanding our analysis from small networks, at the scale of the district, to large

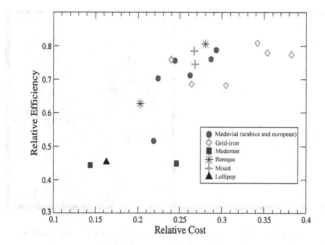

Fig. 6.2 A plot of the relative efficiency, E_{rel}, as a function of the relative cost, W_{rel}, of a city, indicates a correlation between structural properties and a priori known classes of cities (as medieval, grid-iron, modernist, baroque, mixed, and lollipop fabrics). Each point in the plot represents a city. The point of coordinates $(0, 0)$ would correspond to the cost/efficiency of the MST while the point $(1, 1)$ would correspond to the GT network. Irvine 2, having coordinates $(0.175, -0.398)$, i.e. a negative value of relative efficiency, has been plotted instead as having coordinates $(0.175, 0)$

cities and even metropolitan regions. This passage characterised the third phase of our work, and led us to develop the knowledge necessary to deal with another challenge, namely understanding and testing the correlation between centrality and fundamental real-world urban dynamics like the location of economic activities or the real-estate market.

6.2.3 Current Developments: Density of Centrality and Correlation

The problem of correlation had always been well riveted in our mind. After all, the real concern of the urban design side of our team was to develop a tool, and therefore the crucial point was to show that there is a linkage between our model of reality and how things really go out there on the streets. Hillier's work in the last couple of decades and even more, in this sense, has been terrific. The Space Syntax model has been tested widely in a number of cases and correlations between the "*Integration*" (*Closeness*) index and relevant dynamics like pedestrian flows, land use location, crime incidents and others have been established. We had the clear feeling that our MCA model presented a significant number of advantages compared to Hillier's, but this was clearly nothing without evidence of its capacity to capture and explain real dynamics on the ground. However, as always happens, science comes following experience, observation and intuitions; in our case, during the first two phases of this work of research we came across endless testimonies of this capacity. We tested our MCA model extensively on a number of cities, many of which we had

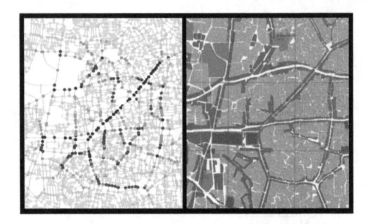

Fig. 6.3 (Color online) Ahmedabad, India. Betweenness centrality C^B (*left*) and land uses (*right*). On-street retail commerce is represented with *blue* in the land-use map

a direct experience of. In other cases, we had documented information of specific dynamics, like land uses. For example, Dr. Shibu Raman, a colleague and friend who conducts research at Oxford Brookes, one day sent an image of Ahmedabad, a map of current land-uses with retail and commerce street fronts highlighted in blue: the visual correlation with our one square mile map of the same place was stunning (Fig. 6.3). In short, "red" (central) streets identified invariably those most popular, evident in the mental maps that everyone forms of the space for navigating it, and especially those around which *the evolution of the city in history* has been unfolding, i.e. the drivers and the backbones of such evolution. Far more than simply a model that predicts where something like the "*community potential*" is (that is an enormous achievement in itself!), MCA appeared as a way for capturing and mapping something even deeper and more fundamental, which is about networks *in time*. Beginning to think about that was very important for us: an entire new strand of research that is grounded on urban morphology and the analogy of urban change with evolution in living organisms and "*morphometrics*" began to take shape within our team, which is currently one of our major areas of investment. One first result of this new strand of research is a brand new surprising model of urban design at the scale of the urban district [21], based on the observation of what appears to be "permanent"—and therefore structural—in cities across time (history) and space (geography). At the same time, we are deeply involved in the morphological analysis of urban blocks and in measuring several of their dominant spatial characters, to bring the study at a lower scale and also to build the ground for a more direct investigation of the evolutionary analogy, beyond the simple conceptual level, which has always been the limit of its use in urban studies. But this is another story that we cannot report here because most of it is still to be done, so let us come back to networks.

We had to substantiate our scattered observations that in space centrality goes with popularity and the potential of places to develop sound urban communities. What we had was a very consistent methodology to map centrality. We also knew that many—if not most—large western municipalities have extensive geo-referenced databases of the location of every single shop or service, so since the very beginning of this research we paid attention to every opportunity in that sense. Soon we came to establish partnerships with two such cities: Bologna, Italy, and Barcelona, Spain. The work with these two cities proceeded slowly and faced many difficulties of different kinds, including the need to increase our computation power in order to jump form the analysis of one square mile samples, which means graphs of the order of hundreds of nodes, to graphs of tens of thousands nodes like those of entire urban regions. However, the greatest difficulties were not merely technical, but, in fact, conceptual.

Firstly, correlation studies of this kind have been seldom produced, and in all cases the procedure implied attributing data of the dynamic under study (for example, shop location, pedestrian flow or crime incidents) to the network's link and then correlating values at the single link level, for example, values of the link, like centrality, with values of the dynamics, like shop location. That was not at all something we were willing to do. It is far too direct and rigid as a method. Again, it was not too rigid in technical terms, but rather in the sense that in all evidence *cities do not leapfrog* in such "binary" way. Cities, in fact, work immersed in a condition that is deeply informed by the laws of *space*, and therefore they work in a quite different way—*smoothly*. If a street is central, its influence is not limited to the street itself and it does not end abruptly at the end of it. If you have one shop in one location, its influence is not just confined to the proper boundaries of its location, but spreads well beyond it to affect what goes on around. Moreover, this influence does not just spread around; it does that *decaying with distance*. This is very fundamental in space, and in urban space in particular. So our methodology had to capture this character of the deep nature of how space works in cities. Secondly, we wanted a methodology that could be applied in the generality of cases, no matter the kind of data that you have. Not always, and to be true not even often, information of social or economic dynamics in cities is provided in a sound geo-referenced way, therefore it is often very difficult, if not impossible, to *realistically* collapse those data on street links. As a result, our methodology of correlation would be the right one only if it could operate in a somehow "looser" way. Thirdly, we still had in front of us the conflict between the multiplicity of centrality, as captured by the different behaviour of its many indices, and the consistency of its influence on urban dynamics and collective behaviours, i.e. the problem presented above, namely how can different centrality indices that distribute spatially in such different ways work together consistently and therefore consistently influence dynamics of urban life? The solution to all these three problems came relatively easy by experimenting the various tools embedded in our GIS software package (ESRI). Studying the package, our attention was grabbed by the very name of a bunch of these tools, a word that was increasingly appearing to our eyes to be a fundamental driver in the history of urban design, a word that is regarded to have countless impact in urban life in a large body of literature ranging from environmental psychology to planning and urban history. A word that was becoming a milestone for us. If, following Martin Heidegger, words do "gather worlds", that word definitely gathered the world of urban history, theory and life altogether. That word is *density*.

Box n.3: Kernel Density Estimation.
A kernel function looks like a bump centred at each point x_i and tapering off to 0 over a bandwidth or window. The kernel density at point x at the centre of a grid cell is estimated to be the sum of bumps within the bandwidth:

$$\hat{f}(x) = \frac{1}{nh} \sum_{i=1}^{n} K\left(\frac{x - x_i}{h}\right)$$

where $K(\cdot)$ is the kernel function, h is the bandwidth, n is the number of points within the bandwidth, and ^{n} is the total number of events. All events x_i within the bandwidth of x generate some bumps reaching the point x, and contribute to the estimated kernel density there. The kernel function $K(y)$ is a function satisfying the normalisation for a two-dimensional vector y such as:

$$\int_{R^2} K(y)\, dy = 1.$$

A regularly adopted kernel is the standard normal curve:

$$K(y) = (2\pi)^{-1/2} \exp\left(-\frac{1}{2}y^2\right).$$

For convenience, our computation in ArcGIS used the following kernel function, as described in [29], p. 76:
One advantage of the equation above is its faster calculation than the regular kernel. As the formula indicates, any activity beyond the bandwidth h from the centroid of the considered cell does not contribute to the summation.

The ArcView GIS package offers a set of tools for implementing spatial smoothing or spatial interpolation techniques [34]. Among them, one is devoted to the Kernel Density Estimation (KDE). The KDE uses the density within a range (window) of each observation to represent the value at the centre of the window. Within the window, the KDE weighs nearby objects more than distant objects, on the basis of a kernel function. By doing so, the KDE generates a density of the events (discrete points) as a continuous field (i.e. a raster), and therefore converts the two datasets to the same raster framework and permits the analysis of relationships between them.

As soon as we discovered this, we got definitely engaged with this method: clearly, that sorted the second of the above-mentioned problems regarding the need of a "looser" procedure in order to deal with the generality of data available on cities. But as we progressed in understanding and using the tool, we found that it equally well sorted the other two. Because of its smoothing effect, KDE perfectly captured the deeper nature of space in cities by actually representing the influence of events as a decaying function within a certain distance, for example, images coming out from our analysis of Barcelona revealed that centrality at street crossings is in any case far higher than that of converging streets, a very well known and all important feature of urban spaces (Fig. 6.4). Finally, we found that while the geography

Fig. 6.4 Barcelona, Spain. Local density ($h = 100$ m) of street centrality, detail of the urban core; straightness centrality C^S

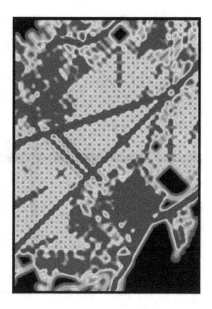

of centrality on streets is very different among the different indices of centrality, the corresponding geographies of *density* of centrality were surprisingly consistent. When we first looked at these results, we could not find an explanation for that, and we even checked accurately our procedure in order to ensure that these results were not the outcome of technical errors. And they weren't. At the end, we became aware of the simple truth—density does not just take into account street centrality, but rather it first and foremost takes into account streets! This means that the very presence and concentration of streets influences the density of street centrality to a great extent. As we discussed in the Barcelona paper, this particular feature of our analysis that might be perceived as a "noise" by geo-computationists is, in fact, probably its strongest point as it captures the deepest nature and somewhat the most mysterious challenge in understanding centrality in cities. Centrality is in itself a multifold and layered phenomenon, but as applied to real urban spaces it gets "tamed" and reduced to consistency by the same presence and concentration of streets. The way streets are laid out and interconnected in a specific case does not just determine to what degree every street is central in terms of the different indices of centrality (every street is likely to be central and marginal at the same time depending on the centrality index you are considering). It also merges the influences of those different ways of being central in a consistent and unitary spatial effect. In other words, because of the properties of the sole street layout, the effect of a variegated distribution of centrality in streets is overall fairly consistent and unitary *in space*.

So looking at a way to correlate street centrality and urban dynamics, we actually got a very relevant achievement in terms of a deeper understanding of the role of streets in cities and the miracle that makes what emerges as diverse at the level of the single part be compounded into a superior whole at the level of the system. That was again very important for us and was immediately exploited in a professional

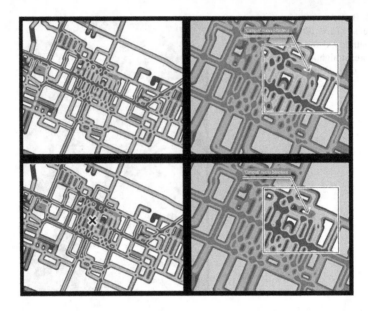

Fig. 6.5 Castelfranco Emilia, Italy. Analysis of the density of betweenness centrality C^B. *Left column*: current situation (*top*); proposed scenario A (disconnection of the Via Emilia) (*bottom*). *Right column* (detail of the new library area): current situation (*top*); proposed reconnection of two local streets with the library area (*bottom*)

task of urban design by deploying maps of density of centrality in the context of a design competition (Fig. 6.5). The occasion arose in 2007 when the municipality of Castelfranco Emilia, a town located between Modena and Bologna in northern Italy, launched an international design competition with the aim of devising architectural solutions that would contribute to the rebuilding of the social and economic fabric of the old city centre along and aside the ancient Roman road named "Via Emilia". The methodology was applied to understand the side effects of small strategic decisions on the connectivity of extant streets, thus guiding an approach that was designed to achieve great results without large public investments. The project was awarded the first prize.

Then we got correlations. So far, we have raised evidence that density of centrality is correlated with three distinct dynamics: location of shops and services at the ground floor [26], location of shops and services at all floors [27] and real estate values [35]. We have done that with studies of entire urban regions, not just neighbourhoods or districts. But there is something subtler: we have shown that *secondary* activities in a large city like Barcelona are not preferentially located close to secondary urban nodes, but they rather tend to concentrate around a primary location in an even stronger way than *primary* activities. By primary and secondary activities we refer here to Jane Jacobs' "classic" taxonomy [16] where the former are land uses that have the capacity to draw people in one place (including industries and nodal activities at metropolitan and regional level like major theatre, stadium, large administrative functions and all other major concentrations of important functions), while the latter are uses that build on the presence of people that is ensured by the former (including all the neighbourhood level functions like groceries, cafés, small pharmacies and retail shops or services to the community). The relevance of this achievement is evident to urban designers, as much of the theories in urban planning since the constitution of our discipline in late nineteenth and early twentieth century have been stating just the opposite, i.e. that primary activities *ought* to be in primary locations and secondary activities in secondary locations. Things, in cities, definitely do not work in separate patches. They work altogether. Or they die.

6.3 Conclusions and Further Research

This paper does not report on a single research work, but rather describes an entire experience of research that stemmed by a partnership between urban designers and physicists for the analysis of complex networks of streets and intersections in cities. Thus the aim of this chapter is to make clear the overall meaning of this effort and to anchor it to its specific achievements across a number of referenced publications. As such, this chapter may be of help for the reader to navigate the research in its entirety and then downscale for the details to specific publications.

Achievements span from the construction of an effective tool for urban design practise, to a deeper understanding of fundamental dynamics in cities that link space and collective behaviours, to a contribution to the reintegration of spatial networks into the broader field of complex network analysis.

The research is all but concluded. New strands include the analysis of how street networks change in time, the development of a tool for computing kernel density along networks rather than in the 2D space, the use of connectivity to describe historical patterns in cities and the impact of transportation on global connectivity [10], and finally the relationship between street centrality and urban morphology at the scale of blocks, streets and lots. Moreover, one effort will be soon directed to the construction of one unique platform for the computation of centrality indices and other graph structural measures in cities.

6.3.1 Crossing the Borders: A Postscript from the First Author

Looking backward to the beginnings of this story, one image that comes to my mind is a lazy, hot summer afternoon in Nervi, a small wealthy suburb near Genoa, Italy. I was taking a rest seeking relief from the oppressive Mediterranean temperature in my uncle place's bedroom, all window shutters closed to keep the glazing out, the sea shining from afar behind them. In the shadowed room space, I could not help approaching a pile of photocopies that had been waiting for me for too long and was now ready at hand in front of me. It was the summer of 2003, and I made those copies five years earlier in Berkeley, but for some reason I never really went through them. But that was the right moment. I wanted to deepen the study of

Hillier's two seminal books on Space Syntax [12, 13]—such was the content of the photocopies—because I just had a rough idea of them.

Months before that, Ombretta Romice, who is now my colleague at UDSU, emailed me the title of a popular book by Mark Buchanan on complex networks [5]. I ordered it on Amazon and after one month I was totally engaged with the theories of "small worlds". An amazing new kind of knowledge—I learned—was increasingly revealing how seemingly different domains of self-organised systems in nature, technology, society and even culture are actually grounded on a similar organisation, or "architecture", which is responsible for the way their constituent parts are connected to each other, no matter the nature of those parts. What really struck me was that those systems were not planned at all, and yet—it turned out—they were all but chaotic; quite on the contrary, they emerged in such a way that they show a *different kind of order*, and that order ensures those systems the capacity to express extraordinary performances. That was the point for me. That was the real point. All that echoed almost literally Jane Jacobs' arguments of half a century ago on the "kind of order a city is" [16, Chap. 22], as the roots of the failure of the "pseudo-science of planning"! She argued, quite simply, that city planning as a discipline just misunderstood the nature of its object of study—the city—which is not a complex-disorganised but, in fact, a complex-organised phenomenon. As such, the many failures of city planning on the ground are not suggesting to embrace an anti-scientific approach, but to apply a different science. That different science was now clearly in front of me: after half a century the promise of Jane Jacobs appeared to have found its way.

Thus, systems that self-organise out of any coordination or control from atop, detached by any form of central authority, do not end up in a bloody mess and eventually in a disaster, but the opposite applies: they gradually form up so that, notwithstanding the lack of any recognisable geometrical structure, an inner and more profound order emerges that rules the way they are internally connected and makes them quicker, stronger and more robust. And for so long I was trying to penetrate this mystery! Cities, in fact, are telling us quite the same tale. I had spent at those times the last years of my post-graduate studies in an effort to free my mind from the ideological pollution of a formal education in Modern Architecture and Urbanism. I had become increasingly aware that city fabrics are by far more liveable still in our days if they had never been planned, and that *adaptability* is key in that. I had begun reading about the many forms of reaction against top-down planning in urban policies and design. I had gone through the study of participatory practises and the theory of argumentative planning and consensus building, and then I came in contact with Christopher Alexander's ideas about generative codes and patterns of change in urban space at the most different scales [1, 2]. A different way of social inclusion in urban processes was proposed in those latter works that I found more convincing. There must be a way—I repeated to myself—to make urban change really democratic, i.e. reflective of the wills of people who use them, well off formal processes of "public participation": such processes, in fact, are too easily tailored on the needs of those who manage the process or just hold key information and, in the end, what kind of democracy do they express? The democracy of those who are present and can speak? With all the problems that representative democracy has in our age, participative democracy is still something I could not see as a real alternative.

As a result, I was beginning to reflect on adaptability in the urban fabric as an inner character of the spatial system. The question was: how can we structure the urban space so that change can actually start happening from the bottom up as it has always been in the history of cities? Buchanan's book was a revelation: here we have a whole theory of self-organisation in complex systems. With this in mind, I rapidly crunched other books and a lot of articles in the theory of the small-worlds. Most of them where highly formal in language, with lots of arcane mathematical terms and formulas that looked like ancient Aramaic to my eyes, that is, completely obscure. However, at the end I could grasp what I wanted, namely a very rough idea of the latest debate around complexity and the use of graphs as the main mathematical tool for the representation and the analysis of the internal structure of systems. I was so excited that I hardly could hold up myself from seeking contact with specialists. It was not time yet, there was one passage I still had to go through. I had to come back to the pot of my discipline and see what I could find of the same kind. Space Syntax immediately came to my mind, but also I knew that graphs are used by traffic engineers for producing simulations of vehicle flows under different scenarios— I knew that very well for I had used some of them professionally in the past. And I also had some clues of the studies in Regional Analysis, which were so popular in the 1960s and 1970s.

Therefore, I spent some time going back to those fields in search of graphs in urban planning, but what I actually found was somewhat surprising: yes, of course, graphs had been used, but nothing really comparable with anything about small-worlds or inner structures. We had regional models where graphs represented communication channels (mainly roads), but in that case the focus of these models was on simulating the overall dynamic of population, production and the market [37]. Here, communication networks where treated just like a substrate in a gigantic effort to embed in the model literally everything that could hold any relevance in urbanisation processes. That was definitely not what I was searching for, there was an evident problem of an epistemological nature: how could we even think of approaching complexity in such a *comprehensive* way? How can we build our way through countless looping relationships in restless transformation with a will to conceptually include all of them in a model? No, we definitely need a synthetic, or better, a *structural* approach. We need to focus on just a tiny section of this complexity on the basis of a reasonable understanding of the whole organisation, so that we are able to identify that section which actually provides structure to the whole. Later on, I will develop all this in a strong interest towards structuralism in social sciences and evolution in biology and the use of it as an analogy to understand non-biological phenomena like dynamics of change in the urban space. But at those times, this was not yet at the horizon; and that was Space Syntax. My very superficial knowledge of Hillier's model, drawn from a few newspaper articles, images grasped on the Internet, a couple of scientific papers and a very quick look at those two monographs were nevertheless enough to raise my interest. That was certainly a structural approach; it was certainly an effort to understand the inner organisation of cities just by handling one section, the street network. Finally,—I thought—that was certainly about urban design. And therefore that was the time to finally get into Hillier's studies beginning from the start, with patience, and with some time ahead. I had patience, and definitely I had some time ahead in that summer afternoon of year 2003, with a pile of photocopies staring at me in the shadows of my uncle's bedroom in Nervi.

It took a while to understand Hillier's model. Later in autumn, when I had my first meeting with Vito in Catania, Sicily, I brought him just a shapeless agglomeration of fuzzy ideas. I wanted to do something on urban street networks, but basically I wanted to do something on applying the small-worlds theory to cities. And that was what I told Vito in the first place; I was really excited and it was not good seeing Vito's face turning to a visible manifestation of boredom. I learned then that Vito's main occupation in recent years had consistently been about kicking off people coming with the idea of finding small worlds in everything from ice cream trading to the reproduction of rabbits in central Australia. Small-worlds were definitely very popular in those years. Vito explained to me that cities are a different class of systems because their nature is *spatial*, and that research in complex networks had mainly focused on non-spatial systems. Spatial networks—he told me—are a very special class of complex networks. They must be described by graphs whose nodes are embedded in a Euclidean space and whose edges do not define relations in an abstract space, such as in networks of acquaintances or collaborations between individuals, but are real physical connections, with an associated length. In spatial networks, speaking of small worlds as in social networks is not entirely appropriate. The topology of spatial graphs is strongly constrained by their spatial embedding. For instance, there is a cost to pay for the existence of long-range connections in a spatial network, this having important consequences on the possibility to observe a small-world behaviour. Moreover, the number of edges that can be connected to a single node is often limited by the scarce availability of physical space, this imposing some constraints on the degree distributions. In a few words, spatial networks are different from other complex networks, and as such they need to be studied in a different way. But Vito insisted that spatial systems are a challenge that interested him exactly because they were still largely to be explored [4]. So, he said, put aside the small worlds and let's go ahead. How would I represent a city and what urban scholars have done so far to understand the structure of space? At that point, I felt lost. With all my knowledge of urban studies, I could hardly answer that question. Believe it or not, urban space has never been central in urban planning and especially not in terms of structure. So I took a pile of photocopies from my bag and displayed them to him. I made those copies from Allan Jacobs' book [15], and this is another interesting short story that it is worth telling.

Five years before my meeting with Vito, I was holding a Visiting Scholar position at Berkeley, CA. There I met Allan Jacobs who on the day of our first appointment waited for me in his office barefoot, white dressed and smiling. One wall of the small hall in front of his office was entirely covered by tens of Letter size sheets. Every sheet reported a one square mile sample of the plan of a city. The graphic was quite straightforward: blocks were represented in black, and spaces between blocks, mostly streets and squares, in white. All maps were represented at the same scale. When Allan came out from his office to let me in, he caught me deeply absorbed in jumping from one map to another, pacing the room across and bending down or stretching up to compare them, to the point that I even did not get aware of him. The fact is—that was a turning point in my intellectual path. From that point on, the enormous power of comparison will be forever unfolded. It was amazing: just representing cities *at the same scale* and with *the same conventional graphics* makes them clearly self-explanatory. Differences where so stunning that you could never even *believe* they were portrayed at the same scale! Part of those drawings had been published in "Great Streets" along with some very fundamental and simple quantitative accounts, for example, the number of street crossings. So I learned that in one square mile of Venice, Italy, you have some 17,000 crossings, while in the same "amount" of Irvine, CA, you can count only 17! Isn't that stunning? How could one even begin stating that this has no impact on urban life or the way people behave collectively in space? Gee, it is 17,000 against 17!! I was amazed comparing cities, comparing their quantities, revealing differences that are so obvious that no one really cares or knows of. My whole contribution to the understanding of cities since then has been reformed by that appointment with Allan Jacobs at Berkeley.

So I displayed copies of those maps to Vito, four years later, in Catania. I said: look, cities can be really different in the way space is configured, and we can quantify that difference to some extent, or at least the exterior manifestation of that difference. But I wanted something more structural. I wanted to capture the more fundamental difference that is so evident looking at the maps but nevertheless so difficult to define. I wanted to do something about the street network because in all evidence it had to do with those fundamentals. Then I began explaining, as an example, Hillier's way to analyse what he calls "integration". It was my "ace in the cuff", my once-and-for-all argument. I thought it would have taken hours to make Vito just grasp the surface of it. To my highest surprise, however, he followed my explanation with a sort of patient relaxation, and soon interrupted me: yes, sure, that is "closeness". Closeness? Closeness. What's closeness? Closeness is one of the most popular indices of centrality in networks as defined since the early 1950s by scientists in structural sociology and then classically established by Freeman in the 1970s [11]. 1950s? 1970s? Vito looked at me patiently in silence while my brain was running at 200 km/h. Then I realised it all at once: my God, *disciplines*!

By meeting Vito, I crossed the borders of my discipline. What I found was that what is mysterious in one field can be nothing less than trivial in another. Mysterious and trivial: the hiatus can be just that wide. Then Vito and I spent the following two days doing just that, crossing the borders. We talked and explained, transferred and asked. And we finally left with one programme of research: I would build the graphs of those maps taken from Allan's book. I would do that in a very straightforward manner: scanning the images, importing them into the Geographic Information System (GIS) environment (GIS was brand new to Vito, my revenge) and then extract the table of connectivity, i.e. the list of all couples of nodes with their coordinates in space and the length of their connecting street. Then I would send them to Vito for analysis. Finally, Vito would send the results back to me, and I would map the results again in GIS. That programme kept both of us, with our collaborators, engaged for the following three years and its developments are still one of the main strands of our research activity.

References

1. Alexander, C.: A city is not a tree. Archit. Forum **122**, 58–62 (1965)
2. Alexander, C., Ishikawa, S., Silverstein, M.: A Pattern Language: Towns, Buildings, Construction. Oxford University Press, New York (1977)
3. Barthelemy, M., Flammini, A.: Modelling urban streets patterns. Phys. Rev. Lett. **100**, 13 (2008)
4. Boccaletti, S., Latora, V., Moreno, Y., Chavez, M., Wang, D.U.: Complex networks: structure and dynamics. Phys. Rep. **424**, 175–308 (2006)
5. Buchanan, M.: Nexus. Small Worlds and the Groundbreaking Science of Networks. Norton, New York (2002)
6. Caniggia, G., Maffei, G.: Composizione Architettonica e Tipologia Edilizia: Lettura Dell'Edilizia di Base. Marsilio, Venezia (1979). English edition: Interpreting Basic Buildings. Alinea, Florence (2001)
7. Cardillo, A., Scellato, S., Latora, V., Porta, S.: Structural properties of planar graphs of urban street patterns. Phys. Rev. E **73**, 066107 (2006)
8. Crucitti, P., Latora, V., Porta, S.: Centrality in networks of urban streets. Chaos **16**, 066107 (2006)
9. Crucitti, P., Latora, V., Porta, S.: Centrality measures in spatial networks of urban streets. Phys. Rev. E **73**, 036125 (2006)
10. Da Fontoura Costa, L., Nassif Travencolo, B.A., Palhares Viana, M., Strano, E.: On the efficiency of underground systems in large cities. arXiv:0911.2028v1 (2009)
11. Freeman, L.: Centrality in social networks: conceptual clarification. Social Networks **1**, 215–239 (1979)
12. Hillier, B.: Space Is the Machine: A Configurational Theory of Architecture. Cambridge University Press, Cambridge (1996)
13. Hillier, B., Hanson, J.: The Social Logic of Space. Cambridge University Press, Cambridge (1984)
14. Hillier, B., Penn, A., Hanson, J., Grajewski, T., Xu, J.: Natural movement: or configuration and attraction in urban pedestrian movement. Environ. Plan. B, Plan. Des. **20**, 29–66 (1993)
15. Jacobs, A.: Great Streets. MIT Press, Cambridge (1993)
16. Jacobs, J.: The Death and Life of Great American Cities. Random House, New York (1961)
17. Jenks, M., Jones, C. (eds.): Dimensions of the Sustainable City. Springer, London (2010)
18. Latora, V., Marchiori, M.: Efficient behavior of small-world networks. Phys. Rev. Lett. **87**, 198701 (2001)
19. Latora, V., Marchiori, M.: A measure of centrality based on the network efficiency. New J. Phys. **9**, 188 (2007)
20. Lopez, M., Van Nes, A.: Measuring spatial visibility, adjacency, permeability and degrees of street life in excavated towns. Paper presented at the CSAAR conference (Amman, 2008)
21. Mehaffy, M., Porta, S., Rofè, Y., Salingaros, N.: Urban nuclei and the geometry of streets: The 'emergent neighborhoods' model. Urban Des. Int. **15**, 22–46 (2010)
22. Newman, P., Kenworthy, J.: Sustainability and Cities. Island Press, Washington (1999)
23. Porta, S., Crucitti, P., Latora, V.: The network analysis of urban streets: a dual approach. Phys. A, Stat. Mech. Appl. **369**, 853–866 (2006)
24. Porta, S., Crucitti, P., Latora, V.: The network analysis of urban streets: a primal approach. Environ. Plan. B, Plan. Des. **33**, 705–725 (2006)

25. Porta, S., Crucitti, P., Latora, V.: Multiple centrality assessment in Parma: a network analysis of paths and open spaces. Urban Des. Int. **13**, 41–50 (2008)
26. Porta, S., Latora, V., Wang, F., Scellato, S.: Street centrality and densities of retail and services in Bologna, Italy. Environ. Plan. B, Plan. Des. **36**, 450–465 (2009)
27. Porta, S., Latora, V., Wang, F., Rueda, S., Cormenzana, B., Cardenas, F., et al.: Understanding urban cores: Geography of street centrality and location of economic activities in Barcelona. Computers, Environment and Urban Systems (2010, in review)
28. Scellato, S., Cardillo, A., Latora, V., Porta, S.: The backbone of a city. Eur. Phys. J. B **50**, 221–225 (2006)
29. Silverman, B.W.: Density Estimation for Statistics and Data Analysis. Chapman and Hall, London (1986)
30. Steadman, P.: The Evolution of Designs. Routledge, Abingdon (2008)
31. The Sustainable Urban Form Consortium: City Form. http://www.city-form.org/uk/ (2006). Accessed 18 Jan 2010
32. Van Nes, A.: Spatial conditions for a typology of shopping areas. In: Proceedings of the 3rd International Space Syntax Symposium, Atlanta (2005)
33. Vragovic, I., Louis, E., Diaz-Guilera, A.: Efficiency of informational transfer in regular and complex networks. Physical Review E **71** (2005)
34. Wang, F.: Quantitative Methods and Applications in GIS. CRC Press, Boca Raton (2006)
35. Wang, F., Antipova, A., Porta, S.: Street centrality and land use intensity in Baton Rouge, Louisiana. Journal of Transport Geography (2010, in press)
36. Wasserman, S., Faust, K.: Social Network Analysis. Cambridge University Press, Cambridge (1994)
37. Wilson, A.G.: Complex Spatial Systems: The Modelling Foundations of Urban and Regional Analysis. Prentice Hall, Upper Saddle River (2000)

Chapter 7
The Structure of Financial Networks

Stefano Battiston, James B. Glattfelder,
Diego Garlaschelli, Fabrizio Lillo,
and Guido Caldarelli

Abstract We present here an overview of the use of networks in Finance and Economics. We show how this approach enables us to address important questions as, for example, the structure of control chains in financial systems, the systemic risk associated with them and the evolution of trade between nations. All these results are new in the field and allow for a better understanding and modelling of different economic systems.

7.1 Introduction

The use of network theory in financial systems is relatively recent, but it has exploded in the last few years, and since the financial crisis of 2008–2009 this topic

S. Battiston (✉) · J.B. Glattfelder
Systemgestaltung, ETH-Zentrum, Zurich, Switzerland
e-mail: sbattiston@ethz.ch

J.B. Glattfelder
e-mail: jglattfelder@ethz.ch

D. Garlaschelli
Said Business School, University of Oxford, Oxford, UK

F. Lillo
Dipartimento di Fisica e Tecnologie Relative, Università di Palermo, Palermo, Italy
e-mail: lillo@unipa.it

F. Lillo
Santa Fe Institute, Santa Fe, USA

G. Caldarelli
Centre SMC, and ISC CNR, Dip. Fisica, University "Sapienza", Piazzale Aldo Moro 5, Rome, Italy
e-mail: Guido.Caldarelli@roma1.infn.it

E. Estrada et al. (eds.), *Network Science*,
DOI 10.1007/978-1-84996-396-1_7, © Springer-Verlag London Limited 2010

has received even more interest. Many approaches have been attempted, and in this
chapter we try to summarise the most interesting and successful of them. This is
only one aspect of the increasing interest in real-world complex networks, indeed
some previous studies revealed unsuspected regularities such as scaling laws which
are robust across many domains, ranging from biology or computer systems to society and economics [40, 63, 68]. This has suggested that universal, or at least generic,
mechanisms are at work in the formation of many such networks. Tools and concepts from statistical physics have been crucial for the achievement of these findings
[13, 28]. From the initial activity, the research in the field of networks evolved so
that three levels of analysis are nowadays possible. The first level corresponds to a
purely topological approach (best epitomised by a binary adjacency matrix, where
links simply exist or not). Allowing the links to carry weights [5], or weights and
direction [66], defines a second level of complexity. Only recent studies have started
focusing on the third level of detail in which the nodes themselves are assigned a degree of freedom, sometimes also called fitness. This is a non-topological state variable which shapes the topology of the network [23, 41, 43]. In this chapter, we shall
try to cover these three aspects by mainly focussing on the methodological aspects,
i.e. which types of networks can be constructed for financial systems, and evaluating the empirical results on networks obtained by investigating large databases of
financial data ranging from individual transactions in a financial market to strategic
decisions at a bank level. Readers have to note that edges and vertices can assume
different meanings according to the system considered. In some situations, we can
have different details of data available, and cannot investigate the three levels of detail in the same way. The cases of study we want to present here are those related
to

- Networks to extract information from *Correlation Matrices*
- Networks of control as, for example, the *Ownership network* and the *Board of Directors* network
- Trading networks as the *World Trade Web* and the *Banks' Credit* networks

Since these fields can be very different, it is important to divide and classify the
networks that we could encounter. An important classification of networks in general, and that will be considered here, is the one that divides networks into similarity
based networks and direct interaction networks. To be specific, consider a network
whose nodes are financial agents: investors, banks, hedge funds, etc. They differ in
the meaning of the links. In similarity-based networks, we draw a link when the
two vertices share some feature: strategy, behaviour, income, etc. In this case, one
needs to assign a criterion to establish whether the similarity between two agents is
relevant enough that we can join the agents with a link. This means that the agents
do not interact with each other, but can be connected if they are similar. Conversely,
in direct interaction networks a link between two nodes signals the presence of an
interaction between the entities represented by the two nodes connected by the link.
In the financial case, the interaction can be a transaction between two agents, an
ownership relation of one node with respect to another, a credit relation, etc. All
these situations are present in real financial networks and we shall analyse various

instances of them. The structure of this chapter reflects the above division of topics so that, Sect. 7.2 overviews the studies of networks in a data mining framework (mostly similarity-based networks). In Sect. 7.3, we analyse the social aspects of the control networks where vertices are real agents or companies, and finally in Sect. 7.4, we analyse some of the most important "trading" webs.

7.2 Similarity-Based Networks

In similarity based networks, a weighted link between two nodes represents a similarity (but not necessarily a direct interaction) between the two nodes. Let us consider a system composed of N elements. Each element is represented by T variables. These variables describe several different properties of the elements (or they can represent values of the variables at different times as it is the case of time series). Typically, one introduces a matrix C describing the various $N \times N$ similarity measurements. We indicate with c_{ij} the generic element of the matrix C. In the language of networks, the matrix C identifies a complete (all edges drawn) weighted network where every of the N elements is represented by a node, and the link connecting nodes i and j is associated to a weight related to c_{ij}. From a purely topological point of view, this does not produce anything usable. In fact, if, for example, we consider the similarities between 1000 different elements, one has to check almost one million entries. The natural choice is then to exploit the extra information embedded in the values of the weights. In other words, it is necessary to filter out the most relevant links of the network. The different methods to perform this filtration give rise to different similarity based networks.

The choice of the similarity measure is also arbitrary. A very common choice is the use of the linear correlation as a measure of similarity. In this case, we have the correlation based networks. The best example of similarity-based networks are correlation based networks. In this case, the similarity between two elements (nodes) of the system is quantified by the linear correlation. The matrix element c_{ij} is the linear (or Pearson's) cross-correlation between element i and j, i.e.

$$c_{ij} = \frac{\langle r_i r_j \rangle - \langle r_i \rangle \langle r_j \rangle}{\sqrt{\langle r_i^2 \rangle - \langle r_i \rangle^2} \sqrt{\langle r_j^2 \rangle - \langle r_j \rangle^2}} \tag{7.1}$$

where r_i and r_j are the investigated variables and the symbol $\langle \ldots \rangle$ is a statistical average defined as

$$\langle r_i \rangle = \frac{1}{T} \sum_{k=1}^{T} r_i(k) \tag{7.2}$$

where $r_i(k)$ is the kth variable of element i. The correlation coefficient has values between -1 and $+1$, corresponding to perfectly anticorrelated and perfectly correlated (i.e. identical) variables, respectively. When the coefficient is zero the variables are not correlated. The correlation coefficient can be associated to a Euclidean distance with the relation [48, 59]

$$d_{ij} = \sqrt{2(1 - c_{ij})}. \tag{7.3}$$

Finally, it is important to stress that correlation coefficients are statistical estimators and therefore are subject to measurement noise. This means, for example, that two variables could be uncorrelated, but their sample correlation coefficient measured over a set of T variables is typically different from zero. Moreover, since one is interested simultaneously in many variables, another common statistical problem, named the curse of dimensionality, is common in correlation based networks. Coming back to our previous example of the correlation matrix, we have $N(N - 1)/2$ distinct elements to be estimated. We remind that each element is represented by T variables so that the number of data points for this estimation is NT. Therefore, unless $T \ll N$, the statistical reliability of the similarity matrix is small because we have a small number of independent measurements per estimated parameter. Therefore, one has to devise a method to reduce the number of variables from the large N^2 value to a subset statistically more significant.

There are many different methods to construct correlation (or similarity) based networks. In this paper, we shall consider two classes, namely threshold networks and hierarchical networks, and we discuss the application of these methods to financial networks.

7.2.1 Threshold Methods

The simplest filtered network is a threshold network. Given the set of correlation or even distances between the vertices, one keeps only those above a determined level of confidence. A suitable choice, based on statistical consideration, could be the following. If the N variables are described by independent Gaussian time series of length T and we use the above defined correlation measure, it is known that for large T the distribution of the sample correlation coefficient of two uncorrelated Gaussian variable can be approximated by a Gaussian distribution with zero mean and standard deviation equal $1/\sqrt{T}$. In this case, a reasonable approach could be to consider a threshold of three standard deviations and to keep the edge values whose associated correlation coefficients are larger in absolute value than $3/\sqrt{T}$. In this way, only links associated with statistically significant correlation are preserved in the filtered network.

Another method for choosing the threshold is to randomise the data by permutation experiments and preserve in the original networks only those links associated to a correlation which is observed in the randomised data with a small probability. In this way, no a priori hypothesis on the probability distribution of data is made, and this approach is very useful especially when data distribution is very different from a Gaussian.

The networks generated with threshold methods are, in general, disconnected. If the system presents a clear cluster organisation, threshold methods are typically able to detect them. On the contrary, if the system has a hierarchical structure, threshold methods are not optimal, and hierarchical methods described below should be preferred.

7.2.2 Hierarchical Methods

A different class of filtering methods are the hierarchical methods. These are devised to detect specifically the hierarchical structure of the data. A system has a hierarchical structure when the elements of the system can be partitioned into clusters which, in turn, can be partitioned into subclusters, and so on up to a certain level. In multivariate statistics, there is a large literature on hierarchical clustering methods [2]. These methods produce dendrograms to describe the hierarchical structure of the system. One interesting aspect for network theory is that hierarchical clustering methods are also often associated with networks which are different from the dendrograms. Here we review the use of these networks as similarity based networks. For a review of the hierarchical methods and their application in finance, see also [76].

One of the most common algorithms to detect a possible hierarchical structure hidden in the data is given by the Minimum Spanning Tree (MST) procedure. The MST is the spanning tree of shortest length. In our case, the length of a link is inversely related to the similarity between the nodes connected by the link. Thus one can either use a relation as the one in (7.3) to obtain a length measure of the links and find the spanning tree of minimum length, or alternatively consider the similarity (or correlation) as "length" and look for the spanning tree of maximum length.

There are several algorithm to extract the MST. A very intuitive one is the following procedure.

- Assign distances between the vertices in such a way that the largest is the correlation between two vertices, while the shortest is the distance.
- Rank these distances from the shortest to the longest.
- Start from the shortest distance and "draw" the edge between the vertices.
- Iterate this procedure until you find an edge that would form a loop. In this case, jump to the next distance (if necessary repeat this operation).
- Stop when all the vertices have been considered.

The resulting graph is the MST of the system and the connected components progressively merging together during the construction of the graph are clusters progressively merging together. The MST is strongly related with a well known hierarchical clustering algorithm, called Single Linkage Cluster Analysis. Recently it has been shown that another network, termed Average Linkage Minimum Spanning Tree, can be associated with the most common hierarchical clustering algorithm, the Average Linkage Cluster Analysis [78].

By using different constraints, it is possible to define other hierarchical networks. The idea is that from the same correlation matrix one can also obtain correlation based networks having a structure more complex than a tree. In the case of Planar Maximally Filtered Graph (PMFG) [3, 77], we can allow loops and cliques by modifying the above algorithm. In particular, you can continue drawing edges, provided that the graph remains planar. That is to say, it should be possible to draw the graph without having to cross two different edges. Since the maximum complete subgraph one can draw with such a feature is K^4, one cannot have cliques of size larger than four in a PMFG. Authors of [3, 77] introduce a correlation based graph obtained by connecting elements with largest correlation under the topological constraint of fixed genus $G = 0$. The genus is a topologically invariant property of a surface defined as the largest number of nonintersecting simple closed curves that can be drawn on the surface without separating it. Roughly speaking, it is the number of holes in a surface. A basic difference of the PMFG with respect to the MST is the number of links which is $N - 1$ in the MST and $3(N - 2)$ in the PMFG. Moreover, the PMFG is a network with loops, whereas the MST is a tree. It is worth recalling that in [77] it has been proven that the PMFG always contains the MST. Thus the PMFG contains a richer structure than the MST (which is constrained by the tree requirement), but the number of links is still $O(N)$ rather than $O(N^2)$ as for the complete graph. Therefore, the PMFG is an intermediate stage between the MST and the complete graph. In principle, this construction can be generalised to a genus $G > 0$, i.e. one adds links only if the graph can be embedded in a surface with genus G.

7.2.3 An Application to NYSE

The main application of similarity based networks to finance has been the characterisation of the cross-correlation structure of price returns in a stocks portfolio. In this case, the nodes represent different stocks or, in general, different assets. The T variables characterising a node are the time series of price return of the associated stock computed over a given time horizon (typically one day, i.e. daily returns). The cross-correlation between stock returns measures how much the price of the two stocks move in a similar way. The characterisation and filtering of the stock return correlation matrix is of paramount importance in financial engineering and specifically in portfolio optimisation.

The threshold method selects the highest correlations and therefore considers the links in the network that are individually more relevant from a statistical point of view. An example of the analysis of the financial correlation matrix with a threshold network was given in [64, 65]. Here the authors computed the price return correlation matrix of a portfolio of $N \simeq 100$ US stocks. The variable considered is the daily price return and they constructed the correlation matrix of these N stocks. The process starts from an empty graph with no edges where the N vertices correspond to stocks. Then they introduced one edge after another between the vertices according to the rank of their correlation strength (starting from the largest value). These "asset graphs" can be studied as the number of links grows when one lowers the threshold. Typically, after a small number of edges (20 for this case study), several cycles appear in the asset graph. As more edges are added, the existing clusters are significantly reinforced and the graph remains disconnected. The graph becomes completely connected, only after a large number of edges are added (typically 1000 for a network of 116 nodes). It is possible to check that even for moderate values of the number of edges added, the connected components (clusters) are quite homogeneous in terms of the industrial sector of the stocks involved. It is also possible to study how the mean clustering coefficient changes when the links are added. Interestingly, three different regimes appear. In the first regime, we have a rapid growth of the clustering coefficient corresponding to an addition of the top 10% of the edges. In other words, the first 10% of the edges add substantial information to the system. In the second regime, when the fraction of added edges is between 10% and 20%, the rate of change of the clustering coefficient starts to slow down and reaches a sort of plateau. Finally, the edges added in the last regime, i.e. having the correlation coefficients with a rank below 30%, have relatively poor information content, and are possibly just noise.

Concerning hierarchical methods, Rosario Mantegna [58, 59] was one of the first to apply this procedure to the price return of a portfolio of stocks. Since this type of analysis has been performed afterwards in many different markets, time periods, and market conditions, the results described below are quite general. At a daily time scale, the MST is able to identify quite clearly the economic sectors of the stocks in the portfolio. Each company belongs to an economic sector (such as Basic Materials, Energy, Financial, Technology or Conglomerates) describing the core activity of the company and assigned by some external company (such as Forbes). The MST shows the presence of clusters of nodes (stocks) which are quite homogeneous in the economic sector. Often the MST displays also a structure in subclusters where nodes are stocks mostly belonging to the same subsector (for example, Communication services and Retail are subsectors of the sector of Services). In this ability of identifying the economic sectors from the correlation matrix, the MST performs typically pretty well when compared with other more traditional methods, such as spectral methods [17]. In this latter procedure, one extracts the eigenvectors of the correlation matrix and identifies sectors as groups of stocks which have a large component (compared to the others) in an eigenvector. Despite the fact that this method gives some useful information [47], the eigenvectors sometimes mix different economic sectors (especially when the eigenvalues are close to each other). A second feature typically found in the MST of daily returns of a portfolio of stocks is the presence of few nodes (stocks) with a very large degree. A typical example is observed in a portfolio of US stocks in the late 1990s. In this case, it has been found that General Electric is a hub in the network, connecting different parts of the tree associated with different economic sectors, but also connecting to leaves, i.e. stocks that are connected to the tree only trough General Electric. General Electric is a conglomerate company, and in the 1990s it was the most capitalised stock in the US financial markets. A conglomerate company is a combination of more firms engaging in entirely different businesses. These two aspects explain why General Electric

138 S. Battiston et al.

was a hub of the network. The fact that hubs are often conglomerates is explained by the fact that a conglomerate company tends to be less affected by industry specific factors and more affected by global market behaviour.

It is interesting to note that when one considers price returns computed on intraday time horizons, the topological structure of the MST changes dramatically [9]. It has been observed that on very short time horizons the MST has roughly a star like structure with the notable exception of the presence of a cluster of technological stocks. As the time horizon used to compute returns is increased, the MST becomes more structured and clusters of stocks belonging to the same economic sector progressively emerge. It is worth noting that the time horizon needed, because a given sector is evident as a cluster in the MST, depends on the considered sector. This has been interpreted as an indication that the market "learns" its cluster structure progressively.

A direct comparison of the MST and an asset graph with $N - 1$ edges (like the MST) shows that the two graphs share only 25% of the edges, i.e. that 75% of the $N - 1$ strongest correlation are not represented in the MST. Therefore, while the MST can inform about the taxonomy of a market, the graph asset built in this way seems to better represent the strongest correlations.

7.2.4 Other Similarity Based Hierarchical Networks in Finance

Hierarchical networks (mainly the MST) have been applied to several other financial variables. These, for example, include: (i) time series of price volatility, (ii) interest rates, (iii) hedge funds' net asset values, and (iv) trading activity of agents. In the first case [60], the investigated variable is the stock price volatility which is a key economic variable measuring the level of price fluctuations, and the MST resembles most of the properties of the price return MST. The interest rates are important economic variables, and the empirical analysis [26] shows that interest rates cluster in the MST and in the PMFG according to their maturity dates. The application of MST to hedge funds' net asset value [61] allows identifying clusters of funds adopting similar strategies (which sometimes are different from the strategies declared by the fund). Finally, the emerging study of networks of agents trading in the market [30] shows that the correlation matrix of the inventory variation of the market members trading a stock in the Spanish Stock Market contains information on the community structure of the investors.

7.3 Control Networks: The Case of Directors and Ownerships

In this case of study, the networks are used to detect chains of control that could be hidden in a traditional analysis. Here the vertices are mainly financial agents, both in the case of Board of Directors where people investigate the relation between different persons and in the case of ownership networks where people want to know about the chains of control behind a particular stock. The physics literature on complex economic networks has previously focused on both of these topics (for the boards of directors, see, for example, [6, 62], while for market investments, see [8, 41]). At the same time, also in economics there is a vast body of literature on corporate control that focuses on corporations as individual units. The research topics this field of study addresses can be grouped into three major categories: firstly, analysing the dispersion or concentration of control [29, 73]; secondly, empirically investigating how the patterns of control vary across countries and what determines them [55, 56]; and thirdly, studying the impact of frequently observed complex ownership patterns [11, 15, 16, 34] such as the so-called pyramids [1] and cross-shareholdings (also known as business groups) [49].

In addition, research in cooperative game theory analysing political voting games has resulted in the development of the so-called power indices [4, 72]. These ideas have been applied to coalitions of shareholders voting at Shareholders Meetings [57].

7.3.1 Stock Ownership Network

It should be noted that most previous empirical studies did not build on the idea that ownership and control define a vast complex network of dependencies. Instead, they selected samples of specific companies and looked only at their local web of interconnections. These approaches are unable to discern control at a global level. This emphasises the fact that the bird's-eye-view given by a network perspective is important for unveiling overarching relationships. Remarkably, the investigation of the financial architecture of corporations in national or global economies taken *as a whole* is just at the beginning [18, 41, 54]. Here we present an analysis based on [45] that allows us to show how control is distributed at the country level, based on the knowledge of the ownership ties.

The dataset considered spans 48 countries and is compiled from Bureau van Dijk's ORBIS database.[1] In this subset, there are a total of 24,877 stocks and 106,141 shareholding entities who cannot be owned themselves (individuals, families, cooperative societies, registered associations, foundations, public authorities, etc.). Note that because the corporations can also appear as shareholders, the network does not display a bipartite structure. The stocks are connected through 545,896 ownership ties to their shareholders. The database represents a snapshot of the ownership relations at the beginning of 2007. The values for the market capitalisation, which is defined as the number of outstanding shares times the firm's market price, are also from early 2007. These values will be our proxy for the size of corporations and hence serve as the non-topological state variables.

The network of ownership relations in a country is very intricate and a cross-country analysis of some basic properties of these networks reveals a great level of

---

[1] http://www.bvdep.com/orbis.html.

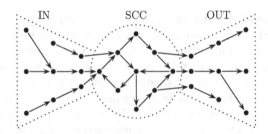

Fig. 7.1 Schematic illustration of a bow-tie topology: the central area is the strongly connected component (SCC) where there is a path from each node to every other node and the *left* (IN) and *right* (OUT) sections contain the incoming and outgoing nodes, respectively

variability. For instance, at the topological level, the analysis of the number and sizes of connected components. Many small components correspond to a fragmented capital market, while a giant and dense component corresponds to an integrated market. It is, however, not very clear what such connected components reveal about the structure and distribution of control. The same pattern of connected components can feature many different configurations of control. Therefore, it makes sense to move on to the next level of analysis by introducing the notion of direction. Now it is possible to identify strongly connected components. In terms of ownership networks, these patterns correspond to sets of corporations where every firm is connected to every other firm via a path of indirect ownership. In particular, these components may form bow-tie structures, akin to the topology of the World Wide Web [12]. Figure 7.1 illustrates an idealised bow-tie topology. This structure is particularly useful to illustrate the flow of control, as every shareholder in the IN section exerts control and all corporations in the OUT section are controlled.

In the above dataset, roughly two thirds of the countries' ownership networks contain bow-tie structures (see also [79]). Indeed, already at this level of analysis, previously observed patterns can be rediscovered. As an example, the countries with the highest occurrence of (small) bow-tie structures are KR and TW, and to a lesser degree JP (the countries are identified by their two letter ISO 3166-1 alpha-2 codes). A possible determinant is the well known existence of the so-called business groups in these countries (e.g. the *keiretsu* in JP, and the *chaebol* in KR) forming a tightly-knit web of cross-shareholdings (see the introduction and references in [49] and [33]). For AU, CA, GB and US, one can observe very few bow-tie structures of which the largest ones, however, contain hundreds to thousands of corporations. It is an open question if the emergence of these mega-structures in the Anglo-Saxon countries is due to their unique "type" of capitalism (the so-called Atlantic or stock market capitalism, see the introduction and references in [27]), and whether this finding contradicts the assumption that these markets are characterised by the absence of business groups [49].

Next to bow-tie structures, we can identify additional structures revealing the chains of control. The simplest way is by considering the core structures of the ownership networks and check the more important vertices in this subset.

The question of the vertices' importance in a network is central in graph theory, and different possibilities have been considered. Traditionally, the most intuitive quantity is the degree k, that is, the number of edges per vertex. If the edges are oriented, one has to distinguish between the in-degree and out-degree, k^{in} and k^{out}, respectively. When the edges are weighted, the corresponding quantity is called *strength* [5]:

$$k_i^w := \sum_j W_{ij}. \tag{7.4}$$

Note that for weighted and oriented networks, one has to distinguish between the in- and out-strengths, $k^{in\text{-}w}$ and $k^{out\text{-}w}$, respectively.

However, the interpretation of $k^{in/out\text{-}w}$ is not always straightforward for real-world networks. In the case of ownership networks, there is no useful meaning associated with these values. In order to provide a more refined and appropriate description of weighted ownership networks, we introduce two quantities that extend the notions of degree and strength in a sensible way.

The first quantity to be considered reflects the relative importance of the neighbours of a vertex. More specifically, given a vertex j and its incoming edges, we focus on the originating vertices of such edges. The idea is to define a quantity that captures the relative importance of incoming edges. When no weights are associated to the edges, we expect all edges to count the same. If weights have a large variance, some edges will be more important than others. A way of measuring the number of prominent incoming edges is to define the *concentration index* as follows:

$$s_j := \frac{(\sum_{i=1}^{k_j^{in}} W_{ij})^2}{\sum_{i=1}^{k_j^{in}} W_{ij}^2}. \tag{7.5}$$

Note that this quantity is akin to the inverse of the Herfindahl index extensively used in economics as a standard indicator of market concentration [50]. Indeed, already in the 1980s the Herfindahl index was also introduced to measure ownership concentration [19]. Notably, a similar measure has also been used in statistical physics as an order parameter [25]. In the context of ownership networks, s_j is interpreted as the effective number of shareholders of the stock j. Thus it can be interpreted as a measure of control from the point of view of a stock.

The second quantity to be introduced measures the number of important outgoing edges of the vertices. For a given vertex i with a destination vertex j, we first define a measure which reflects the importance of i with respect to all vertices connecting to j:

$$H_{ij} := \frac{W_{ij}^2}{\sum_{l=1}^{k_j^{in}} W_{lj}^2}. \tag{7.6}$$

This quantity has values in the interval $(0, 1]$. For instance, if $H_{ij} \approx 1$ then i is by far the most important destination vertex for the vertex j. For our ownership network,

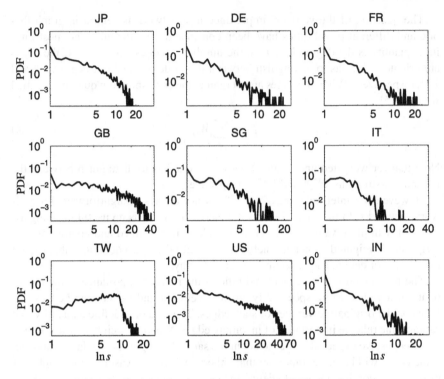

Fig. 7.2 Probability distributions of s_j for selected countries; PDF in log–log scale

H_{ij} represents the *fraction of control* shareholder i has on the company j. In a next step, we then define the *control index*:

$$h_i := \sum_{j=1}^{k_i^{\text{out}}} H_{ij}.$$ (7.7)

This quantity is a way of measuring how important the outgoing edges of a node i are with respect to its neighbours' neighbours. Within the ownership network setting, h_i is interpreted as the effective number of stocks controlled by shareholder i.

7.3.1.1 Distributions of s and h

The above defined measures can provide insights into the patterns of how ownership and control are distributed at a local level. In particular, Fig. 7.2 shows the probability density function (PDF) of s_j for a selection of nine countries. There is a diversity in the shapes and ranges of the distributions to be seen. For instance, the distribution of GB reveals that many companies have more than 20 leading shareholders, whereas in IT few companies are held by more than five significant shareholders. Such country-specific signatures were expected to appear due to the differences in

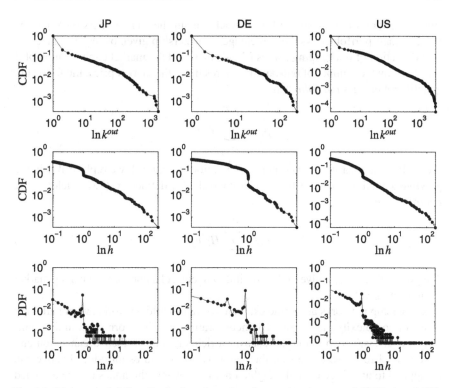

Fig. 7.3 Various probability distributions for selected countries: (*top panel*) CDF plot of k_i^{out}; (*middle panel*) CDF plot of h_i; (*bottom panel*) PDF plot of h_i; all plots are in log–log scale

legal and institutional settings (e.g. law enforcement, protection of minority shareholders [55], etc.).

On the other hand, looking at the cumulative distribution function (CDF) of k_i^{out} (shown for three selected countries in the top panel of Fig. 7.3) a more uniform shape is revealed. The distributions range between two to three orders of magnitude. Indeed, some shareholders can hold up to a couple of thousand stocks, whereas the majority have ownership in less than ten. Considering the CDF of h_i, seen in the middle panel of Fig. 7.3, one can observe that the curves of h_i display two regimes. This is true for nearly all analysed countries, with a slight country-dependent variability. Notable exceptions are FI, IS, LU, PT, TN, TW, VG. In order to understand this behaviour, it is useful to look at the PDF of h_i, shown in the bottom panel of Fig. 7.3. This uncovers a new systematic feature: the peak at the value of $h_i = 1$ indicates that there are many shareholders in the markets whose only intention is to control one single stock.

The quantities defined in (7.5) and (7.7) rely on the direction and weight of the links. However, they do not consider non-topological state variables assigned to the nodes themselves. In our case of ownership networks, a natural choice is to use the market capitalisation value of firms in thousand USD, v_j, as a proxy for their sizes. Hence v_j will be utilised as the state variable in the subsequent analysis. In a first step, we address the question of how much wealth the shareholders own, i.e. the value in their portfolios. As the percentage of ownership given by W_{ij} is a measure of the fraction of outstanding shares i holds in j, and the market capitalisation of j is defined by the number of outstanding shares times the market price, the following quantity reflects i's *portfolio value*:

$$p_i := \sum_{j=1}^{k_i^{out}} W_{ij} v_j. \tag{7.8}$$

Extending this measure to incorporate the notions of control, we replace W_{ij} in the previous equation with the fraction of control H_{ij}, defined in (7.6), yielding the *control value*:

$$c_i := \sum_{j=1}^{k_i^{out}} H_{ij} v_j. \tag{7.9}$$

A high c_i value is indicative of the possibility to control a portfolio with a big market capitalisation value.

Ownership networks are prime examples of real-world networks, where all three levels of complexity play a role. By incorporating all this information in their empirical analysis, it is possible to discover a rich structure in their organisation and unveil novel features. Moreover, the new network measures introduced above can be applied to any directed and weighted network, where the nodes can be assigned an intrinsic value.

7.3.2 Board of Directors

Another class of financial networks tracks the structure of the control of the companies by considering the people sitting on the board of directors. This is an example of a bipartite graph, that is to say, a graph that can be divided in two nontrivial subsets such that the edges connect one element of the first set with an element in the second one. The first set of nodes is composed of the companies, while the other set is composed of the people who sit in at least one board of directors. A link between a person and a company exists if that person sits on the board of directors of that company. As in all bipartite networks, it is possible to extract two graphs. In the first case, the nodes are the companies and a link exists if two companies share at least one common director (boards network). In the second case, the nodes are the directors, and a link exists if two directors sit together on at least one board (directors network). The empirical analysis of real data (see [20] for US companies and [7] for US and Italian companies) revealed that the networks display small world properties, are assortative and clustered. Table 7.1 shows some summary statistics from the empirical analysis of these networks. These empirical results strongly indicate the presence of lobbies of directors sitting on the same boards. Moreover, the

Table 7.1 The first three columns report data for the Boards (B) network in Italy in 1986 (B 86), in Italy in 2002 (B 02), and in USA in 1999 (B US). The last three columns report the data for the Directors (D) network in the same cases (1986, 2002 in Italy and USA in 1999)

	B 86	B 02	B US	D 86	D 02	D US
N	221	240	916	2,378	1,906	7,680
M	1,295	636	3,321	23,603	12,815	55,437
Nc/N	0.97	0.82	0.87	0.92	0.84	0.89
k/kc (%)	5.29	2.22	1.57	0.84	0.71	0.79
b/N	0.736	0.875	1.08	1.116	1.206	1.304
$\langle C \rangle$	0.356	0.318	0.376	0.899	0.915	0.884
$\langle d \rangle$	3.6	4.4	4.6	2.7	3.6	3.7
r	0.12	0.32	0.27	0.13	0.25	0.27

assortative character of the network indicates that directors that sit on many boards (and are therefore very influential) tend to sit on the same boards (more than what is expected from a random null model).

7.4 Transaction Networks: Interbank Networks and Bank–Firm Networks

The most immediate application of networks to finance and economics is given whenever we have a transaction between two agents. The latter are the vertices and the transaction is the edge between them. In particular, many theoretical and empirical studies have considered the networks where the nodes are the banks and a link represents a possible (directed and weighted) relation between banks. For this system, two types of networks have been considered, the interbank market and the payment system. Boss et al. [10] were among the first to study the interbank market with concepts and tools of modern network theory. They empirically studied the complete Austrian interbank market composed of around 900 banks in the years 2000–2003. The interbank market is described as a network where the vertices given by the banks are nodes and the claims and liabilities between them are described as links. The interbank market is therefore a weighted and directed network. Following a rule similar to that of food webs, the direction of the link goes from the bank having a liability to the bank claiming the liability. The weight is the amount (in money) of the liability. Authors investigated the community structure of this network by applying the Girvan–Newman algorithm based on link betweenness [44]. They found that the sectoral organisation of the banking industry (in terms of saving banks, agricultural banks, joint stock banks, etc.) is rediscovered by the community detection algorithm with a 97% precision, showing that the network structure brings information on the real sectoral organisation of the banking sector. The study of the topology of the network shows that it can be modelled as a scale-free network. In fact, both the in-degree and the out-degree probability density functions display a clear power-law behaviour with a tail exponent equal to 1.7 and 3.1, respectively. The clustering coefficient of the undirected graph is equal to 0.12 and this low value has been associated to the community organisation of the network. On the other hand, the average path length is 2.59, showing a clear small-world effect. The analysis of the interbank market is important in the framework of the quantification of systemic risk [21], the risk of collapse of an entire financial system. In fact, scale-free networks are typically robust with respect to the random breakdown of nodes and fragile with respect to intentional attack against the hubs. A proper characterisation of the interbank network topology is potentially useful in determining the criticality of the financial system. Sorämaki et al. [74] have investigated the daily network of the Fedwire R Funds Service, which is a gross settlement system operated by the Federal Reserve System (USA). Today almost 10,000 participants initiate funds transfer through Fedwire for the settlement of different operations, such as the trading of federal funds, securities transactions, real estate transactions, etc. The daily value exchanged is close to $ 3 trillion. The network describing the fund transfers in a day is clearly a directed and weighted (either in terms of value or in terms of number of transfers) network. There is typically a giant undirected connected component which accounts for almost all the nodes. Inside this component, authors studied the giant strongly connected component, which comprises all the nodes that can reach each other through a directed path. This component has typically 5,000 nodes (in the investigated year 2004) and contains roughly 80% of all the nodes in the giant undirected component. The connectivity, i.e. the probability that two nodes share a link, is very low and close to 0.3%, indicating that the network is extremely sparse. The reciprocity, i.e. the fraction of links for which there is a link in the opposite direction, is 22%, even if large links (either in terms of value or in term of volume) are typically reciprocal, probably as a result of complementary business activity or the risk management of bilateral exposure. Authors also studied the dynamics of the network and found that during days of high activity in the system, the number of nodes, links, and connectivity increases, while the reciprocity is not affected. The in-degree and out-degree of the network is power law distributed with an exponent close to two, indicating a scale-free behaviour. The network is disassortative. As in the Austrian interbank market, the average path length is between two and three, suggesting a small-world behaviour. However, differently from the previous case, the mean clustering coefficient is quite large (0.53), even if the distribution of clustering coefficients across nodes is very broad, and for one fifth of the nodes the clustering coefficient is equal to zero. There is a nice scaling relation between the out-degree of a node and its strength (defined as the total volume or value exchanged transferred by the node) with an exponent 1.2–1.9. This means that more connected nodes transact a higher volume or value than would be suggested by the degree. Finally, they consider as an important case study the change in the payment network topology due to the terrorist attack of September 11th, 2001, when some infrastructure of the system was destroyed with a clear occurrence of a liquidity crisis. They found that the network became smaller, less connected, and with a larger average path length than in a typical trading day. Another type of interbank market recently investigated in the framework of network theory is the Italian interbank money market [23, 52, 53]. In order to buffer liquidity shocks, the European Central Bank requires that on average 2% of all deposits and debts owned by banks are stored at national central banks. Given this constraint, banks can exchange excess reserves on the interbank market with the objective to satisfy the reserve requirement and in order to minimise the reserve implicit costs. Authors investigated the Italian electronic broker market for interbank deposits e-MID in the period 1999–2002. They constructed a network where the nodes are the banks. For every pair of banks i and j, there is an oriented edge from i to j, if bank j borrows liquidity from bank i. The mean number of banks (nodes) active in a day is 140 and the mean number of links is 200. As in the previous bank networks, authors found that the in- and out-degree are described by a distribution with a power law tail with an exponent between two and three. They also found that the network is disassortative and that the clustering coefficient of a node decreases with its degree as a power law. The various banks operating in a market can be divided into different groups roughly related to their size, i.e. the volume of their transaction. Smaller banks make few operations and on average lend or borrow money from larger banks. The latter ones have many connections with each other, making many transactions, while the small banks do not. A visualisation of the network in a typical day shows that the core of the structure is composed of the big banks. There is also a tendency for small banks to be mostly lenders, while large banks are more likely to be borrowers. All the above quantities can be reproduced by means of a suitable model of network growth [14]. The idea is that the vertices representing the banks are defined by means of an intrinsic character that could, for example, be their size. Edges are then drawn with a probability proportional to the sizes of the vertices involved. The community analysis of the network based on the cross-correlation of the signed traded volume confirms the presence of two main communities, one mainly composed by large banks and the other composed mainly by small banks [23]. By looking at the network dynamics, the authors of this set of studies found a clear pattern where the network degree increases and the strength decreases close to the critical days when the reserves are computed. All the above studies found that the banking system is highly heterogeneous with large banks borrowing from a high number of small creditors. Iori et al. [51] showed in an artificial market model that when banks are heterogeneous high connectivity increases the risk of contagion and systemic failure.

7.4.1 Credit Networks

A different and interesting type of financial networks describes the complex credit relation between firms and banks. The reasons for a credit relation between a bank and a firm are the following. The bank supplies credit to the firm in anticipation of interest margin, while the firm borrows money form the bank in order to financing the growth of its business. A credit relation, thus, creates a strong dependence between a firm and a bank. The credit network between firms and banks is important for the understanding and quantification of systemic risk of the economic and financial system [21]. In fact, the failure of a big firm may have a strong effect on the balance sheet of a bank and the insolvency of a firm may lead many banks to fail or to change their credit policy, by increasing the interest rates or by reducing the supply of loans. This, in turn, may lead other firms to failure, which creates more financial distress among banks and so on, in a sort of domino effect affecting the whole system. An example of such scenario happened in Japan during the 1990s. A way of studying the mutual interdependency between banks and firms is through the investigation of the credit network [22, 24, 35]. In an empirical study of the Japan credit network [24, 35], roughly 200 banks and 2, 700 publicly quoted firms were considered. The credit network is a typical case of bipartite network where the two types of nodes correspond to banks and firms and a weighted link exists between bank i and firm j if, at the considered time, there is a credit relation between i and j. The weight of the link is the amount of money firm j borrows from bank i. The average degree of firms is 8, while the average degree of banks is 120. Both the degree distributions of firms and banks are fat tailed, possibly consistent with a scale-free network, and the fitted tail exponent for the cumulative distribution is around 1 for banks and 2.5 for firms. The weights in the network are highly heterogeneous, and there is a scaling relation between the degree of a node and its strength (i.e. the total amount of money borrowed or lent by the node), indicating that the average loan is larger for a larger degree (typically, larger banks). A widely discussed topic in the economics of credit is the existence of two models of credit. In Anglo-Saxon countries, firms typical establish credit relationship with few banks, while in countries such as Japan, Germany, and Italy a firm borrows moneys from more banks. The theory of optimal number of bank relationships is quite complicated because different choices have different advantages and disadvantages. The question can be investigated empirically by measuring the participation ratio of node i

$$Y_i = \sum_j \frac{w_{ij}}{s_i} \tag{7.10}$$

where w_{ij} is the weight of the link between i and j and s_i is the strength of node i. In the case of full homogeneity, the participation ratio is the inverse of the degree of node i. In a multiple bank scenario, the participation ratio is much higher, since one bank dominates the credit of firm i. The analysis of the Japan dataset confirms that large firms tend to have a participation ratio different from the inverse of the degree, i.e. large firms tend to establish credit relations with many banks. From any bipartite network, it is possible to extract two projected networks. In the bank network, two banks are linked if they share at least one borrower, while in the firm network, two firms are linked if they have at least one common lender. The weight of the links is the number of common borrowers/lenders. The authors of [24] extracted the MST from these projected networks. They found that the bank network is characterised by large hubs, and the cluster structure of this network is largely explained by the geographic region where the banks operate. In other words, banks in the same geographic region tend to lend money to the same firms, probably from the same region. The analysis of the MST of the firms in the same economic sector shows that each firm is connected to many others and that there are no communities. This is probably due to the fact that lending is not sectoral. Moreover, in almost all the investigated sectoral networks, a large hub is observed. Finally, in [35], a linear analysis of the same dataset was performed in order to measure a set of scores related to the financial fragility. It was found that these scores were statistically significant with respect to a random network and that there were periods when the structure was stable or unstable. Drastic changes were observed in the late 1980s when the bubble started in Japan. Moreover, the set of regional banks had large values of the fragility score.

7.5 The World Trade Web

The world economy is a tightly interconnected system of mutually dependent countries, and one of the dominant channels mediating international interactions is trade. When countries are represented as vertices, and their trade relations as connections, the world trade system appears as an intricate network, known in the literature as the International Trade Network or World Trade Web (WTW). The recent advances in network theory have renewed the analysis of the trade system from a perspective that fully takes into account its global topology [31, 32, 37, 42, 43, 69–71]. Indeed, traditional macroeconomic approaches have extensively addressed the empirical patterns of trade by considering the pairwise interactions involved locally between countries, but have placed much less emphasis on the analysis of higher-order properties obtained considering indirect interactions embedded in the whole international network. On the other hand, the globalisation process of the economy highlights the importance of understanding the large-scale organisation of the WTW and its evolution.

In what follows, we present some of the recent research results obtained in the analysis of the global trade network. The WTW has many possible network representations. In particular, it can be either directed or undirected, and either weighted (by taking into account the magnitude of trade flows) or unweighted. The properties of the WTW as a weighted network (where trade volumes are explicitly taken into account) are of great importance, as link intensities are extremely heterogeneous and are found to change significantly the picture obtained in the binary case [31, 32, 69, 71]. On the other hand, if regarded as a binary network (thus ignoring the magnitude of trade links), the WTW is found to be one of the few real networks whose topology can be modelled in detail using simple ideas that have been developed recently [37, 42, 43]. This implies that, besides its importance for understanding the global economic system, the WTW is particularly interesting for network theory. By contrast, unfortunately no complete model of the weighted WTW has been proposed, at least not reaching the same level of detail as its binary counterpart. At present, the only available weighted models of trade are the so-called *gravity models* which aim at predicting the observed magnitude of trade fluxes in terms of a few explanatory factors, but fail to explain their topology. So it appears that our current understanding of the trade system requires a combination of both approaches, and that the definition of a complete and satisfactory model of the WTW is still an open problem. For this reason, since here we are particularly interested in the data-driven problem of modelling the international trade network, we briefly present gravity models first, and then report in more detail various empirical properties and models of the WTW

only at a purely topological level. For weighted analyses, the reader is referred to
the relevant literature [31, 32, 69, 71].

7.5.1 Gravity Models

The so-called 'gravity models', first introduced by Tinbergen [75] and then
rephrased in various extended or alternative forms, are the earliest econometric
models of trade. Their name originates from a loose analogy with Newton's law of
gravitation, where the magnitude of the force attracting two objects carrying mass
is completely determined by the two masses involved and the distance separating
them. Similarly, gravity models assume that the volume of trade between any two
countries can be traced back to a suitable measure of the 'mass' of the two countries
(representing their intrinsic economic size) and to some 'distance' between them
(representing a combination of factors determining the overall resistance to trade).
The economic 'mass' of a country is customarily identified with its total Gross Do-
mestic Product (GDP in the following). Also, geographic distance is the main factor
expected to determine trade resistance. However, additional factors may be incorporated in the models, having either a positive or negative effect on the volume of
trade. In the simple case where one additional factor coexists with geographical distance as an explanator of trade, the gravity model predicts that the volume of trade
from country i to country j in a given year is

$$w_{ij} = \beta_0 w_i^{\beta_1} w_j^{\beta_2} d_{ij}^{\beta_3} f_{ij}^{\beta_4} \qquad (7.11)$$

where w_i is the total GDP of country i in the year considered, d_{ij} is the geographic
distance between countries i and j, and f_{ij} is an additional factor either favouring
or suppressing trade between i and j. The various factors expected to determine w_{ij}
are controlled by the associated parameters $\{\beta_0, \dots, \beta_4\}$, which are global and do
not depend on the two countries involved. Usually, a Gaussian error term is added
to the above equation, allowing to employ standard statistical techniques to fit the
model to the empirical (nonzero) trade flows and obtain the corresponding values
of $\{\beta_0, \dots, \beta_4\}$. These analyses have been applied extensively on different datasets,
and the general result is that β_1 and β_2 are positive and of the same order (both close
to one), confirming the expectation that larger GDPs imply more trade. Similarly,
empirical analyses provide evidence for a negative value of β_3, confirming a negative effect of geographic distance on trade. Depending on the nature of the additional
factor f_{ij}, the parameter β_4 can be either positive or negative. Positive effects are
found to be associated to two countries being members of the same economic group,
having signed a trade agreement, or sharing geographic borders. By contrast, negative effects are found in presence of embargo, trade restrictions or other conditions
representing a trade friction.

Gravity models have been tested extensively on many case studies reporting trade
volumes, either at a global or regional level. In general, they make very good predictions of the magnitude of nonzero trade flows. However, they do not predict zero

Fig. 7.4 Time evolution of the connectance c in the undirected WTW

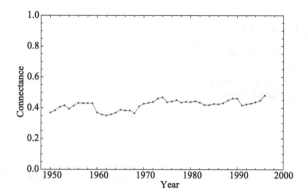

volumes, which means that they always generate a complete weighted graph where all pairs of countries exchange goods in both directions. As we now show, this is in sharp contrast with what is empirically observed. Indeed, recent analyses of the WTW have revealed that its topology is highly structured, and have thus highlighted a previously unrecognised drawback of gravity models.

7.5.2 The Heterogeneous Topology of Trade Neighbourhoods

In what follows, we show some empirical properties of the WTW topology and discuss a modelling framework that has been proposed to reproduce them. Data on the WTW topology can be obtained from the dataset [46], where annual snapshots of the network are available for all years from 1950 to 2000. We first report the properties of the WTW as an undirected network, and address its directed structure later on.

A key observation regards the heterogeneity of the number of trade partners (the degree k_i) of world countries. If only the average degree $\bar{k}$ of the WTW is considered, or equivalently the connectance $c \equiv \bar{k}/(N-1)$, then the WTW is found to display an almost constant temporal behaviour [37] (see Fig. 7.4). However, this regularity hides an intrinsic variability in the degrees. Indeed, it is found that the degree k_i of a country is positively correlated with both the total GDP and the per capita GDP of that country [43, 70]. If the total GDP w_i is considered, the relation is particularly strong [43], as shown in Fig. 7.5 for both raw and logarithmically binned data. For brevity, here and in what follows we only show the results obtained for a particular snapshot (the year 1995). These results have been shown to be robust in time through the entire period covered by the database [37]. The above result means that, on average, higher-income countries have a larger number of trade partners. And, since the total GDP is broadly distributed across world countries, this also means that one expects the number of trade partners to be broadly distributed as well. Similarly, one expects many other topological quantities, especially those involving the degree explicitly, to be strongly dependent on the GDP. As we show later on, empirical analyses have shown that this is exactly the case. These considerations

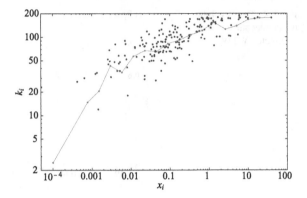

Fig. 7.5 Degree k_i as a function of the rescaled GDP $x_i \equiv w_i/\overline{w}$ in the undirected version of the WTW (year 1995): (*isolated points*) raw data; (*joined points*) logarithmically binned data

immediately imply that gravity models, which trivially produce a complete network of trade irrespective of the GDP values, are bad models of the WTW topology. This motivates the introduction of models that explicitly address the heterogeneity of trade neighbourhoods, i.e. who trades with whom in the world. We first describe one such class of models that has been proposed, before comparing its predictions to real trade data.

7.5.3 The Fitness Network Model

In the popular random graph model by Erdős and Rényi, all pairs of vertices are independently connected with probability p with an undirected edge. This is known to generate an ensemble of graphs where all vertices are statistically equivalent. For instance, the degree distribution is sharply peaked about the expected value $\langle k \rangle = p(N - 1)$, where N is the number of vertices. More recently, a generalised class of random graphs, known as the *hidden variable* or *fitness* model, has been defined [14]. This model can incorporate a high degree of heterogeneity in the statistical properties of vertices. To this end, an arbitrary distribution $\rho(x)$ is specified, from which a value x_i is assigned to each vertex i. This value, interpreted as a fitness affecting the connectivity patterns of vertices differentially, is treated as a hidden variable responsible for the topological properties of the network. In particular, a link between any two vertices i and j is drawn with probability $p_{ij} = p(x_i, x_j)$. Thus $p(x_i, x_j)$ and $\rho(x)$ determine the topology of the network in a way that is simple enough to be controlled analytically, and yet allows very complex structural properties to be generated [14].

When applied to the WTW, the fitness model is a minimal model that allows to retain the basic ingredient of gravity models, i.e. that the GDP is the main factor determining trade, to the different purpose of modelling the topology, rather than the magnitude, of trade flows. Indeed, as we discussed, the degree of a vertex in the WTW is empirically found to be dependent on the GDP of the corresponding country. This finding can be exploited by defining a fitness model where the hidden variable x_i is taken to be a function of the total GDP of country i, that we denoted as w_i [43]. This means $x_i = f(w_i)$, and implies that the distribution $\rho(x)$ is no longer arbitrary, but empirically accessible. Still, one needs to specify the connection probability $p(x_i, x_j)$. The simplest nontrivial choice is one where x_i controls the degree k_i, but not other properties directly. This does not mean that other topological properties (besides k_i) will not depend on x_i, but rather that they will depend on x_i as a result of their being dependent on k_i, which is constrained directly by x_i. In more formal words, this scenario in one where the network generated by $p(x_i, x_j)$ has a specified degree sequence $\{k_i\}$ (determined by $\{x_i\}$), and is maximally random otherwise. It is known [67] that this scenario corresponds to the particular choice

$$p(x_i, x_j) = \frac{\delta x_i x_j}{1 + \delta x_i x_j} \tag{7.12}$$

where δ is a global parameter controlling the expected total number of links, and the $\{x_i\}$ distribute these links among vertices heterogeneously. The above considerations result in a model for each yearly snapshot of the WTW, where two countries are connected with probability given by (7.12), where $x_i = f(w_i)$ [43]. By assuming the simplest form of dependence, i.e. a linear relation, and reabsorbing the coefficient of proportionality in δ, then for a given year one can define x_i as an adimensional rescaled variable representing the GDP relative to the average GDP in the same year:

$$x_i \equiv \frac{w_i}{\sum_{j=1}^{N} w_j / N} \tag{7.13}$$

(note that the number of independent world countries N depends on the particular year considered). This specifies the model completely, and leaves δ as the only free parameter to be tuned in each snapshot of the network. By applying the maximum likelihood principle to the model [39], one can show that the optimal choice is the value δ^* such that

$$L = \sum_i \sum_{j<i} \frac{\delta^* x_i x_j}{1 + \delta^* x_i x_j} \tag{7.14}$$

where L is the observed number of links in that particular snapshot of the network.

After this simple parameter choice is made, one can check the predictions of the model against real data [43]. In particular, one can obtain the explicit dependence of the degrees on the GDP predicted by the model. The average degree of a vertex having fitness x_i is simply

$$\langle k_i \rangle = \sum_{j \neq i} p_{ij} \tag{7.15}$$

which is an increasing function of x_i, since p_{ij} is an increasing function of both x_i and x_j. The resulting predicted curve [43] is shown in Fig. 7.6, where the empirical (logarithmically binned) trend shown previously in Fig. 7.5 is reported again.

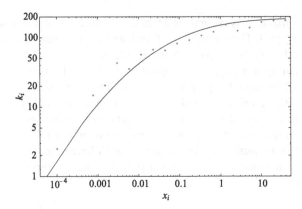

Fig. 7.6 Degree k_i as a function of the rescaled GDP $x_i \equiv w_i/\overline{w}$ in the undirected version of the WTW (year 1995): (*points*) real data (logarithmically binned); (*solid line*) theoretical prediction of the fitness model

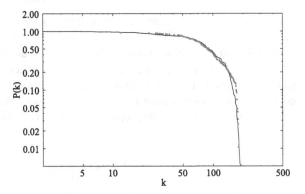

Fig. 7.7 Degree distribution in the undirected WTW (year 1995): (*points*) real data; (*solid line*) theoretical prediction of the fitness model

The agreement between empirical data and the model is very good. One can thus proceed in testing the prediction of the model against other empirical topological properties. As mentioned, the degree distribution of the WTW is found to be highly heterogeneous [43, 70]. We now describe it in more detail and show it in Fig. 7.7. One can see that there is indeed a huge variability in the number of trade partners of world countries. However, unlike other real-world networks, this variability is not captured by a scale-free distribution, as one observes an accumulation of degrees close to the maximum possible value $N - 1$, which results in a strong cut-off in the right tail of the distribution [43]. The reason for this cut-off is the saturation effect shown in Fig. 7.6, i.e. the convergence of k_i to values close to $N - 1$ when x_i increases. This behaviour is well reproduced by the model, and indeed the predicted degree distribution (which is shown in Fig. 7.7 superimposed to the empirical one) is in very good accordance with the data.

Additional properties of the WTW include higher-order patterns. An important one is the correlation between the average degree k_i^{nn} of the neighbours of vertex i and the degree k_i. This property is shown in Fig. 7.8. The observed decreasing trend means that, on average, highly connected countries trade with poorly connected countries, and that trade between countries of the same level of connectivity

Fig. 7.8 Average nearest neighbour degree k_i^{nn} versus degree k_i in the undirected WTW (year 1995): (*points*) real data; (*solid line*) theoretical prediction of the fitness model

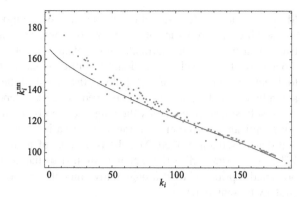

Fig. 7.9 Clustering coefficient c_i versus degree k_i in the undirected WTW (year 1995): (*points*) real data; (*solid line*) theoretical prediction of the fitness model

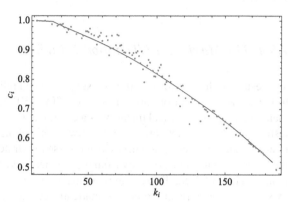

is suppressed. One can test the model prediction by calculating the expected average nearest neighbour degree as

$$\langle k_i^{nn} \rangle = \frac{\sum_{j \neq i} \sum_{k \neq j} p_{ij} p_{jk}}{\sum_{j \neq i} p_{ij}}. \tag{7.16}$$

As Fig. 7.8 shows, the resulting curve represents again a very good prediction [43].

Finally, we report the behaviour of the clustering coefficient c_i, defined as the fraction of realised triangles originating at vertex i. This is shown in Fig. 7.9. Again, one finds a decreasing trend signalling that highly connected countries have on average poorly interconnected neighbours, while poorly connected countries have on average tightly interconnected neighbours. The model prediction can in this case be derived using the formula

$$\langle c_i \rangle = \frac{\sum_{j \neq i} \sum_{k \neq j,i} p_{ij} p_{jk} p_{ki}}{\sum_{j \neq i} \sum_{k \neq j,i} p_{ij} p_{ki}} \tag{7.17}$$

which, as shown in Fig. 7.9, is once again found to be in remarkable agreement with real data [43].

The above results suggest that the model reproduces the basic properties of the WTW, and traces them back to the heterogeneity in the GDPs of world countries.

Moreover, the simple assumptions at the basis of the model offer an interpretation for the observed properties of the WTW topology. In particular, the accordance between real data and the particular form of the model suggest that, once the heterogeneity at the level of individual countries is taken into account and assumed to directly affect the degrees $\{k_i\}$ alone, then most of the other network properties are indirectly and automatically explained [43]. An independent finding confirming this result comes from studies showing that the observed topology of the WTW is not significantly different from randomised variants obtained by keeping the original degree sequence fixed. Yet, the behaviour of higher-order properties such as k_i^{nn} and c_i, even if directly explained by that of the degrees, could not be simply predicted a priori without a quantitative model. This adds value to the modelling strategy presented here.

7.5.4 The Maximum Likelihood Principle

The results of the previous section are supported and refined by an inverse approach to the extraction of information from the WTW [39]. On a general ground, rather than assuming an empirical quantity as a candidate for the hidden variables $\{x_i\}$ and testing whether the networks generated with this choice are indeed similar to the real-world network considered, one can reverse the strategy and extract the values of the hidden variables $\{x_i\}$ directly from the real network. Then one can compare these unique values with candidate empirical quantities, to check whether a relation really exists. This comparison would automatically provide the form of the dependence between $\{x_i\}$ and the empirical quantities.

A way to realise this approach is provided by the Maximum Likelihood (ML) principle, a procedure commonly used in statistics whose use can be easily extended to networks [39]. Rather than requiring the values of model parameters as the input and generating an ensemble of possible networks as the output, the ML principle requires one particular real-world network as the input and provides the corresponding optimal parameter values $\{x_i^*\}$ as the output. *Optimal* stands for the parameter values that maximise the likelihood (or equivalently its logarithm) to obtain the particular real-world network under the model considered.

In the hidden variable model, the empirical input quantities are the rescaled GDP values $\{x_i\}$, which are fixed by observation, while the output values are the expected degrees $\{\langle k_i \rangle\}$. These expected values, and any other expected topological property, can then be compared with (but not fitted to) the empirical values $\{k_i\}$. By contrast, in the maximum likelihood approach the empirical input quantities are the degrees $\{k_i\}$, while the $\{x_i^*\}$ are output values depending uniquely on the observed degree sequence. In this case too, these output values can be compared with (but not fitted to) the empirical rescaled GDPs $\{x_i\}$ [39]. This comparison is shown in Fig. 7.10 where for consistency the parameter δ^* used in the hidden variable model and the same parameter used in the maximum likelihood approach have been both reabsorbed in the variables $\{x_i\}$ by redefining the latter as $x_i \rightarrow x_i \sqrt{\delta}$. One finds that the fitness values determined using only topological information are indeed proportional to the empir-

Fig. 7.10 Scatter plot of the likelihood-maximising values $\{x_i^*\}$ versus the rescaled GDP values $\{x_i\}$ (*isolated points*) and linear fit (*solid line*) for the undirected WTW in the year 2000

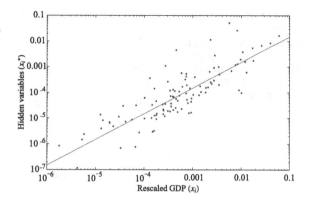

ical GDPs of world countries, and therefore that the maximum likelihood approach successfully identifies the GDP as the hidden variable shaping the topology of the WTW. Note that the two sets of values are, in principle, completely independent.

7.5.5 The WTW as a Directed Network

We now consider the topological properties of the WTW as a directed network. In any directed graph, the following relation exists between the entries $\{a_{ij}\}$ of its adjacency matrix and the entries $\{b_{ij}\}$ of the adjacency matrix of the same graph if regarded as undirected:

$$b_{ij} = a_{ij} + a_{ji} - a_{ij}a_{ji}. \tag{7.18}$$

Consequently, a relation is implied between the directed in- and out-degrees ($k_i^{\text{in}} = \sum_{j \neq i} a_{ji}$ and $k_i^{\text{out}} = \sum_{j \neq i} a_{ij}$) and the undirected degrees k_i observed on the two different representations of the same network:

$$k_i = k_i^{\text{in}} + k_i^{\text{out}} - k_i^{\leftrightarrow} \tag{7.19}$$

where $k_i^{\leftrightarrow} = \sum_{j \neq i} a_{ij}a_{ji}$ is the number of reciprocated connections incident at vertex i (the number of neighbours connected to i by incoming and outgoing links simultaneously), i.e. the reciprocated degree of vertex i.

The above relations indicate that, in principle, many different directed graphs can have the same undirected projection, making the latter not completely representative of an intrinsically directed network. However, the WTW has been found to display a peculiar structure that allows recovering significant information about its directed properties from the knowledge of the undirected ones [36, 37]. In particular, this is possible due to two empirically observed patterns. The first one is that on average $k_i^{\text{in}} \approx k_i^{\text{out}}$, i.e. a country generally has similar numbers of exporters and importers. The second one, shown in Fig. 7.11, is that the reciprocated degree $k_i^{\leftrightarrow}$ is proportional to the total degree $k_i^{\text{T}} \equiv k_i^{\text{in}} + k_i^{\text{out}}$

$$k_i^{\leftrightarrow} \approx \frac{r}{2} k_i^{\text{T}} \tag{7.20}$$

Fig. 7.11 Reciprocated degree $k_i^{\leftrightarrow}$ as a function of the total degree k_i^{T} in various directed snapshots of the WTW (from bottom to top: 1975, 1980, 1985, 1990, 1995, 2000)

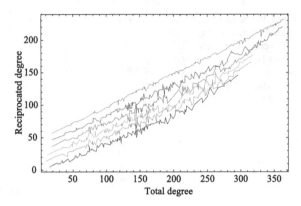

where r is the *reciprocity* defined as the ratio between the number $L^{\leftrightarrow}$ of reciprocated links and the number L of directed links,

$$r \equiv \frac{L^{\leftrightarrow}}{L} = \frac{\sum_i \sum_{j \neq i} a_{ij} a_{ji}}{\sum_i \sum_{j \neq i} a_{ij}}. \tag{7.21}$$

The latter relation means that the number of simultaneous exporters and importers of a country is an approximately constant fraction of the total number of importers and exporters of the same country.

Combining the two observations mentioned above, it is possible to simply relate many directed properties of the WTW to its undirected ones [37]. For instance, the directed degrees can be expressed in terms of the undirected ones as

$$k_i^{\mathrm{in}} \approx k_i^{\mathrm{out}} \approx \frac{k_i^{\mathrm{T}}}{2} \approx \frac{k_i}{2 - r}. \tag{7.22}$$

Similarly, the number L of directed links can be related to the number L^{u} of undirected links as follows:

$$L = \sum_i k_i^{\mathrm{in}} = \sum_i k_i^{\mathrm{out}} \approx \frac{\sum_i k_i}{2 - r} = \frac{2L^{\mathrm{u}}}{2 - r}. \tag{7.23}$$

Thus, the knowledge of the reciprocity r alone allows in many cases recovering the directed structure of the WTW from the undirected one. Note that this is a peculiar property of the WTW, as for a generic network no clear relation exists between the two representations, and a substantial loss of information may be associated with the undirected projection. Importantly, the above results hold for every analysed snaphot of the WTW [36] (see, for instance, Fig. 7.11). Therefore, the directedness of the network is easily monitored in terms of the time evolution of the reciprocity $r(t)$ [37]. The latter is shown in Fig. 7.12 together with a different measure of the reciprocity [36], i.e. the quantity

$$\rho \equiv \frac{r - c}{1 - c}. \tag{7.24}$$

The index ρ is an alternative and more refined definition that allows consistent comparisons of the reciprocity across networks of different sizes and connectances [36].

Fig. 7.12 Evolution of the reciprocity indices r (*top curve*) and ρ (*bottom curve*) in the directed WTW

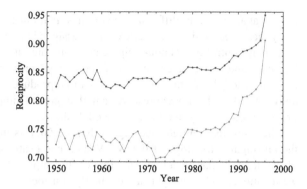

Indeed, since the null value of r expected in the uncorrelated case (where there is no tendency towards either favouring or avoiding the formation of reciprocated links) is c itself, then r alone cannot be used to compare networks with different values of c. Thus, even if c displays small variations in time (as we showed in Fig. 7.4), these variations does not allow to assess the evolution of the reciprocity of the WTW on the basis of r alone. As Fig. 7.12 shows, both r and ρ display small fluctuations up to the early 1980s, and then increase rather steadily. However, the increase of ρ is steeper than that of r, signalling that (once density effects are taken into account) a rapid reciprocation process occurred in the WTW starting from the 1980s. It is instructive to combine this result with the approximately constant trend of the connectance in the undirected version of the WTW. As at the undirected level, there is no increase of link density, the rapid increase of reciprocity signals many new directed links being placed between countries that had already been trading in the opposite direction, rather than new pairs of reciprocal links being placed between previously non-interacting countries. In other words, many pairs of countries that had previously been trading only in a single direction have been establishing also a reverse trade channel, and this effect dominates on the formation of new bidirectional relationships between previously non-trading countries.

Since the directedness of the WTW can be significantly recovered from its undirected description in terms of the reciprocity parameter, and since the undirected network is excellently reproduced by the fitness model, a natural question is whether the model can be simply extended in order to reproduce the directed structure of the WTW. In the simplest case, the fitness model can be generalised to the directed case by introducing two fitness values $\{x_i, y_i\}$, separately controlling the out-degree and the in-degree of every vertex i. This allows to draw a directed link from i to j with an asymmetric probability $p_{ij} = p(x_i, y_j) \neq p_{ji}$. However, in this simple extension the presence of a link from i to j is statistically independent from the presence of the reciprocal link from j to i. This implies that, in contrast with what empirically observed, the reciprocity coefficient ρ is trivially zero, or in other words that there is no interesting reciprocity structure. Non-trivial reciprocity can only be generated by a more refined extension of the fitness model where mutual links are statistically dependent on each other. A way to do this is by drawing, for each single vertex pair (i, j), a single link from i to j, a single link from j to i, two reciprocal links, or no link at all with four different probabilities (that must sum up to one) [36, 38]. In this generalised model, each vertex is now assigned three fitness values $\{x_i, y_i, w_i\}$, separately controlling its non-reciprocated outgoing links, non-reciprocated incoming links, and reciprocated links going both ways, respectively [38]. When applied to the directed WTW, this model turns out to reproduce all the properties discussed above. Notably, the model preserves a high degree of simplicity, as the three values $\{x_i, y_i, w_i\}$ are all again related to the GDP alone.

These results highlight once again that the GDP is the main factor underlying the unweighted topology of the WTW, and that a satisfactory and detailed model of the network can be defined in terms of the empirical GDP values. However, as we mentioned, when weights are explicitly considered a range of new possibilities emerge, as relations that are indistinguishable at a topological level may be strongly heterogeneous at the weighted level. As we discussed, while nonzero weights are well reproduced by gravity models of trade, there is currently no model that allows to simultaneously capture the topology and the weighted architecture of the real WTW. This implies that one important open problem to address in the future is the definition of a unified framework where network models and gravity models are reconciled. This is likely to involve joint efforts from the different scientific communities of trade economists and network theorists.

References

1. Almeida, H., Wolfenzon, D.: A theory of pyramidal ownership and family business groups. J. Finance **61**(6), 2637–2680 (2006)
2. Anderberg, M.R.: Cluster Analysis for Applications. Academic Press, New York (1973)
3. Aste, T., Di Matteo, T., Hyde, S.: Complex networks on hyperbolic surfaces. Physica A **346**, 20–26 (2005)
4. Banzhaf, J.F.: Weighted voting doesn't work: A mathematical analysis. Rutgers Law Rev. **19**, 317–343 (1965)
5. Barrat, A., Barthelemy, M., Pastor-Satorras, R., Vespignani, A.: The architecture of complex weighted networks. Proc. Natl. Acad. Sci. USA **101**, 3747 (2004)
6. Battiston, S., Catanzaro, M.: Statistical properties of corporate board and director networks. Eur. Phys. J. B **38**(2), 345–352 (2004)
7. Battiston, S., Catanzaro, M.: Statistical properties of corporate board and director networks. Eur. Phys. J. B **38**, 345–352 (2004)
8. Battiston, S., Rodrigues, J.F., Zeytinoglu, H.: The network of inter-regional direct investment stocks across Europe. Adv. Complex Syst. **10**(1), 29–51 (2005)
9. Bonanno, G., Vandewalle, N., Mantegna, R.: Taxonomy of stock market indices. Phys. Rev. E **62**, 7615–7618 (2000)
10. Boss, M., Elsinger, H., Summer, M., Thurner, S.: Network topology of the interbank market. Quant. Finance **4**, 677–684 (2004)
11. Brioschi, F., Buzzacchi, L., Colombo, M.: Risk capital financing and the separation of ownership and control in business groups. J. Bank. Finance **13**(1), 747–772 (1989)
12. Broder, A., Kumar, R., Maghoul, F., Raghavan, P., Rajagopalan, S., Stata, R., Tomkins, A., Wiener, J.: Graph structure of the web. Comput. Netw. **33**, 309–320 (2000)
13. Caldarelli, G.: Scale-Free Networks: Complex Webs in Nature and Technology. Oxford University Press, Oxford (2007)

14. Caldarelli, G., Capocci, A., De Los Rios, P., Munoz, M.A.: Scale-free networks from varying vertex intrinsic fitness. Phys. Rev. Lett. **89**, 258702 (2002)
15. Chapelle, A.: Separation of ownership and control: Where do we stand? Corp. Ownersh. Control **15**(2) 91–101 (2005)
16. Chapelle, A., Szafarz, A.: Controlling firms through the majority voting rule. Physica A **355**, 509–529 (2005)
17. Coronnello, C., Tumminello, M., Lillo, F., Micciche, S., Mantegna, R.: Sector identification in a set of stock return time series traded at the London stock exchange. Acta Phys. Pol. B **36**, 2653–2679 (2005)
18. Corrado, R., Zollo, M.: Small worlds evolving: Governance reforms, privatizations, and ownership networks in Italy. Ind. Corp. Change **15**(2), 319–352 (2006)
19. Cubbin, J., Leech, D.: The effect of shareholding dispersion on the degree of control in British companies: Theory and measurement. Econ. J. **93**(370), 351–369 (1983)
20. Davis, G.F., Yoo, M., Baker, W.E.: The small world of the corporate elite, 1982–2001. Strateg. Organ. **1**, 301–326 (2003)
21. De Bandt, O., Hartmann, P.: Systemic risk: a survey. CEPR Discussion Paper No. 2634 (2000)
22. De Masi, G., Gallegati, M.: Debt-credit economic networks of banks and firms: The Italian case. In: Chatterjee, A., Chakrabarti, B.K. (eds.) Econophysics of Markets and Business Networks. Springer, Berlin (2007)
23. De Masi, G., Iori, G., Caldarelli, G.: Fitness model for the interbank money market. Phys. Rev. E **74**, 066112 (2006)
24. De Masi, G., Fujiwara, Y., Gallegati, M., Greenwald, B., Stiglitz, J.: An analysis of the Japanese credit network (2009). arxiv:0901.2384
25. Derrida, B., Flyvbjerg, H.: Multivalley structure in Kauffman's model: Analogy with spin glasses. J. Phys. A **19**, 1003–1008 (1986)
26. Di Matteo, T., Aste, T., Hyde, S., Ramsden, S.: Interest rates hierarchical structure. Physica A **335**, 21–33 (2004)
27. Dore, R.: Stock market capitalism vs. welfare capitalism. New Polit. Econ. **7**(1), 115–127 (2002)
28. Dorogovtsev, S.N., Mendes, J.F.F.: Evolution of Networks: From Biological Nets to the Internet and WWW. Oxford University Press, Oxford (2003)
29. Eisenhardt, K.M.: Agency theory: An assessment and review. Acad. Manag. Rev. **14**(1), 57–74 (1989)
30. Lillo, F., Moro, E., Vaglica, G., Mantegna, R.N.: Specialization and herding behavior of trading firms in a financial market. New J. Phys. **10**, 043019 (2008)
31. Fagiolo, G., Reyes, J., Schiavo, S.: World-trade web: Topological properties, dynamics, and evolution. Phys. Rev. E **79**, 036115 (2009)
32. Fagiolo, G., Reyes, J., Schiavo, S.: On the topological properties of the world trade web: A weighted network analysis. Physica A **387**, 3868–3873 (2008)
33. Feenstra, R.C., Yang, T.H., Hamilton, G.G.: Business groups and product variety in trade: evidence from South Korea, Taiwan and Japan. J. Int. Econ. **48**(1), 71–100 (1999)
34. Flath, D.: Indirect shareholding within Japan's business groups. Econ. Lett. **38**(2), 223–227 (1992)
35. Fujiwara, Y., Aoyama, H., Ikeda, Y., Iyetomi, H., Souma, W.: Structure and temporal change of the credit network between banks and large firms in Japan. Economics **3**, 2009-7 (2009)
36. Garlaschelli, D., Loffredo, M.: Fitness-dependent topological properties of the world trade web. Phys. Rev. Lett. **93**, 268701 (2004)
37. Garlaschelli, D., Loffredo, M.: Structure and evolution of the world trade network. Physica A **355**, 138–144 (2004)
38. Garlaschelli, D., Loffredo, M.: Multispecies grand-canonical models for networks with reciprocity. Phys. Rev. E **73**, 015101 (2006)
39. Garlaschelli, D., Loffredo, M.: Maximum likelihood: extracting unbiased information from complex networks. Phys. Rev. E **78**, 015101 (2008)
40. Garlaschelli, D., Caldarelli, G., Pietronero, L.: Universal scaling relations in food webs. Nature **423**(6936), 165–168 (2003)

41. Garlaschelli, D., Battiston, S., Castri, M., Servedio, V.D.P., Caldarelli, G.: Detecting communities in large networks. Physica A **350**, 491–499 (2005)
42. Garlaschelli, D., Di Matteo, T., Aste, T., Caldarelli, G., Loffredo, M.: Interplay between topology and dynamics in the world trade web. Eur. Phys. J. B **57**, 159 (2007)
43. Garlaschelli, D., Loffredo, M.I.: Fitness-dependent topological properties of the world trade web. Phys. Rev. Lett. **93**(18), 188701 (2004). doi:10.1103/PhysRevLett.93.188701
44. Girvan, M., Newman, M.E.J.: Community structure in social and biological networks. Proc. Natl. Acad. Sci. USA **99**, 7821–7826 (2002)
45. Glattfelder, J.B., Battiston, S.: Backbone of complex networks of corporations: The flow of control. Phys. Rev. E **80**(3), 36104 (2009)
46. Gleditsch, K.: Expanded trade and GDP data. J. Confl. Resolut. **46**, 712–724 (2002)
47. Gopikrishnan, P., Rosenow, B., Plerou, V., Stanley, H.: Quantifying and interpreting collective behavior in financial markets. Phys. Rev. E **64**, 035106 (2001)
48. Gower, J.: Some distance properties of latent root and vector methods used in multivariate analysis. Biometrika **53**, 325–338 (1966)
49. Granovetter, M.: Coase revisited: Business groups in the modern economy. Ind. Corp. Change **4**, 93–130 (1995)
50. Herfindahl, O.: Copper Costs and Prices: 1870–1957. John Hopkins University Press, Baltimore (1959)
51. Iori, G., Jafarey, S., Padilla, F.: Systemic risk on the interbank market. J. Econ. Behav. Organ. **61**, 525–542 (2006)
52. Iori, G., Renó, R., De Masi, G., Caldarelli, G.: Trading strategies in the Italian interbank market. Physica A **376**, 467–479 (2007)
53. Iori, G., De Masi, G., Precup, O., Gabbi, G., Caldarelli, G.: A network analysis of the Italian overnight money market. J. Econ. Dyn. Control **32**, 259–278 (2008)
54. Kogut, B., Walker, G.: The small world of Germany and the durability of national networks. Am. Sociol. Rev. **66**(3), 317–335 (2001)
55. La Porta, R., de Silanes, F.L., Shleifer, A.: Corporate ownership around the world. J. Finance **54**(2) 471–517 (1999)
56. La Porta, R., de Silanes, F.L., Shleifer, A., Vishny, R.: Law and finance. J. Polit. Econ. **106**(6), 1113–1155 (1998)
57. Leech, D.: The relationship between shareholding concentration and shareholder voting power in British companies: A study of the application of power indices for simple games. Manag. Sci. **34**(4), 509–527 (1988)
58. Mantegna, R.: Hierarchical structure in financial markets. Eur. Phys. J. B **11**, 193–197 (1999)
59. Mantegna, R., Stanley, H.: An Introduction to Econophysics: Correlations and Complexity in Finance. Cambridge University Press, Cambridge (2000)
60. Miccichè, S., Bonanno, G., Lillo, F., Mantegna, R.: Volatility in financial markets: stochastic models and empirical results. Physica A **314**, 756–761 (2003)
61. Miceli, M., Susinno, G.: Using trees to grow money. Risk 11–12 (November 2003)
62. Newman, M., Strogatz, S., Watts, D.: Random graphs with arbitrary degree distributions and their applications. Phys. Rev. E **64**(2), 26118 (2001)
63. Newman, M., Watts, D., Strogatz, S.: Random graph models of social networks. Proc. Natl. Acad. Sci. USA **99**, 2566–2572 (2002)
64. Onnela, J.P., Kaski, K., Kertesz, J.: Clustering and information in correlation based financial networks. Eur. Phys. J. B **38**, 353–362 (2004)
65. Onnela, J.P., Chakraborti, A., Kaski, K., Kertesz, J., Kanto, A.: Asset trees and asset graphs in financial markets. Phys. Scr. T **106**, 48–54 (2003)
66. Onnela, J.P., Saramäki, J., Kertész, J., Kaski, K.: Intensity and coherence of motifs in weighted complex networks. Phys. Rev. E **71**(6), 065103 (2005)
67. Park, J., Newman, M.: Properties of highly clustered networks. Phys. Rev. E **68**, 026112 (2003)
68. Pastor-Satorras, R., Vázquez, A., Vespignani, A.: Dynamical and correlation properties of the Internet. Phys. Rev. Lett. **87**(25), 258701 (2001)

69. Serrano, M.: Phase transition in the globalisation of trade. J. Stat. Mech. Theory Exp. (2007). doi:10.1088/1742-5468/2007/01/L01002
70. Serrano, M., Boguñá, M.: Topology of the world trade web. Phys. Rev. E **68**(1), 15101 (2003)
71. Serrano, M.A., Boguñá, M., Vespignani, A.: Patterns of dominant flows in the world trade web. J. Econ. Interact. Coord. **2**, 111–124 (2007)
72. Shapley, L.S., Shubik, M.: A method for evaluating the distribution of power in a committee system. Am. Polit. Sci. Rev. **48**(3), 787–792 (1954)
73. Shleifer, A., Vishny, R.W.: A survey of corporate governance. J. Finance **52**(2), 737–783 (1998)
74. Sorämaki, K., Bech, M., Arnold, J., Glass, R., Beyeler, W.: The topology of the interbank payment flows. Physica A **379**, 317–333 (2007)
75. Tinbergen, J.: Shaping the World Economy: Suggestions for an International Economic Policy. The Twentieth Century Fund, New York (1962)
76. Tumminello, M., Lillo, F., Mantegna, R.N.: Correlation, hierarchies, and networks in financial markets. Journal of Economic Behavior and Organization **75**, 40–58 (2010)
77. Tumminello, M., Aste, T., Di Matteo, T., Mantegna, R.: A tool for filtering information in complex systems. Proc. Natl. Acad. Sci. USA **102**, 10421–10426 (2005)
78. Tumminello, M., Coronnello, C., Lillo, F., Miccichè, S., Mantegna, R.: Spanning trees and bootstrap reliability estimation in correlation-based networks. Int. J. Bifurc. Chaos Appl. Sci. Eng. **17**, 2319–2329 (2007)
79. Vitali, S., Glattfelder, J.B., Battiston, S.: The map of the global corporate control network. Working paper (2008)

Chapter 8
A Hierarchy of Networks Spanning from Individual Organisms to Ecological Landscapes

Ferenc Jordán, Gabriella Baranyi,
and Federica Ciocchetta

Abstract Living systems are hierarchically organised. A number of components are linked by the multiplicity of interactions at each level (from organisms to species to ecosystems). This kind of compositional and hierarchical complexity is a computational and conceptual challenge. We need new approaches to determine the key components of large interaction networks and we need to better understand how they influence the system dynamics horizontally (at the same level) and vertically (between organisational levels). We provide examples for various interaction networks (animal social group, food web, landscape) and discuss how to dynamically link them.

8.1 Introduction

Biological systems are composed of a large number of various components, like millions of molecules in a cell, thousands of cells in an organism, hundreds of individuals in a population and dozens of species in an ecological system. Yet, biosystems are complex not primarily because of the number of components but rather because of composition: the multiplicity of interactions among similar components and the hierarchical, nested nature of different kinds of components at several organisational levels. These components are composed of subsystems as well as compose larger systems, and all layers have been coevolved in evolution. The value of a molecular

F. Jordán (✉) · F. Ciocchetta
Centre for Computational and Systems Biology, The Microsoft Research-University of Trento,
Povo-Trento, Italy
e-mail: jordan@cosbi.eu

F. Ciocchetta
e-mail: ciocchetta@cosbi.eu

G. Baranyi
Institute of Environmental Studies, Eötvös University, Budapest, Hungary

E. Estrada et al. (eds.), *Network Science*,
DOI 10.1007/978-1-84996-396-1_8, © Springer-Verlag London Limited 2010

mutation is realised via the success of the organism that must be well positioned within the population of a species that are successful on the ecological theatre. Understanding this kind of hierarchical, compositional complexity is a much greater challenge than simply facing large numbers of any kind of units.

The history of systems thinking is surprisingly old, even if modern systems biology is considered to have originated only in the computer age. Modelling the morphological evolution of organisms by coordinate systems [126], describing an island ecosystem by a graph [125] or metaphorising animal development by a slope where a ball rolls down (i.e. the embryo [134]) are early and fine examples for systems-related problems and approaches in biology. In most of these examples, and in nearly all of the more recent ones, network representations also appear. This indicates that understanding relevant interactions among units is of key importance at all levels as well as between different levels. According to some authors, understanding interactions may be even more important than understanding the components themselves [129, 130]. Also, because of the relevance of interaction structures, effects among components can be transmitted, and indirect determination can be thought as even more important than the simple direct interactions among components [102, 103]. For example, the indirect effect between two particular species can be even stronger than the direct one (see an experimental example with direct predation and indirect trophic cascade [100]).

This chapter is not long enough to cover the whole spectrum of biological networks at all organisational levels but aims to overview and link the highest organisational levels, from individuals to landscape ecology, from a network perspective. We discuss the role of network analysis, overview old and new methods and give examples for hierarchical biological networks ranging from the individual to the landscape level. We note that hierarchical organisation is meant here in a biological sense [3], not in a topological one [115].

8.2 The Network Perspective

The key message of the network perspective is that in order to understand the behaviour of a dynamical system, it is important to study how changes in individual components influence the system (from local to global, bottom-up) and how system-level changes influence the constituting components (from global to local, top-down). Taking an ecological example, the extinction of a species may have a cascading effect on the whole ecosystem, while climate change drives the ecosystem and provokes a response at individual species. Networks describe how the parts form the whole [45], so network analysis can be regarded as a hard kind of holism [67]: it makes it possible to quantify and predict the "everything is connected to everything else" interactions and to make a difference between "only theoretical" and "also practical" effects.

8.3 Network Data

There is a wealth of data for supraindividual-level biological networks. Depending on the type of network (organisational level), network nodes represent individual organisms (in social networks), species (in food webs) or habitat patches (in landscape graphs), while links correspond to various interactions, most typically to expression of dominance, prey–predator interaction and migration, respectively. Network links can be directed (asymmetrical) or undirected (symmetrical) and weighted or unweighted (binary). In some cases, we are able to study also signed networks where each link is either positive or negative (see [43] for an application in a somewhat different context). For example, if wolf eats hare, it can be measured how much carbon is transferred (link weight), whether the hare also eats wolf (link direction) and that it is a negative effect on hare population size (sign).

8.3.1 Animal Social Network Data

Various animal groups are well described: from dolphins [75, 76] to guppies [22] and from wasps [39] to marmots [5] and primates [38]. In most cases, interactions are physical or chemical communication, weighted by frequency or strength. However, an interaction can also be defined simply as spatial closeness [22]. These interactions are characteristically directed in case of social hierarchies (e.g. pecking orders) but can be symmetrical otherwise.

8.3.2 Community Food Web Data

Different coexisting species also interact by means of interspecific interactions. The most widespread representation of these is the food web of the community [21, 28, 105, 106]. Other kinds of interspecific interactions are described by host/parasitoid [89], plant/pollinator [62] or competitive [99] interaction networks. All these networks can be weighted [6] as well as binary [80]. As for material flows, the food web contains mostly directed links with only a few exceptions (e.g. [7]), however, if "effects" are understood in a broader sense, undirected links also make sense: the prey and the predator both influence the other (and the relative importance of top-down and bottom-up effects may be close to equal, see also [110]). (It is noted that "bottom-up" is used here clearly in a different sense than in the Introduction: it means the direction of material flows instead of organisational levels.) Spatial [135, 140] and temporal [48, 49, 135, 140] food web series are only sporadic but their analysis will be crucial in future studies, as they may provide the most realistic basis for testing dynamical simulations. An even harder problem is how to define network nodes: several arguments suggest not representing species in food webs but, instead, ecologically relevant functional groups (either below or above the species level). Functional aggregation is the key of food web studies. Note that the strength and especially the symmetry of trophic links depend on the resolution of the network. For example, at the species level, nearly all adult marine fish are able to eat the larvae of the others. Directed trophic links only emerge if we only consider adults of each species (or life stages, with no respect to taxonomy).

8.3.3 Landscape Graph Data

Local communities, represented by food webs, are connected at larger spatial scales [108]: individuals of a population may migrate among suitable habitat patches, across ecological corridor-like spatial elements, creating one-species metapopulation and multi-species metacommunity dynamics. In a landscape graph, nodes and links represent habitat patches and ecological corridors, respectively [16, 127, 131]. For single-species systems, there is a wealth of landscape ecological studies describing habitat use and spatial movement [9, 41, 59, 60, 118]. However much fewer, but we have both abstract [8] and data-driven [84] models for better understanding meta-communities [46]. Spatial considerations are essential in order to better understand local communities: [23] presents an example where landscape processes (shrubland fragmentation) have major community-wide effects (mesopredator release, trophic cascade, secondary extinction). Subsidisation is also a key phenomenon in several ecosystems [107]: systems boundaries are not easy to find if the significance of spatial dynamics is temporarily variable. Metacommunity dynamics describes how spatial phenomena influence interacting sets of species.

8.4 Understanding Complexity

There are several ways how to better understand complex networks. The "statistical physicist" approach prefers to characterise the network by its macroscopic properties. For example, the degree distribution [92, 120], the small world property [87, 137] or the diameter [1, 139] of the network are simple descriptions condensing information and simplifying complexity. The hope here is that these properties can be used as proxies for predicting network functioning. For example, it can be argued that a certain degree distribution can imply vulnerability against attacks but resistance against errors [2]. These kinds of macroscopic approaches were favoured also in classical systems ecology, providing thermodynamical (e.g. exergy [63]) or information theoretical (e.g. ascendency [129]) indicators.

The "ecologist" approach provides two alternatives, both focusing on data transformation. First, complexity is easier to understand if the network is made smaller, for example, by aggregating food web nodes into larger groups. The aggregated form of the network can be easier to analyse, model and understand. Some Eco-Path models describe highly aggregated ecological networks (see [18]). Instead of speciose food webs, these trophic networks typically contain larger functional groups. This level of resolution is not inferior to species-level description, only provides different kind of information. The former may be better if we need to analyse the effects of a species-specific poison, while the latter can be favoured if the maturity of an ecosystem is to be evaluated, based on the extent of cycling. Second, in many cases it is reasonable to focus on a subgraph of the community food web. It can be either a small network module (e.g. [15]) or a larger, well-defined subsystem (e.g. a host/parasitoid network [116]). Massive experimental field work [85] as well as novel theoretical [73] and multidisciplinary research [86] focus on smaller subgraphs as the building blocks of complex networks. The main question here is additivity: whatever information we get about isolated modules, whether it is still relevant in the context of the whole network. Otherwise the distribution of different kinds of modules provides only little information. In social networks, for example, a clique can also be a functional unit but it is a question how to evaluate several cliques being close to each other or even overlapping. In this case, probably the most important functional consequences of cliquishness disappear: it is not a dense subgraph, being relatively isolated from the rest of the graph anymore. Thus, a simple statistics of how many of a given module can be counted in a complex network is just of very little functional meaning.

Finally, the "sociologist" approach is to focus on the key nodes of complex networks and try to understand group dynamics based on their study. This approach may stem from the paradigm of (human) "social stars" and their trivially large role in shaping group dynamics. It is noted, however, that the anisotropic nature of trophic networks [78, 79], the concept of alpha males in animal groups or geographical hot spots for diversity also imply the different relative importance of key network elements in particular ecological networks. This approach suggests that roles (functions) depend on positional importance in the system. The following section overviews how to quantify structural key nodes in networks.

8.5 Key Positions in Networks

According to the simplest definition, key nodes are the ones with the largest number of neighbours (highest degree). However, it can be demonstrated in nearly all biological systems that important positions may not necessarily mean a large number of neighbours. This is because of indirect effects and the significance of the larger neighbourhood [30, 141–143]. In most biological (and other) networks, effects spread from node to node in several steps (otherwise it is a question whether the network model is reasonable). Thus, conclusions based on node degree and degree distribution can be limited, however, serve well as a simple, preliminary analysis. The importance of considering indirect effects is larger as information changes more while being transmitted in the network (organisms can be metaphorised as semi-conductors, because of the flow-component interaction [79]). In ecology, the first (indirect) positional measurement for network nodes was developed for directed acyclic graphs (net status, [42, 44]; see also keystone index, its ecological adaptation [58]). Centrality indices imported from sociology [136] provided alternatives for measuring the position (structural importance) of network nodes. These include closeness centrality, betweenness centrality, information centrality and eigenvalue centrality [136]. Some of these indices have already been used for social animals [138], ecosystems [32, 54] as well as ecological landscape graphs [33]. More sophisticated tools are, for example, communicability betweenness for measuring betweenness by considering all pathways weighted by length [34], or topological importance [56] for measuring indirect interactions of length up to a given maximum. Beyond using a growing number of topological measurements also in biology, it is also becoming clearer what is the relationship between the above indices, how much they differ from each other [33, 54]. This can be measured based on the similarity of different node ranks they provide for the same network or based on the similarity of different index value distributions [10].

Apart from evaluating the network centrality of individual nodes, it is also of interest which set of n nodes is most central in a network [35]. Based on two alternative approaches (considering either fragmentation or reachability), key player sets can be determined for a given n number of nodes [14]. From a biological viewpoint, it is of interest how nested are these sets. In the case of a particular network, if the smaller set is generally a subset of the larger one, i.e. key player sets are nested, the integrity of the network is easier to control (or manage). On the contrary, if the most central n nodes are not elements of the most important $n + m$ nodes, network topology constrains the efficiency of network management [11].

Functionally important nodes can also be of low centrality. Alternative nodal metrics provide other tools for quantifying, for example, the uniqueness of the neighbourhood of different nodes. Regular equivalence (REGE) identifies classes of nodes of similar neighbourhood [74], while topological overlap (TO) quantifies the structural redundancy of neighbourhoods [55]. Clearly, even if not central, a node in a highly unique position can also be of key interest for group dynamics (its absence may be critical), and vice versa, a highly central node may play a less important role if there is another node of a largely overlapping neighbourhood (redundancy makes functional replacement easier). The TO index is based on considering indirect effects in a larger neighbourhood, while other overlap indices are based on shared direct neighbours [121] or maximal cliques [26].

Particular positions in networks, let them be central or unique, are likely to indicate nodes of outstanding functional importance. These anisotropies in networks can be largely responsible for higher-level system properties, providing the link to the higher organisational level.

8.6 Hierarchical Organisation of Networks

There are several examples for the outstanding role of structural key player positions in social networks (both human and animal, see [27]). Even if wolves may be the textbook example for social hierarchy, the perfect example is provided by invertebrates. The tropical paper wasp species *Ropalidia marginata* lives in small colonies, where individuals show no morphological caste differentiation (they are all similar-looking), but there is behavioural caste differentiation (showing statistically clearly different behavioural patterns, [39, 112]). If the queen dies in the colony, a new queen will appear within one day's time. Under laboratory conditions, individuals may be marked and pairwise interactions can be observed and registered. Thus, accurate social networks can be produced (where nodes are individual wasps and links are dominant/subordinate interactions). In these social networks, the position of the reigning queen is nothing particular [124]. However, the new queen (called post-queen) is generally of extreme centrality. It can also happen that all individuals are directly linked to the new queen and there is no other interaction among them (100% network centralisation, i.e. a perfect "star" topology, [12]). The functional significance of the queen is trivial; it acts as the pacemaker of the colony, controlling all activities. It is also of interest that as the colony becomes mature, the position of the queen is less and less central, and finally she can become even an isolated graph node.

The social interaction networks of yellow-bellied marmots (*Marmota flaviventris*) are similarly heterogeneous. Here, links mean more like communication than expression of dominance. Some individuals are less reliable, giving lower-quality signals, and their social position (status, prestige) mirrors this. In marmot networks, information coming from central individuals are more accepted by the others, so these individuals have larger role in shaping group dynamics [13, 91]. The success of the group, as a whole, mostly depends on the behaviour of these key nodes in the social network [138]. Figure 8.1 presents the social network of a yellow-bellied marmot group [13, 91]. Nodes correspond to individuals and links correspond to their interactions. Links can be symmetric or asymmetric, as well as weak and strong (in terms of frequency). Some individuals are isolated from the rest, while others are of much higher centrality in the interaction network (in the figure, node size is proportional to betweenness centrality). Group performance (e.g. predator avoidance) can correlate to social network structure.

To what extent a wasp colony is prone to the attack of predators or how quickly a marmot group realise the eagle matters a lot. Social network structure influences the strength of interspecific interactions (e.g. predation pressure). In principle, what is a macroscopic indicator at the highest level in animal sociology (e.g. network centralisation) can be a subtle parameter in an ecosystem model (e.g. the rate of a prey–predator interaction). In the top-down direction, if predators kill the *Ropalidia marginata* wasp queen, social network centralisation will dramatically increase soon. But it is also known that community-level patterns influence species dynamics, for example, extinction chance depends on food web topology [50, 104], and all these changes have group dynamics as the mechanistic background.

A food web can be simply defined as the collection of all populations in an ecosystem and all the feeding (prey–predator) interactions among them. Here, we do not discuss resolution and aggregation (nodes can be also lower and higher-level groups, like "0–1 years old herring" or "fungivore nematodes"), do not consider alternative interactions (e.g. mutualism, competition, facilitation) and assume that interactions can be perfectly an unambiguously documented (there is no missing

Fig. 8.1 Social network of a yellow-bellied marmot group. Some individuals can be isolated from the rest, while others are of much higher importance in the interaction network (node size is proportional to betweenness centrality). Data from [91], drawing by CoSBiLab Graph [132]

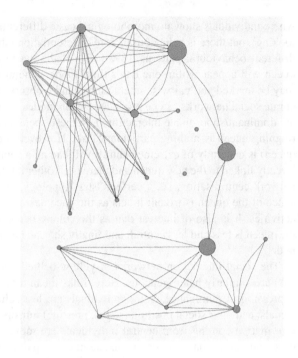

link caused by measurement error). With these simplifications, we can say that food web position of a species can differ and can be correlated to functional importance within the community. Some species are really richly linked to others, like small pelagics (sardine, anchovy [24, 119]) or copepods [122] in the wasp-waist position of marine food webs [24]. These species are of relatively high functional importance, as they serve as prey as well as predator for many other organisms. In other cases, functional importance is encoded in the rich indirect interaction pattern. The very first definition of keystone species [97, 98] (but see also [64, 69, 111]) discusses the disproportionate importance of the seastar *Pisaster*. This is a top predator that has only a few prey "neighbours" in the food web but one of them is richly linked. Thus, *Pisaster* has a number of second neighbours. Its importance is mechanistically realised by a type of indirect effect called "keystone predation" [85]: its dominant prey is a superior dominant competitor on rocky shores, and without the top-down control of *Pisaster*, it can competitively exclude the weaker competitors. Species in these particular and similar network positions are largely responsible for the higher-level system properties of ecological communities (local ecosystems). The extinction of keystone species may trigger cascades, like in the case of the Californian sea otter [31]. Also, there is increasing evidence that the "well-being" of copepods is the proxy for the "health" of marine ecosystems. These structural keystone species are to a large extent responsible for the stability, invadibility and resilience of ecosystems [81, 105, 106]. These macroscopic, ecosystem-level properties, and other indicators (like the Finn Cycling Index [37]) determine the functioning of local ecosystems within the context of larger-scale ecological landscapes.

Fig. 8.2 The Prince William Sound food web: node size correlates with betweenness centrality (**a**) and stochastic simulation-based community importance (**b**). Larger nodes are more important structurally (**a**) or dynamically (**b**). Data from [95], drawing by CoSBiLab Graph [132]

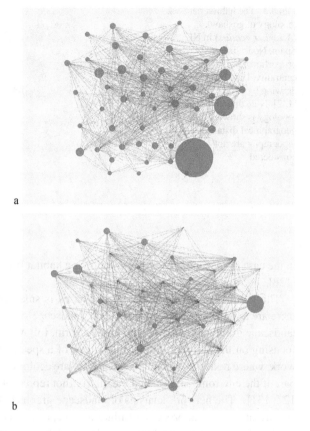

a

b

Figure 8.2(a) presents the food web of Prince William Sound, Alaska. Nodes represent species (or other functional groups) and links represent trophic interactions (prey–predator). In this figure, node size correlates with a topological (betweenness centrality, Fig. 8.2(a)) and a dynamical (Hurlbert response to perturbation, Fig. 8.2(b); see more below) measure of community importance. Food web topology determines how to link the part to the whole, i.e. which species may have outstanding effects on the community. In particular, importance indices inform on which species mostly affect ecosystem functioning, stability, vulnerability and other macroscopic properties.

Whether a local ecosystem can develop a rich cycling structure, or whether it is able to keep its resistance against invasions will determine large-scale ecological processes, like subsidisation [107], the extent of dispersal or the source-sink metapopulation dynamics of species. Macroscopic indicators of ecosystem structure (e.g. FCI) can be subtle parameters in a landscape-level metacommunity model (e.g. low ecotrophic efficiency may make the local habitat patch a source patch, increasing emigration rates and decreasing immigration rates). In the top-down direction, landscape-level changes may also influence local community dynamics, like

Fig. 8.3 The habitat network
topology of goshawk
(*Accipiter gentilis*) in NE
Spain. Node size is
proportional to betweenness
centrality. Data from [144],
drawing by CoSBiLab Graph
[132]. Note that only
topology is shown,
geographical distances and
topography are not
considered

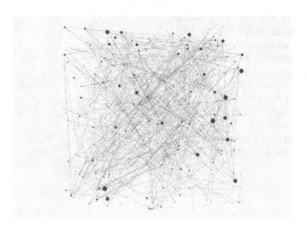

in the case of mesopredator release following habitat fragmentation [23] or invasion
[128].

The number of metacommunity databases is small (one example is [84]), but
there are a lot of data for species-specific landscape studies [33, 59, 60, 101]. These
landscape graph models, in their simplest form, follow the patch/corridor paradigm
focusing on the assumption that the habitat of a species can be described as a network, where nodes are habitat patches, links are ecological corridors and every other
part of the environment is called the matrix (not represented in the graph model [16,
127, 131]). The network analysis of landscape graphs helps to reveal the structural
constraints on spatial processes (migration, dispersal, gene flow) and provides tools
to identify key patches and key corridors mostly responsible for maintaining connectivity (hence, providing quantitative priorities for conservation practise, [117]).

Figure 8.3 presents the habitat network topology of goshawk (*Accipiter gentilis*)
in NE Spain. Nodes represent forest habitat patches and links represent ecological corridors. The graph is a complete graph theoretically, i.e. migration is possible
between each pair of patches, with different probability (it is a realistic approach to
birds and other flying organisms). However, cut-off values render network topology.
Corridors are defined here as transition probabilities over a threshold value (here
0.999 was used, otherwise the network is too dense for visualisation). Node size
is proportional to betweenness centrality [136]. Highly central habitat patches are
of critical importance in maintaining landscape connectivity, making thus dispersal and gene flow possible. The fragmentation of natural habitats is an increasingly
dangerous process, especially because it is combined with local increased distur-
bance: climatic changes may force populations to move, but in a fragmented habitat
it may not be possible. Climate change and fragmentation, separately, would probably mean much less danger. In the case of several species, maintaining landscape
connectivity seems to be the key to survival, because they approach the brink of
extinction and small, isolated populations are at extreme risk.

8.7 Dynamics

Since biological systems are in continuous change, social animal networks, food webs and landscape graphs are dynamical, both in terms of macroscopic properties and at the local level. Understanding this dynamics is a challenge in itself, but also because predictions (results of network analysis) concerning the topology/functioning relationship need to be tested. Centrality and overlap indices are useful only if we see their predictive power. Network dynamics can be studied in a descriptive way and by simulations of generative as well as quasi-equilibrium models.

8.7.1 Descriptive Network Dynamics

Describing time series of food webs [6, 135] is a straightforward way to understand the phenology of the community. Based on the statistical analyses of these series, it is possible to determine which components are mostly variable and which network properties are most stable. Another question is how sensitive different network analytical indices are to temporal aggregation (lumping). For example, [53] found that certain properties of lumped food webs are really around the average of the seasonal values, while other network indices may show extreme values for the lumped version (in this case, their use is clearly misleading). Also, based on statistical observations, various causal relationships have been suggested between topology and network behaviour. In food webs, triangularity and boxicity have been related to invadibility and prohibited species combinations [106, 123]. In signed social networks, tension caused by negative loops was used to explain the tendency for structural balance [43, 52].

8.7.2 Simulating Network Dynamics

Generative network models may explain the origin of ecological networks. Here, for example, game theory-based rules and graph grammars can be combined in order to provide network time series possibly reproducing real trajectories [17]. However, it is noted that network "generation" is the exception in most ecological systems, while the rule is network transformation. Ecological networks are not built up step by step from one-node stages, but rather change with the continuous transformation of earlier networks. In a sense, today's food webs are the "same" ones as the food webs of the primordial soup; they have just been being continuously modified by a (fairly large) number of compositional changes. It is very exceptional (e.g. following a volcano eruption) that a food web needs to be built up "from zero". Despite of these serious limitations, generative models can be of extreme use, as they may simulate systems behaviour far from equilibrium.

The approach using the most data and providing the most detailed mechanistic information on network dynamics is quasi-equilibrium simulation. ODE-based, deterministic models (e.g. EcoSim [19]) have been used, for example, to develop dynamical community importance (keystoneness) indices for species [95, 96]. These importance indices are based on the sensitivity analysis of the dynamical system simulated close to equilibrium. Comparison of these functional keystone nodes and topological keystones suggests that (1) network dynamics is easier to predict based on the structural analysis of weighted (i.e. not binary) graphs and (2) network dynamics is easier to predict by nodal indices considering also indirect (i.e. not only local) effects [61]. This may be important information, considering that one of the key tools in modern complex network analysis is determining degree distribution that is local and binary (hence, may not be very informative and predictive). Other approaches investigated the relationship between network position and extinction risk [29, 57, 114] and the effect of network topology on species substitution (regime shift) in model marine food webs [88].

Several properties of biological systems call for stochastic dynamical models [40, 65, 82, 109]. Stochastic, individual-based simulations of ecosystems by appropriate algorithms (e.g. [25]) may provide results different from both topological and deterministic dynamical results [72]. Such a simulation of the Prince William Sound ecosystem, Alaska [95] makes it possible to quantify the relative community importance of species based on sensitivity analysis (considering Hurlbert response, see [47]). Figure 8.2 shows the relative importance of species in the Prince William Sound food web, based on topology (betweenness centrality, Fig. 8.2(a)) and based on sensitivity analysis of stochastic simulation (Hurlbert response, Fig. 8.2(b)). The difference may be due to several reasons but illustrates also that a simple topological index hardly can be used as a proxy for predicting ecosystem dynamics.

Finally, Fig. 8.4 presents a conceptual and stochastic modelling framework for connecting the three studied organisational levels [20]. Here, individuals form a social network, species of different social networks are linked to each other in food webs and food webs are linked to each other by spatial dynamics. Parameters describing food web dynamics are sensitive to both lower (social network density) and higher-level (patch centrality) processes. The multi-level, hierarchical sensitivity analysis (structural and dynamical) of this model provides some insight into the interplay of processes within social networks, food webs and landscape graphs. For example, a general problem is to determine under which parameter combinations food webs are more sensitive to the group dynamics of the constituent species than to spatial processes in the landscape. One question to address by this model is whether to control natural enemies or help the other local populations in the landscape if a particular population needs to be protected.

8.8 Outlook

Focusing on the hierarchical organisation of supraindividual biology, we emphasised a "vertical" integration of various types of biological networks (social network,

Fig. 8.4 The scheme of the hierarchical network simulation model by [20]. Five interacting species (A, B, C, D and E) form local communities in four habitat patches (1, 2, 3 and 4), connected by ecological corridors in a spatial ecosystem model (a metacommunity). Each species is composed of interacting individuals forming a social network (illustrated in patch 2)

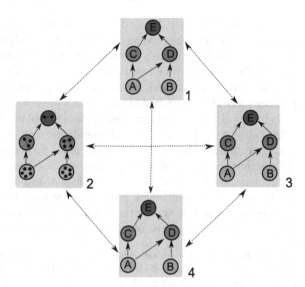

food web, landscape graph). Apart of this, a "horizontal" approach is also possible, and this latter one has longer traditions [36]: this would mean the comparison of different networks at similar levels of organisation. For example, comparing social networks (e.g. guppies to dolphins) to each other, the comparison of community networks (food webs, social networks, e.g. [12, 83]) to each other, the integration of ecological and economic network models [90] or, for example, the integration of landscape graph models with certain social networks (like transportation networks, see [133]).

Beyond biological networks at supraindividual organisational levels, the study of key nodes in interaction networks is an increasingly relevant issue also in molecular systems biology [71] and system-based medicine [93]. These applications follow the same logic and they are natural extensions of the above vertical scenario. Beyond biological networks, network centrality analysis is applied for different kinds of social networks [136], like transportation networks [51], terrorist networks [66] or international relations networks [77]. In general, network analysis has deep traditions in several fields of natural and human sciences (see, for example, [68, 70, 94]). The study of central nodes is generally a relevant issue but their role in linking subsystems to high-level systems may be more or less exclusive to biological systems, considering that hierarchical organisational is a feature of natural, not necessarily of human systems.

8.9 Closing Remarks

One way to better understand complex networks is to identify and study their particular nodes, let them be in central, unique or some other kind of critical positions (e.g. [4]). We begin to understand the relationship between various topological indices as well as between topology and dynamics. Studying key nodes in networks, if they are suitably identified, may provide a lot of information about the modelled system. This is helpful for better understanding the system itself, making predictions about its behaviour and, for our particular present interest, understand the link between hierarchically embedded networks.

In the unrealistically extreme case, we aim to find the conditions for the situation when killing an alpha male in a wolf population may alter dispersal patterns in the landscape, through changing the structure of the particular wolf population, altering the consumption rate of this top predator species, that cascades down in the food web, alters relative abundances and the habitat use of several other species, and finally changes the source-sink patterns in the metacommunity [113]. In a sense, this line of research would be the extension of the environ theory [102] towards several organisational levels. But this task is still very far away.

Acknowledgements For animal social network data, we are grateful to Daniel Blumstein and Tina Wey (marmots) as well as Professor Raghavendra Gadagkar and Anindita Bhadra (wasps). In research of food webs, we are mostly grateful to Thomas Okey, Barbara Bauer, Wei-chung Liu, István Scheuring and János Podani for cooperation and help. In research in landscape networks, we acknowledge Santiago Saura and Lucia Pascual-Hortal for providing data and discussions. The work of FJ was partly supported by Society in Science: The Branco Weiss Fellowship, ETH, Zürich.

References

1. Albert, R., Jeong, H., Barabási, A.L.: Diameter of the world-wide web. Nature **401**, 130–131 (1999)
2. Albert, R., Jeong, H., Barabási, A.L.: Error and attack tolerance of complex networks. Nature **406**, 378–382 (2000)
3. Allen, T.F.H., Starr, T.B.: Hierarchy: Perspectives for Ecological Complexity. University of Chicago Press, Chicago (1982)
4. Allesina, S., Bodini, A.: Who dominates whom in the ecosystem? Energy flow bottlenecks and cascading extinctions. J. Theor. Biol. **230**, 351–358 (2004)
5. Armitage, K.: Evolution of sociality in marmots. J. Mammal. **80**, 1–10 (1999)
6. Baird, D., Ulanowicz, R.E.: The seasonal dynamics of the Chesapeake Bay ecosystem. Ecol. Monogr. **59**, 3234 (1989)
7. Barkai, A., McQuaid, C.: Predator–prey role reversal in a marine benthic ecosystem. Science **242**, 62–64 (1988)
8. Bascompte, J., Solé, R.: Effects of habitat destruction in a prey–predator metapopulation model. J. Theor. Biol. **195**, 383–393 (1998)
9. Baudry, J., Burel, F.: Trophic flows and spatial heterogeneity in agricultural landscapes. In: Polis, G., Power, M., Huxel, G. (eds.) Food Webs at the Landscape Level, pp. 317–332. University of Chicago Press, Chicago (2004)
10. Bauer, B., Jordán, F., Podani, J.: Node centrality indices in food webs: rank orders versus distributions. Ecol. Complex. (2010). doi:10.1016/j.ecocom.2009.11.006
11. Benedek, Z., Jordán, F., Báldi, A.: Topological keystone species complexes in ecological interaction networks. Community Ecol. **8**, 1–8 (2007)
12. Bhadra, A., Jordán, F., Sumana, A., Deshpande, S., Gadagkar, R.: A comparative social network analysis of wasp colonies and classrooms: linking network structure to functioning. Ecol. Complex. **6**, 48–55 (2009)

13. Blumstein, D.T., Runyan, A., Seymour, M., Nicodemus, A., Ozgul, A., Ransler, F., Im, S., Stark, T., Zugmeyer, C., Daniel, J.C.: Locomotor ability and wariness in yellow-bellied marmots. Ethology **110**, 615–634 (2004)
14. Borgatti, S.P.: Identifying sets of key players in a social network. Comput. Math. Organ. Theory **12**, 21–34 (2006)
15. Brose, U., Berlow, E., Martinez, N.: Scaling up keystone effects from simple to complex ecological networks. Ecol. Lett. **8**, 1317–1325 (2005)
16. Cantwell, M., Forman, R.: Landscape graphs: ecological modelling with graph theory to detect configurations common to diverse landscapes. Landsc. Ecol. **8**, 239–255 (1993)
17. Cavaliere, M., Csikász-Nagy, A., Jordán, F.: Graph transformations and game theory: a generative mechanism for network formation. Technical Report TR-25-2008, CoSBi, Trento (2008)
18. Christensen, V., Pauly, D. (eds.): Trophic Models of Aquatic Ecosystems. ICLARM, Manila (1993)
19. Christensen, V., Walters, C.: Ecopath with ecosim: methods, capabilities and limitations. Ecol. Model. **172**, 109–139 (2004)
20. Ciocchetta, F., Jordán, F.: Modelling and analysing hierarchical ecological systems in BlenX. Technical Report TR-1-2010, CoSBi, Trento (2010)
21. Cohen, J.: Food Webs and Niche Space. Princeton University Press, Princeton (1978)
22. Croft, D.P., James, R., Thomas, P.O.R., Hathaway, C., Mawdsley, D., Laland, K.N., Krause, J.: Social structure and co-operative interactions in a wild population of guppies (*Poecilia reticulata*). Behav. Ecol. Sociobiol. **59**, 644–650 (2006)
23. Crooks, K.R., Soulé, M.E.: Mesopredator release and avifaunal extinctions in a fragmented system. Nature **400**, 563–566 (1999)
24. Cury, P., Bakun, A., Crawford, R., Jarre, A., Quinones, R., Shannon, L., Verheye, H.: Small pelagics in upwelling systems: patterns of interaction and structural changes in "wasp-waist" ecosystems. J. Mar. Sci. **57**, 603–618 (2000)
25. Dematté, L., Priami, C., Romanel, A.: The Beta Workbench: a computational tool to study the dynamics of biological systems. Brief. Bioinform. **9**, 437–449 (2008)
26. Doreian, P.: Analyzing overlaps in food webs. J. Soc. Biol. Struct. **9**, 115–139 (1986)
27. Croft, D., James, R., Krause, J.: Exploring Animal Social Networks. Princeton University Press, Princeton (2007)
28. Dunne, J.: The network structure of food webs. In: Pascual, M., Dunne, J. (eds.) Ecological Networks: Linking Structure to Dynamics in Food Webs, pp. 27–86. Oxford University Press, Oxford (2006)
29. Eklof, A., Ebenman, B.: Species loss and secondary extinctions in simple and complex model communities. J. Anim. Ecol. **75**, 239–246 (2006)
30. Elton, C.: Animal Ecology. University of Chicago Press, Chicago (1927)
31. Estes, J., Tinker, M., Williams, T., Doak, D.: Killer whale predation on sea otters linking oceanic and nearshore ecosystems. Science **282**, 473–476 (1998)
32. Estrada, E.: Characterisation of topological keystone species: local, global and "meso-scale" centralities in food webs. Ecol. Complex. **4**, 48–57 (2007)
33. Estrada, E., Bodin, O.: Using network centrality measures to manage landscape connectivity. a short path for assessing habitat patch importance. Ecol. Appl. **18**, 1810–1825 (2008)
34. Estrada, E., Higham, D.J., Hatano, N.: Communicability betweenness in complex networks. Physica A **388**, 764–774 (2009)
35. Everett, M., Borgatti, S.: The centrality of groups and classes. J. Math. Sociol. **23**, 181–201 (1999)
36. Faust, K., Skvoretz, J.: Comparing networks across space and time, size and species. Sociol. Method. **32**, 267–299 (2002)
37. Finn, J.: Measures of ecosystem structure and function derived from analysis of flows. J. Theor. Biol. **56**, 363–380 (1976)
38. Flack, J., Krakauer, D., de Waal, F.: Robustness mechanisms in primate societies: a perturbation study. Proc. R. Soc. Lond. B, Biol. Sci. **272**, 1091–1099 (2005)

39. Gadagkar, R.: The Social Biology of *Ropalidia marginata*. Harvard University Press, Cambridge (2001)
40. Gard, T.: Persistence in stochastic food web models. Bull. Math. Biol. **46**, 357–370 (1984)
41. Haddad, N., Browne, D., Cunningham, A., Danielson, B., Levey, D., Sargent, S., Spira, T.: Corridor use by diverse taxa. Ecology **84**, 609–615 (2003)
42. Harary, F.: Status and contrastatus. Sociometry **22**, 23–43 (1959)
43. Harary, F.: A structural analysis of the situation in the Middle East in 1956. J. Confl. Resolut. **5**, 167–178 (1961)
44. Harary, F.: Who eats whom? Gen. Syst. **6**, 41–44 (1961)
45. Higashi, M., Burns, T.: Theoretical studies of ecosystems—the network perspective (1991)
46. Holyoak, M., Leibold, M., Holt, R.: Metacommunities: Spatial Dynamics and Ecological Communities. University of Chicago Press, Chicago (2005)
47. Hurlbert, S.: Functional importance vs keystoneness: reformulating some questions in theoretical biocenology. Aust. J. Ecol. **22**, 369–382 (1997)
48. Jarre, A., Muck, P., Pauly, D.: Two approaches for modelling fish stock interactions in the Peruvian upwelling ecosystem. ICES Mar. Sci. Symp. **193**, 171–184 (1991)
49. Jarre-Teichmann, A.: The potential role of mass balance models for the management of upwelling ecosystems. Ecol. Appl. **8**, 93–103 (1998)
50. Jonsson, T., Karlsson, P., Jonsson, A.: Food web structure affects the extinction risk of species in ecological communities. Ecol. Model. **199**, 93–106 (2006)
51. Jordán, F.: Predicting target selection by terrorists: A network analysis of the 2005 London underground attacks. Int. J. Crit. Infrastructures **4**, 206–214 (2008)
52. Jordán, F.: Children in time: community organisation in social and ecological systems. Curr. Sci. **97**, 1579–1585 (2009)
53. Jordán, F., Osváth, G.: The sensitivity of food web topology to temporal data aggregation. Ecol. Model. **220**, 3141–3146 (2009)
54. Jordán, F., Benedek, Z., Podani, J.: Quantifying positional importance in food webs: a comparison of centrality indices. Ecol. Model. **205**, 270–275 (2007)
55. Jordán, F., Liu, W.C., Mike, A.: Trophic field overlap: a new approach to quantify keystone species. Ecol. Model. **220**, 2899–2907 (2009)
56. Jordán, F., Liu, W.C., van Veen, F.: Quantifying the importance of species and their interactions in a host-parasitoid community. Community Ecol. **4**, 79–88 (2003)
57. Jordán, F., Scheuring, I., Vida, G.: Species positions and extinction dynamics in simple food webs. J. Theor. Biol. **215**, 441–448 (2002)
58. Jordán, F., Takács-Sánta, A., Molnár, I.: A reliability theoretical quest for keystones. Oikos **86**, 453–462 (1999)
59. Jordán, F., Magura, T., Tóthmérész, B., Vasas, V., Ködöböcz, V.: Carabids (Coleoptera: Carabidae) in a forest patchwork: a connectivity analysis of the Bereg Plain landscape graph. Landsc. Ecol. **22**, 1527–1539 (2007)
60. Jordán, F., Báldi, A., Orci, K., Rácz, I., Varga, Z.: Characterizing the importance of habitat patches and corridors in maintaining the landscape connectivity of a *Pholidoptera transsylvanica* (*Orthoptera*) metapopulation. Landscape Ecology, 83–92 (2003)
61. Jordán, F., Okey, T., Bauer, B., Libralato, S.: Identifying important species: a comparison of structural and functional indices. Ecol. Model. **216**, 75–80 (2008)
62. Jordano, P.: Patterns of mutualistic interactions in pollination and seed dispersal: connectance, dependences, asymmetries and coevolution. Am. Nat. **129**, 657–677 (1987)
63. Jørgensen, S., Nielsen, S., Mejer, H.: Emergy, exergy and ecological modelling. Ecol. Model. **77**, 99–109 (1995)
64. Kareiva, P.M., Levin, S.A.: The Importance of Species. Princeton University Press, Princeton (2003)
65. Kazanci, C., Matamba, L., Tollner, E.: Cycling in ecosystems: an individual based approach. Ecol. Model. **220**, 2908–2914 (2009)
66. Krebs, V.: Mapping terrorist networks. Connections **24**, 43–52 (2002)
67. László, E.: Nonlocal coherence in the living world. Ecol. Complex. **1**, 7–15 (2004)

68. Leontief, W.: The Structure of American Economy 1919–1939. Oxford University Press, New York (1963)
69. Libralato, S., Christensen, V., Pauly, D.: A method for identifying keystone species in food web models. Ecol. Model. **195**, 153–171 (2006)
70. Liljeros, F., Edling, C., Amaral, L.: Sexual networks: implications for the transmission of sexually transmitted infections. Microbes Infect. **5**, 189–196 (2003)
71. Liu, W.C., Lin, W., Davis, A.J., Jordán, F., Yang, H., Hwang, M.: A network perspective on the topological importance of enzymes and their phylogenetic conservation. BMC Bioinform. **8**, 121 (2007)
72. Livi, C.M., Jordán, F., Lecca, P., Okey, T.A.: Identifying keystone species in ecosystems with stochastic sensitivity analysis. Ecological Modelling, under review
73. Loreau, M.: Ecosystem development explained by competition within and between material cycles. Proc. R. Soc. Lond. B, Biol. Sci. **265**, 33–38 (1998)
74. Luczkovich, J., Borgatti, S., Johnson, J., Everett, M.: Defining and measuring trophic role similarity in food webs using regular equivalence. J. Theor. Biol. **220**, 303–321 (2003)
75. Lusseau, D.: The emergent properties of a dolphin social network. Proc. R. Soc. Lond. B, Biol. Sci. **270**, 186–188 (2003)
76. Lusseau, D., Newman, M.: Identifying the role that animals play in their social networks. Proc. R. Soc. Lond. B, Biol. Sci. **271**, 477–481 (2004)
77. Maoz, Z., Terris, L., Kuperman, R., Talmud, I.: International relations: a network approach. In: Mintz, A., Russett, B. (eds.) New Directions for International Relations. Lexington Books, Lanham (2004)
78. Margalef, R.: Perspectives in Ecological Theory. University of Chicago Press, Chicago (1968)
79. Margalef, R.: Networks in ecology. In: Higashi, M., Burns, T.P. (eds.) Theoretical Studies of Ecosystems—The Network Perspective, pp. 41–57. Cambridge University Press, Cambridge (1991)
80. Martinez, N.: Artifacts or attributes? Effects of resolution on the Little Rock lake food web. Ecol. Monogr. **61**, 367–392 (1991)
81. May, R.: Stability and Complexity in Model Ecosystems. Princeton University Press, Princeton (1973)
82. McKane, A., Newman, T.: Predator–prey cycles from resonant amplification of demographic stochasticity. Phys. Rev. Lett. **94**, 218102 (2005)
83. McMahon, S., Miller, K., Drake, J.: Networking tips for social scientists and ecologists. Science **293**, 1604–1605 (2001)
84. Melian, C., Bascompte, J., Jordano, P.: Spatial structure and dynamics in marine food webs. In: Belgrano, A., Scharler, U., Dunne, J., Ulanowicz, R. (eds.) Aquatic Food Webs. Oxford University Press, Oxford (2005)
85. Menge, B.: Indirect effects in marine rocky intertidal interaction webs: patterns and importance. Ecol. Monogr. **65**, 21–74 (1995)
86. Milo, R., Shen-Orr, S.S., Itzkovitz, S., Kashtan, N., Chklovskii, D., Alon, U.: Network motifs: simple building blocks of complex networks. Science **298**, 824–827 (2002)
87. Montoya, J., Solé, R.: Small world patterns in food webs. J. Theor. Biol. **214**, 405–412 (2002)
88. Móréh, A., Jordán, F., Szilágyi, A., Scheuring, I.: Overfishing and regime shifts in minimal food web models. Community Ecol. **10**, 234–241 (2009)
89. Müller, C., Adriaanse, I., Belshaw, R., Godfray, H.: The structure of an aphid-parasitoid community. J. Anim. Ecol. **68**, 346–370 (1999)
90. Mullon, C., Shin, Y., Cury, P.: NEATS: A network economics approach to trophic systems. Ecol. Model. **220**, 3033–3045 (2009)
91. Nanayakkara, D.D., Blumstein, D.T.: Defining yellow-bellied marmot social groups using association indices. Oecol. Mont. **12**, 7–11 (2003)
92. Newman, M.E.J.: The structure and function of complex networks. SIAM Rev. **45**(2), 167–256 (2003)

93. Nguyen, T., Jordán, F.: A quantitative approach to study indirect effects among disease proteins in the human protein interaction network. BMC Syst. Biol. **4**, 103 (2010)
94. Odum, H.: Ecological and General Systems. University Press of Colorado, Boulder (1994)
95. Okey, T.A.: Shifted community states in four marine ecosystems: some potential mechanisms. PhD thesis, University of British Columbia, Vancouver (2004)
96. Ortiz, M., Avendaño, M., Cantillañez, M., Berrios, F., Campos, L.: Trophic mass balanced models and dynamic simulations of benthic communities from la Rinconada Marine Reserve off northern Chile: network properties and multispecies harvest scenario assessments. Aquat. Conserv. Mar. Freshw. Ecosyst.. **20**, 58–73 (2009)
97. Paine, R.: Food web complexity and species diversity. Am. Nat. **100**, 65–75 (1966)
98. Paine, R.: A note on trophic complexity and community stability. Am. Nat. **103**, 91–93 (1969)
99. Paine, R.: Ecological determinism in the competition for space. Ecology **65**, 1339–1348 (1984)
100. Palomares, F., Gaona, P., Ferreras, P., Delibes, M.: Positive effects on game species of top predators by controlling smaller predator populations: an example with lynx, mongooses, and rabbits. Conserv. Biol. **9**, 295–305 (1995)
101. Pascual-Hortal, L., Saura, S.: Comparison and development of new graph-based landscape connectivity indices: towards the prioritization of habitat patches for conservation. Landsc. Ecol. **21**, 959–967 (2006)
102. Patten, B.: Environs: the superniches of ecosystems. Am. Zool. **21**, 845–852 (1981)
103. Patten, B.C.: Network ecology: indirect determination of the life-environment relationship in ecosystems. In: Higashi, M., Burns, T. (eds.) Theoretical Studies of Ecosystems—The Network Perspective, pp. 288–351. Cambridge University Press, Cambridge (1991)
104. Pimm, S.: Food web design and the effect of species deletion. Oikos **35**, 139–149 (1980)
105. Pimm, S.: Food Webs. Chapman and Hall, London (1982)
106. Pimm, S.: The Balance of Nature? University of Chicago Press, Chicago (1991)
107. Polis, G.A., Hurd, S.D., Jackson, T., Sanchez Piñero, F.: ElNino effects on the dynamics and control of an island ecosystem in the Gulf of California. Ecology **78**, 1884–1897 (1997)
108. Polis, G., Anderson, W., Holt, R.: Toward an integration of landscape and food web ecology: the dynamics of spatially subsidized food webs. Ann. Rev. Ecolog. Syst. **28**, 289–231 (1997)
109. Powell, C., Boland, R.: The effects of stochastic population dynamics on food web structure. J. Theor. Biol. **257**, 170–180 (2009)
110. Power, M.: Top-down and bottom-up forces in food webs: do plants have primacy? Ecology **73**, 733–746 (1992)
111. Power, M., Tilman, D., Estes, J., Menge, B., Bond, W., Mills, L., Daily, G., Castilla, J., Lubchenco, J., Paine, R.: Challenges in the quest for keystones. Bioscience **46**, 609–620 (1996)
112. Premnath, S., Sinha, A., Gadagkar, R.: Dominance relationships in the establishment of reproductive division of labour in a primitively eusocial wasp (*Ropalidia marginata*). Behav. Ecol. Sociobiol. **39**, 125–132 (1996)
113. Pulliam, H.: Sources, sinks, and population regulation. Am. Nat. **132**, 652–661 (1988)
114. Quince, C., Higgs, P., McKane, A.: Deleting species from model food webs. Oikos **110**, 283–296 (2005)
115. Ravasz, E., Barabási, A.: Hierarchical organisation in complex networks. Phys. Rev. E **67**, 026112 (2003)
116. Rott, A., Godfray, H.: The structure of a leafminer-parasitoid community. J. Anim. Ecol. **69**, 274–289 (2000)
117. Saura, S., Pascual-Hortal, L.: A new habitat availability index to integrate connectivity in landscape conservation planning: comparison with existing indices and application to a case study. Landsc. Urban Plan. **83**, 91–103 (2007)
118. Selonen, V., Hanski, I.: Movements of the flying squirrel Pteromys volans in corridors and in matrix habitat. Ecography **26**, 641–651 (2003)
119. Shannon, L.J., Cury, P.: Indicators quantifying small pelagic fish interactions: application using a trophic model of the southern Benguela ecosystem. Ecol. Indic. **3**, 305–321 (2003)

120. Solé, R., Montoya, J.: Complexity and fragility in ecological networks. Proc. R. Soc. Lond. B, Biol. Sci. **268**, 2039–2045 (2001)
121. Solé, R., Valverde, S., Rodriguez-Caso, C.: Modularity in biological networks. In: Képès, F. (ed.) Biological Networks. World Scientific, Singapore (2007)
122. Stibor, H., Vadstein, O., Diehl, S., Gelzleichter, A., Hansen, T., Hantzsche, F., Katechakis, A., Lippert, B., Loseth, K., Peters, C., Roederer, W., Sandow, M., Sundt-Hansen, L., Olsen, Y.: Copepods act as a switch between alternative trophic cascades in marine pelagic food webs. Ecol. Lett. **7**, 321–325 (2004)
123. Sugihara, G.: Graph theory, homology and food webs. Proc. Symp. Appl. Math. **30**, 83–101 (1984)
124. Sumana, A., Gadagkar, R.: *Ropalidia marginata*—a primitively eusocial wasp society headed by behaviourally non-dominant queens. Curr. Sci. **84**, 1464–1468 (2003)
125. Summerhayes, V., Elton, C.: Contributions to the ecology of Spitsbergen and Bear Island. J. Ecol. **11**, 214–268 (1923)
126. Thompson, D.W.: On Growth and Form. Cambridge University Press, Cambridge (1917)
127. Tischendorf, L., Fahrig, L.: How should we measure landscape connectivity? Landsc. Ecol. **15**, 633–641 (2000)
128. Torchin, M., Lafferty, K., Kuris, A.: Release from parasites as natural enemies: increased performance of a globally introduced marine crab. Biol. Invasions **3**, 333–345 (2001)
129. Ulanowicz, R.: Growth and Development—Ecosystems Phenomenology. Springer, Berlin (1986)
130. Ulanowicz, R.: On the importance of higher-level models in ecology. Ecol. Model. **43**, 45–56 (1988)
131. Urban, D., Keitt, T.: Landscape connectivity: a graph-theoretic perspective. Ecology **82**, 1205–1218 (2001)
132. Valentini, R., Jordán, F.: CoSBiLab Graph: the network analysis module of CoSBiLab. Environ. Model. Softw. **25**, 886–888 (2010)
133. Vasas, V., Magura, T., Jordán, F., Tóthmérész, B.: Graph theory in action: evaluating planned highway tracks based on connectivity measures of a fragmented forest landscape. Landsc. Ecol. **24**, 581–586 (2009)
134. Waddington, C.: The Strategy of the Genes. Allen & Unwin, London (1957)
135. Warren, P.: Spatial and temporal variation in the structure of a freshwater food web. Oikos **55**, 299–311 (1989)
136. Wasserman, S., Faust, K.: Social Network Analysis. Cambridge University Press, Cambridge (1994)
137. Watts, D.J., Strogatz, S.H.: Collective dynamics of 'small-world' networks. Nature **393**, 440–442 (1998)
138. Wey, T., Blumstein, D., Shen, W., Jordán, F.: Social network analysis of animal behaviour: a promising tool for the study f sociality. Anim. Behav. **75**, 333–344 (2008)
139. Williams, R., Berlow, E., Dunne, J., Barabási, A., Martinez, N.: Two degrees of separation in complex food webs. Proc. Natl. Acad. Sci. USA **99**, 12913–12916 (2002)
140. Winemiller, K.: Factors driving temporal and spatial variation in aquatic floodplain food webs. In: Polis, G., Winemiller, K. (eds.) Food Webs: Integration of Patterns and Dynamics, pp. 298–312. Chapman and Hall, London (1996)
141. Wootton, J.: The nature and consequences of indirect effects in ecological communities. Ann. Rev. Ecolog. Syst. **25**, 443–466 (1994)
142. Yodzis, P.: Diffuse effects in food webs. Ecology **81**, 261–266 (2000)
143. Yodzis, P.: Must top predators be culled for the sake of fisheries? Trends Ecol. Evol. **16**, 78–84 (2001)
144. Estrada, J., Pedrocchi, V., Brotons, L., Herrando, S. (eds.) Atles dels Ocells Nidificants de Catalunya 1999–2002. Lynx Edicions, Barcelona (2004)

Chapter 9
Revealing Structure of Complex Biological Systems Using Bayesian Networks

V. Anne Smith

Abstract Bayesian networks represent statistical dependencies among variables; they are able to model multiple types of relationships, including stochastic, non-linear, and arbitrary combinatoric. Such flexibility has made them excellent models for reverse-engineering structure of complex networks. This chapter reviews the use of Bayesian networks for probing structure of biological systems. We begin with an introduction to Bayesian networks, addressing especially issues of their interpretation as relates to understanding system structure. We then cover how Bayesian network structures are learned from data, considering a popular scoring metric, the BDe, in detail. We finish by reviewing the uses of Bayesian networks in biological systems to date and the concurrent advances in Bayesian network methodology tailored for use in biology.

9.1 Introduction

Bayesian networks are a powerful statistical methodology, representing dependencies and conditional relationships among a set of variables in a graphical format [65]. The idea of presenting statistical relationships using graphs can be traced to Sewall Wright's development of path analysis early in the twentieth century [93]. In the 1980s, the use of directed acyclic graphs (DAGs) grew for the representation of probabilistic contingencies [43, 91], and were first called *Bayesian networks* by Pearl in 1985 [64].

Bayesian networks (BNs) were initially used as *expert systems* [65]: human experts would be consulted to determine contingencies between a set of variables, and the resulting Bayesian network would be used to make predictions. As such, early learning in BNs concentrated on learning the *parameters* of a given structure [65].

V.A. Smith (✉)
School of Biology, University of St Andrews, St Andrews, Fife KY16 9TH, UK
e-mail: anne.smith@st-andrews.ac.uk

E. Estrada et al. (eds.), *Network Science*,
DOI 10.1007/978-1-84996-396-1_9, © Springer-Verlag London Limited 2010

For, while a doctor might be able to indicate which symptoms were associated with what disease, the precise nature of the probabilistic relationship was more accurately assessed from data. Learning the *structure* of Bayesian networks initially arose from the problem: if experts provide conflicting sets of relationships, how do we determine which is more accurate? To answer this problem, methods were developed to score provided structures, and thus compare between them [6, 78]. However, once a method of scoring existed, it was then a short step to dispensing with the expert altogether: one could apply machine learning to search through possible networks and find the best structure to explain a given data set [13, 79, 81].

Learning the structure of BNs from data has been applied in a number of domains, from finding lost people [86] to understanding the interplay of variables that lead to efficient transport systems [28]. It is based on the concept that dynamic interactions within a network will leave traces in statistical dependence among variables; recovering these dependence relationships thus reveals the underlying network dynamics. BNs have become particularly useful for probing the structure of biological systems, and it is these applications upon which this chapter concentrates. We will begin with an introduction to the theory behind Bayesian networks, address methods of structure learning, and survey BNs' applications—and consequent developments—across a number of biological systems.

9.2 Theory of Bayesian Networks

9.2.1 Definition

A Bayesian network is a graphical representation of a joint probability distribution over a set of variables $\chi = \{X_1, \ldots, X_n\}$. A BN is specified by a pair $\langle G, \Theta \rangle$. G represents a directed graph whose nodes correspond to the variables $X_1, \ldots, X_n$; links between nodes indicate that the child variable is statistically dependent on its parent. Conditional independence among variables is read from the graph structure: a variable X_i is conditionally independent of all of its non-descendants given its parents in G, $Pa(X_i)$ (Fig. 9.1). The parameters Θ specify the probabilistic relationship of each node to its parents, $P(X_i|Pa(X_i))$. For example, in a discrete Bayesian network, where all variables take on discrete values, Θ consists of a collection of $\theta_{x_i|pa(X_i)} = P(X_i = x_i|Pa(X_i) = pa(X_i))$ for each variable X_i, denoting the probability of X_i taking on the discrete state x_i given its parents $Pa(X_i)$ having the state set $pa(X_i)$. The joint probability distribution specified by $\langle G, \Theta \rangle$ is thus:

$$P(X_1, \ldots, X_n) = \prod_{i=1}^{n} P(X_i|Pa(X_i)). \tag{9.1}$$

This definition leads to a number of features. First, because a BN represents a minimal set of dependencies coded in a particular factoring (equation (9.1)) of a joint probability distribution, the graph G is restricted to be acyclic; thus BNs are

Fig. 9.1 Example Bayesian network. The node D is conditionally independent of its non-descendants (white nodes) given its parent, B. The joint probability distribution specified by this BN is $P(A, B, C, D, E) = P(A)P(B|A)P(C|B) \times P(D|B)P(E|D)P(F|D)$

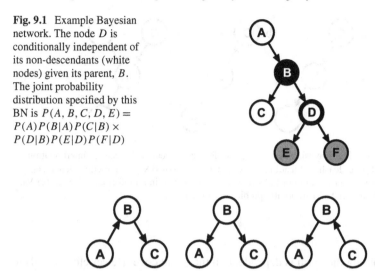

Fig. 9.2 Equivalence classes in Bayesian networks. Three BNs forming an equivalence class are shown; each BN represents a different factoring of the same joint probability distribution

always DAGs. Second, because a given joint probability distribution might have multiple mathematically equivalent factorings that represent the same dependence and conditional independence relationships, one probability distribution can be represented with equal validity by multiple BNs; these BNs differ only in the direction of (some of) their links. A collection of BNs representing the same joint probability distribution is known as an equivalence class (Fig. 9.2). A third feature relates to discrete BNs: because each parameter $\theta_{x_i|pa(X_i)}$ in a discrete BN can be specified independently, the statistical relationship between a child and its parents is represented by arbitrary combinatorics; thus, modelling non-linear and non-additive relationships is just as simple as any other. This ability to model statistical relationships without the need to specify the form of the dependency is one of the reasons that discrete BNs have been used in so many different domains.

9.2.2 Interpretation

To gain a more intuitive sense of what a Bayesian network means, we will take a simple example. Consider a dog owner, who when he is able, and usually on sunny, pleasant days, takes his dog for long walks in the park; consider three variables that we might measure about the dog and his owner in their home: cloudiness of the sky outside (cloud, C), whether the man is holding the dog's leash (leash, L), and the level of the dog's excitement (excitement, E). We can draw a BN among these variables as seen in Fig. 9.3(a): the dog's excitement is dependent on his owner holding the leash (holding the leash leads to higher probability of excitement), and

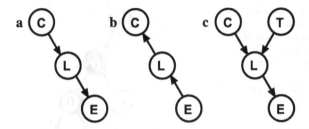

Fig. 9.3 Dog-walking Bayesian networks. (**a**) BN congruent with causal interpretation of clouds (*C*) leading to leash (*L*) leading to excitement (*E*). (**b**) BN of same equivalence class as in (**a**), highlighting interpretation of links in a BN as predictive in an informative sense. (**c**) Variables cloud (*C*) and tired (*T*) are jointly predictive of leash (*L*)

the owner holding the leash is dependent on the cloud cover (fewer clouds leads to higher probability of holding the leash). Links in a BN are most usefully translated to the phrase "is useful for predicting"; so here, we may say cloud is useful for predicting leash, and leash is useful for predicting excitement.

The BN in Fig. 9.3(b) represents these variables using another member of the same equivalence class: we see how the links are all in the opposite direction. Considering the interpretation of this network addresses an important point in BNs. While in some cases it is possible to infer causality from links in a Bayesian network [66], in most situations links in a BN refer to prediction in an informative, rather than causal, sense. So, from the BN in Fig. 9.3(b) we see that excitement is useful for predicting leash—this is true, because were you to observe the dog's excitement, you could then infer that the owner is holding the leash. The dog's excitement did not *cause* the owner to hold the leash (at least in our toy example here); however, it is a useful informative cue to make a prediction about the other variable. A similar situation occurs with the common co-occurrence of rain and open umbrellas. While it is the presence of rain that causes people to walk about with open umbrellas, it is possible to correctly infer that it is raining outside from the observation that people are carrying umbrellas.

In Fig. 9.3(c), we add one more variable to our example, how tired the dog owner currently is (tired, *T*). We do this to make a particular point: when a BN contains multiple parents for one variable, all parents of a variable must be included when interpreting dependencies. For example, from the structure in Fig. 9.3(c), we say that cloud and tired together are useful for predicting leash; one would not want to say only that cloud is useful for predicting leash, because it may only be useful in the context of tired (e.g. low cloudiness may only be predictive of holding the leash when the owner is not tired). This would be a combinatoric, non-additive relationship among parents. Only with knowledge of the parameters can one say whether multiple parents in a BN act independently or not. And in all cases they act *together*:

the minimal set of dependencies in this probability distribution requires knowledge of both tired and cloud in order to predict leash.[1]

9.2.3 Dynamic Bayesian Networks

As noted above, Bayesian networks are acyclic; thus, a basic BN cannot represent cyclic features in a system like feedback loops. Because feedback loops are an expected feature of many biological systems, this has often been cited as a limitation of BNs as applied to biology. However, if the dimension of time is considered, loops can be modelled using dynamic Bayesian networks (DBNs) [59].

DBNs represent all variables at two (or more) points in time. In the most basic case, there are two *time slices*: t and $t + \Delta t$; the only links allowed are those from variables in t to those in $t + \Delta t$, and all variables in t are linked to themselves in $t + \Delta t$. In this way, cyclic dependencies over time can be represented (Fig. 9.4(a)–(b)). Such a DBN makes a first-order Markov assumption: the DBN can be conceptually "rolled out" to represent more than one time slice (Fig. 9.4(c)); doing so, we can read conditional independence from the BN structure and see that all variables in one time slice, given their parents in the most recent time slice, are conditionally independent of all previous times. Multi-order DBNs (Fig. 9.4(d)) and DBNs with intra-slice connections (Fig. 9.4(e)) are also possible; these latter, of course, need to maintain acyclicity among variables within a time slice.

Another advantage that DBNs have over static BNs—in addition to modelling loops—is that equivalence classes cease to present a problem for causal interpretation of links. While an equivalence class member of a DBN structure may exist with links reversed in time,[2] and while it may be true that knowledge of a variable at $t + \Delta t$ may be useful for predicting its past value at t, the only possible causal interpretation of the DBN is that variables in t have causal influence on variables in $t + \Delta t$. The problem of accuracy of this causal interpretation is transferred to those shared by any inference based on observation of sequential events: did one directly cause the other, is there an indirect relationship through an unobserved variable, or are there unmeasured factors that contributed independently to both? When using DBNs to model a system, in most cases the goal is to include all relevant variables in the model; links are thus usually interpreted to represent direct causation. The possibility of unmeasured intermediates or common influences, however, is always prudent to keep in mind.

---

[1]It is worth noting that the addition of tired has formed a *v-structure* [60] that has no other equivalence class representation; this thus uniquely orients all links in the BN, enabling causal interpretation.

[2]Note that with basic DBNs, which include self-links from a variable in one time to itself in the next, the only link reversals would be those to variables in $t + \Delta t$ without influence from different variables in t: the convergence of self-links and links from other variables creates a combinatoric v-structure (as in Fig. 9.3(c)).

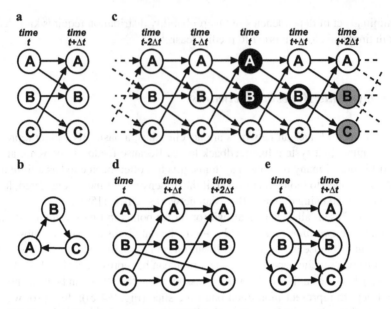

Fig. 9.4 Dynamic Bayesian networks. (**a**) DBN representing a cycle over time among variables A, B, and C. (**b**) Cycle represented by DBN in (**a**). (**c**) DBN of (**a**) "rolled out" in time. Variable B at time $t + \Delta t$ is conditionally independent of its non-descendents (*white nodes*) given its parents in time t; this conditional independence includes all variables prior to time t, demonstrating the first-order Markov assumption. (**d**) Second-order DBN. (**e**) DBN with intra-time slice connections

An important consideration when modelling a system with a DBN is the validity of the Markov assumption. If higher-order Markov relationships are called for, it is a relatively simple matter to use DBNs with more time slices; a more serious problem that can be encountered is when the time resolution measured from the system is less fine than the underlying causal dynamics. For example, if measuring the number of cars at various city intersections, it would be a reasonable assumption that the volume of cars at one intersection could be useful for predicting the volume of cars one block away and a few minutes in the future: such dependence would have the direct causal interpretation that the cars from one intersection travelled the intervening distance during that time, and were now contributing to the count of cars one block away. However, if instead of every few minutes, traffic density at each intersection was measured at 9 a.m. every day, it is a less reasonable assumption that the volume of cars at one intersection could be useful for predicting the volume of cars at another intersection *the following day*. One could still build a DBN to represent this data, and perhaps even find statistical structure in it. The interpretation of links in such a DBN would not be nearly so straightforward, and might involve more complicated relationships mediated by features such as individuals' expectation of better commuting routes based on their experiences the previous day.

Thus, in systems where time series data are available, DBNs are useful for modelling loops and for facilitating causal interpretation. However, when interpreting these networks, the level of coverage of relevant variables and the time scale of samples as related to system dynamics should be kept in mind.

9.3 Structure Learning in Bayesian Networks

9.3.1 Overview

When using Bayesian networks to probe biological systems, the building of a fully parameterised BN capable of making predictions is not necessarily the goal; it is the dependency structure among variables that is of paramount interest. Identification of these dependencies requires only determination of the graphical structure of the BN that describes the joint probability distribution of variables in one's data set. This is known as *structure learning* of BNs.

It is generally considered that BN structure learning can be done from one of two perspectives: (1) performing tests to identify all conditional independence relationships among measured variables (e.g. [2, 11, 52, 79]) or (2) using a score, which indicates how well a particular BN structure describes a given data set, as the criteria in a search to identify the best BN structure (e.g. [35]). However, Cowell [15] has shown that the two methods can be mathematically equivalent. The scoring method has been most commonly applied in biological systems [24, 53].

Scoring methods require heuristic search, since finding the BN with the highest score is NP-complete [12]. A variety of search techniques are used in biological applications, such as greedy search [96], simulated annealing [34, 89, 96], or genetic algorithms [1, 96]. Additionally, model averaging approaches have been developed to either provide a summary of "best" solutions from a heuristic search [34] or, as is becoming more popular, to provide a fully Bayesian picture of the probability of each link being in the solution [25, 37, 51].

BN scores can be subdivided into those aiming to provide a most concise description of both the model and the data (MDL: minimum description length [46, 81]; MML: minimum message length [87]), and those calculating a Bayesian scoring metric (BSM) that estimates the probability of the graph given the data, $P(G|D)$ [2, 6, 13, 26, 35, 39, 78]. Again, there is mathematical equivalence between the two types of scores [23]; here, we concentrate on scores calculating a BSM. The BSM is generally represented as a log of $P(G|D)$, and, expanded via Bayes' rule, can be written as:

$$BSM(G:D) = \log P(G|D) = \log P(D|G) + \log P(G) - \log P(D). \quad (9.2)$$

In practise, $P(D)$ is left as an uncalculated constant. The prior over graphs, $P(G)$, can be used to incorporate prior knowledge about network structure. We will cover usage of $P(G)$ tailored for biological systems later; here we address the basic situation when there is no reason to prefer some structures over others, and $P(G)$, too, is left uncalculated. This leaves $P(D|G)$ to be either calculated or approximated. As an example, we describe the direct calculation of $P(D|G)$ using the BDe score (Bayesian Dirichlet equivalent) [6, 13, 35, 78], which has been widely applied to biological systems.

9.3.2 Bayesian Dirichlet Equivalent Score

The BDe calculates the marginal probability $P(D|G)$ for a discrete Bayesian network by integrating over all possible parameter settings Θ for graph G:

$$P(D|G) = \int_{\Theta} P(D|G, \Theta) P(G|\Theta) \, d\Theta. \qquad (9.3)$$

This integration provides an inherent penalty for complexity of G; this is in contrast to, for example, the BIC score (Bayesian Information Criterion) which asymptotically approximates $P(G|D)$ and includes an explicit penalty for complexity based on the dimensionality of Θ [35]. The integral of (9.3) is solvable, if the prior over parameters $P(G|D)$ is assumed to be distributed in a Dirichlet manner. Details of this derivation can be found in Heckerman [35]; here, we simply present the solution:

$$P(D|G) = \prod_{i=1}^{n} \prod_{j=1}^{q_i} \left\{ \frac{\Gamma(\alpha_{ij})}{\Gamma(\alpha_{ij} + N_{ij})} \prod_{k=1}^{r_i} \frac{\Gamma(\alpha_{ijk} + N_{ijk})}{\Gamma(\alpha_{ijk})} \right\}, \qquad (9.4)$$

where n is the number of variables X_i in the set χ, q_i is the number of possible instantiations of parent states $pa(X_i)$ of the parents of X_i, r_i is the number of value states x_i of X_i, $\Gamma(\cdot)$ is the gamma function (continuous extension of the factorial), α_{ij} and α_{ijk} are equivalent sample size statistics of the Dirichlet prior distribution, and N_{ij} and N_{ijk} are counts in D of the number of times the parents of X_i take on instantiation j, and the number of times the variable X_i takes on value k with parents in instantiation j, respectively. The BDe score is then calculated from these values in the data as the log of this probability.

Inspection of (9.4) can assist in understanding how the BDe score relates to the data. The rightmost term, $\Gamma(\alpha_{ijk} + N_{ijk})/\Gamma(\alpha_{ijk})$, is higher when the counts N_{ijk} for the jth parent state of the ith node are concentrated in a particular child value. Thus, the score is higher when a particular parent state is more useful for predicting a particular child state: this matches the definition of statistical dependence. The leftmost term, $\Gamma(\alpha_{ij})/\Gamma(\alpha_{ij} + N_{ij})$, is higher when (1) the counts N_{ij} are distributed evenly across parent states j and (2) there are fewer possible parent states. The first feature simply indicates that higher scoring networks are possible when the data set includes equal numbers of examples showing outcome across possible combinations of parent states. The second feature is the inherent penalty for complexity: more complex networks can only increase the score if the detriment from more parents (leftmost term) is counterbalanced by increased predictive value for the child (rightmost term) [95].

Two other considerations affect the value of the BDe score: the number of discrete states q_i for each variable and the value of the Dirichlet distribution's equivalent sample size (ess; used to calculate α_{ij} and α_{ijk}). In systems with actual discrete variables, there is little the user can do to modify the effect of number of discrete states; however, BNs are often applied to systems with continuous variables that are then discretized for analysis. In such situations, or in ones where many states may be collapsed into fewer, the following implications of number of discrete states are of interest. More discrete states maintains more information present in original continuous data; fewer discrete states masks noise. More discrete states can lead to more predictive power from parent to child (rightmost term in (9.4)); fewer discrete states leads to greater statistical power to find relationships (leftmost term). Thus, choosing the number of levels for discretisation represents finding a balance between opposing influences on the accuracy of results.

In practical application in biology, a relative low number of discretisation levels is usually chosen, e.g. two to four, corresponding to concepts such as "on/off" or "low/medium/high". Yu et al. [96] did simulation studies identifying three states as optimal for gene regulatory networks; however, the generalisability of this result to more complicated gene regulation or beyond genetic systems is unclear. Additionally, because statistical power for finding relationships is increased with equal examples of parent states (leftmost term in (9.4)), using a discretisation strategy that results in equal distribution across states is desirable. However, care must be taken to consider the biological meaning behind values. For example, while in genetic systems, the difference between no transcripts of a gene and one transcript (or even a few hundred) may be of no consequence, making it is reasonable to lump zero and other values together as "low", in ecological systems, the difference between no predators and a single predator can be highly biologically significant [57]. Thus, knowledge of the system must be combined with that of the score's properties to choose appropriate discretisation methods.

The contribution of the Dirichlet's ess to the BDe score is usually conceptualised as how many data points worth of belief one has that "anything can happen": the higher the ess, the less statistical dependence required between variables for a link to increase the score [80], and thus the easier it is for any link to be found. Low values of ess (e.g. one or two) are thus used to put a high burden on the data for providing evidence for relationships. While this is true, to gain a more detailed understanding of the effect of the ess—and to avoid pitfalls blind extensions of this concept can create—it is worthwhile to return to the step between (9.3) and (9.4) above. This step is the assumption of the prior over parameters, $P(G|\Theta)$, to be distributed as a Dirichlet.

The Dirichlet distribution is the extension of the beta distribution to the multivariate domain [45], and takes the form:

$$\text{Dirichlet}(\theta_1, \ldots, \theta_r; \alpha_1, \ldots, \alpha_r) = \frac{\Gamma(\sum_{k=1}^{r} \alpha_k)}{\prod_{k=1}^{r} \Gamma(\alpha_k)} \prod_{k=1}^{r} \theta_k^{\alpha_k - 1}, \tag{9.5}$$

for r variables $\theta_1, \ldots, \theta_r$ with parameters (or hyperparameters, in the context of a prior) $\alpha_1, \ldots, \alpha_r$.

The first issue to address is precisely what we are assuming follows a Dirichlet distribution. Recall that in a discrete BN, Θ consists of a collection of $\theta_{x_i|pa(X_i)}$ for each variable X_i. These $\theta_{x_i|pa(X_i)}$ form a conditional probability table (CPT) relating the probability of X_i taking on any of its values given a particular parent instantiation; each element of this table can also be referred to as θ_{ijk}, related to $\theta_{x_i|pa(X_i)}$ for the probability of the ith node taking on the kth value x_i for the jth parent instantiation $pa(X_i)$. It is a single row of this CPT that we assume is distributed as a Dirichlet: the prior over parameters is a Dirichlet over the variables $\theta_{ij1}, \ldots, \theta_{ijr}$,

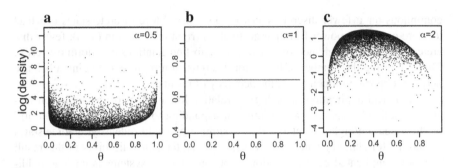

Fig. 9.5 Dirichlet distribution. Projection of log-probability density for 10,000 random deviates of the three-variable Dirichlet distribution with equal hyperparameters $\alpha_1 = \alpha_2 = \alpha_3 = \alpha$ onto one of the variables θ for (**a**) $\alpha = 0.5$, (**b**) $\alpha = 1$, and (**c**) $\alpha = 2$. Note differing scales of y-axes; log of probability density is plotted to emphasise curvature

corresponding to the parameters θ_{ijk} for each of the r possible child states in the jth row of node i's CPT. This Dirichlet's hyperparameters, $\alpha_{ij1}, \ldots, \alpha_{ijr}$, correspond to the α_{ijk} in (9.4); α_{ij} in (9.4) is simply a shorthand for the sum $\alpha_{ij} = \sum_{k=1}^{r} \alpha_{ijk}$.

Now that we know what we assume is distributed as a Dirichlet, it is necessary to cover how the ess relates to the hyperparameters of this distribution. In the most common form of the BDe score, the BDeu (Bayesian Dirichlet equivalent uniform) [35], the hyperparameters α_{ijk} are calculated from the ess to be equal for all r child states and q parent instantiations of node i: $\alpha_{ijk} = ess/rq$, i.e. all hyperparameters are equal in each Dirichlet distribution, and each row of the CPT for a node is assumed to follow the same Dirichlet distribution.

With this knowledge, we can consider implications of modifying the values of the ess. At the simplest level, we note that the higher the ess, the higher are the α_{ijk} and α_{ij} values in (9.4). But it is more instructive to consider how adjustment to the ess modifies the prior. The typical low values of ess lead to α_{ijk}'s that are less than one; the Dirichlet corresponding to these hyperparameters is a U-shape (Fig. 9.5(a)). Thus, our prior belief of the parameters in G is that the CPT table of a child node contains probabilities which follow a U-shaped distribution: they are likely to be very low, or very high, but less likely to be medial values. Because the distribution is defined across a row of the CPT and is constrained to sum to one, this means our prior belief is that any given row of the CPT most likely contains a mix of high and low values. Such a prior is reassuringly sensible: the assumption is that if a link exists in G, then given a parent state j, we expect some child values k to be more probable than others, i.e. the parents are useful for predicting the child.

As we increase the ess, the camber of the Dirichlet's U decreases until at $\alpha_{ijk} = 1$ it reaches a straight line (Fig. 9.5(b)). For $\alpha_{ijk} > 1$, the Dirichlet forms a hump (Fig. 9.5(c)); the prior assumption is now that if a link exists in G, then given a parent state j, we expect the child values k to have similar, medial probabilities. This means that we assume the parents are of no use for predicting the child! Thus, increasing the ess in the hope of finding more links—following the logic that a higher ess makes links easier to reveal—can backfire, as at some point this will change the nature of the prior belief behind the meaning of a link in the graph. This occurs simultaneously with increasing this prior's strength and thus its contribution to the posterior. Therefore, it is prudent to choose an ess which maintains $\alpha_{ijk} < 1$.

As can be seen by the above discussion, the score used for identifying the best BN to describe a data set can have a number of implications involving choices made by the user as well as features of the data itself; much of the work in BNs applied to biological systems relates to developing modifications to the score to take advantage of biological knowledge (e.g. calculation of $P(G)$ [4, 40]) or the development of new scores tailored to the statistical properties of a system [19].

9.4 Bayesian Networks in Biology

9.4.1 Complex Biological Systems

Biology is rife with complex systems formed of networks of interacting variables; in many cases the identities of the partners in these interactions are both unknown and of great interest to discover. Thus, structure learning of Bayesian networks can be a powerful tool for understanding biological systems.

The "genomic revolution" led to BNs entering biology through attempts to make sense of the large amounts of data suddenly available in molecular biology, and particularly gene expression measured by microarrays. Molecular biology remains the area of most popular application of structure learning of BNs in biology, despite some rather drastic mismatches between the requirements of BNs and the available data; instead of stymying progress in this area, these challenges have lead to a number of advances in BN methodology applied to molecular systems. BNs have recently gained use in neuroscience, where the needs of BNs and the available data are more congruent; additionally, the theory that neurons in fact perform Bayesian inference [73] suggests that BNs may be highly suited to modelling this biological domain. One more biological application of BNs is in ecology; research here is in very early stages, but the need to understand interactions within ecological systems in the context of outside of influence from human activities and global climate change [71] means that ecology is a very promising area for BN analysis.

9.4.2 Molecular Biology

Friedman et al. [27] first applied Bayesian networks to gene expression microarray data with the intent to recover transcriptional regulatory networks. This was quickly followed by a number of similar applications [33, 34, 38, 63, 68, 69].

BNs were seen to be well suited for gene regulation, for unlike other modelling frameworks, they are capable of capturing many types of relationships expected in molecular systems; for example, gene expression is known to be stochastic [55] and expected to contain non-linear features such as non-monotonic (where both high and low levels may have suppressive effects) and non-additive (where all elements of regulatory complex are required to be present for gene activation) relationships. Early on, Murphy and Mian [59] suggested that DBNs could overcome the perceived limitation of BNs' cyclicity constraint for genetic systems, in which feedback loops are expected to be major components. This was supported by simulation studies and successful applications [51, 70, 76, 96]. Thus, many researchers have gone on to develop and improve BNs and DBNs specifically for application to gene expression data.

Because a natural question of gene regulatory interactions is whether they are activating or suppressing, researchers developed methods of annotating links in BNs with directional semantics. Hartemink et al. [33] enabled identification of up-regulatory (+), down-regulatory (–), or non-monotonic links. Yu et al. [96] expanded on this to provide an influence score giving both the sign (+/–) and magnitude (scaled 0–1) of the relationship between two genes.

A major challenge for learning structure of BNs from microarray data is that the data amount is relatively limited: at most several hundred data points, often around 20–50, are available. Friedman et al.'s initial application [27] used 76 gene expression data points to find static BNs; Ong et al.'s later work [63] recovered DBNs from only 12! Because structure learning in BNs performs poorly with low data amount [35, 88, 96], much work in the molecular realm has been geared towards enabling more accurate recovery of BNs from limited data. Using only provided microarray data, one can post-process links based on magnitude of influence score [96], interpolate in time series [96], limit the number of parents per variable considered [31, 95], and use conditional independence tests to provide better starting networks for heuristic search [88]. Other methods take advantage of biological intervention experiments (e.g. mutations, knockouts, over-expression, drug interference, etc.), and develop BSMs and search techniques tailored for these types of experiments [14, 18, 68, 69, 83, 94].

The large body of genomics and bioinformatics data provides an additional avenue to improving BN representation of gene regulation through the prior over graphs $P(G)$. For example, ChIP-chip (chromatin immunoprecipitation on a gene chip) data provides information about where on a genome particular proteins bind; this information can be used to suggest gene regulatory interactions if a transcription factor (a protein which influences gene expression) binds upstream of a gene. Such data can be used to rule out interactions which are not supported [34], adjust $P(G)$ to give a higher probability to supported interactions while still allowing novel interactions given strong evidence from the data [40], and even model confidence in the original ChIP-chip data using $P(G)$ [4]. $P(G)$ can incorporate other types of biological knowledge such as the location of binding motifs, sequences of DNA to which a transcription factor is known to bind [40, 82, 84], and outcome of prior intervention experiments [41]. Werhli and Husmeier [90] have developed an extensible framework to incorporate multiple sources of prior biological knowledge into a $P(G)$ value simultaneously.

Other imaginative methods of incorporating prior biological knowledge into BNs have been developed, ranging from creation of nodes representing protein complexes [40, 62] to simplifying the heuristic search [17, 47]. With all of these developments tailoring BNs to gene expression data, BNs are now being employed to discover novel biological knowledge: for example, exploring networks related to specific biological functions [99], identifying candidate genes for disease [50, 54], and even using BN structure to assist in identifying binding motifs [9].

In addition to gene expression, more types of molecular data are now available in high-throughput quantities. Metabolic flux, protein expression, and phosphoprotein expression have been used to discover networks representing signalling pathways [30, 49, 74]. Of particular note is Sachs et al. [74], who used phosphoprotein and phospholipid expression to recover known signalling pathways, as well as validated novel predicted interactions. Many of these newer molecular data types, such as the flow cytometry measurements used by Sachs et al. [74], come in much greater quantities (e.g. thousands of data points), and are expected to be more even more amenable to BN analysis. Thus, molecular biology is a continuing area for development and application of BNs.

9.4.3 Neuroscience

Neuroscience burst onto the Bayesian network structure learning scene in 2006 with three independent applications of BNs to neural data [77, 97, 98]. Two analysed fMRI (functional magnetic resonance imaging) data, which uses magnetic signals from haemoglobin to measure blood flow to—and thus infer neural activity of—regions in the brain [97, 98]; one analysed extracellular, multi-unit electrophysiology data, which uses implanted electrodes to record action potentials from nearby neurons, providing an activity level measure for a brain region [77].

Both Zhang et al. [97] and Zheng and Rajapakse [98] applied the BIC score for static, continuous Gaussian BNs to recover networks among brain areas from fMRI data of humans performing cognitive tasks. Smith et al. [77] used the BDe score to learn discrete DBNs from electrophysiology of the auditory regions of songbirds; theses DBNs were compared to known anatomical structure of the auditory system, enabling evaluation of accuracy of the results. In contrast to a previous, linear-based method of recovering neural information flow (partial directed coherence: PDC [75]), the DBN recovered only accurate connections, corresponding to neural information flow along physical connections in the brain [77]. This work thus gave confidence for the ability of BNs to accurately reveal pathways of neural information flow.

Further work analysing fMRI data has introduced the use of DBNs [7, 72]. In all these fMRI applications, much care has been taken in the interpretation of networks due to issues related to the time scales involved (as discussed in Sect. 9.2.3): fMRI measures blood flow, assumed to be a proxy for neural activity, on a time scale of seconds; however, neural activity travels between brain regions in milliseconds. Thus, DBNs built from fMRI data cannot have the direct causal interpretation of neural information flow from action potentials travelling down axons; instead the connections are interpreted as reflective of slower mental dynamics [7, 72, 97, 98].

Further work analysing electrophysiology data has concentrated on applying BNs to spike train data; spike trains are recordings of action potentials of, not groups, but individual neurons. The goal with electrophysiology continues to be to find BNs that can be interpreted as direct neural signals travelling between nodes. Spike trains have two major issues for BNs: (1) potential irregularity of the lag between the signal from one neuron and the response of another, due to neural integration of signals over time and variations in transmission time along axons and (2) a distribution across the discrete states of firing versus not firing that is heavily biased towards not firing.

Eldawlatly et al. [20–22] applied the BDe to find DBNs from simulated spike train data, showing improved recovery of DBNs over static BNs and other neural information flow methods: PDC [75] and generalised linear models (GLM) [85]. Multiple potential time-lags between neurons were incorporated using high-order Markov models in the DBNs [22]. Jung [42] also used the BDe on simulated spike trains, addressing both issues presented by spike train data by recovering static BNs with spike frequency calculated in large time bins (e.g. 150 ms). The large time bins were expected to contain influences between neurons across multiple possible time delays (which only range on the order of around ten or less milliseconds), and thus result in statistical dependencies between simultaneously sampled bins; additionally, the frequency transformation enabled discretisation of a now-continuous value [42].

Echtermeyer et al. [19] directly addressed the two issues facing spike train data for BNs by developing a new score: the Snap Shot Score (SSS). The SSS is a likelihood score capturing probability of firing due to excitatory influences. It avoids artefacts due to biased distribution of discrete states by assigning semantics and treating firing and not firing states differently; it explicitly includes multiple time lags through a time-averaged transformation of parent spike trains. The SSS was shown to perform well on simulated spike trains, including with only partial observability of the simulated circuit: a highly likely situation for real data [19].

All BN applications to spike trains have thus far only evaluated accuracy in simulations; however, given the growing popularity of BNs in neuroscience, applications to real spike train data cannot be far away. Curiously, the only other BN application to electrophysiology data to date has been in fact not to neurons, but to muscles: Li [48] used the BIC to recover Gaussian BNs based on surface electromyograms (sEMG), which measure electrical signals from contracting muscles using electrodes on the skin. BNs among muscles were interpreted to be reflective of interactions among their driving neural processes [48].

Because neural data can come in quantities of thousands, to tens or hundreds of thousands, of data points, neural systems are well-suited to data-hungry BN structure learning. Other types of neural data exist: for example, calcium imaging of individual cells, which measures the calcium influx related to neural firing [29]; electroencephalography (EEG), which measures electrical signals of neurons from scalp electrodes; magnetoencephalography (MEG), which measures magnetic fields produced by action potentials in the brain using superconducting quantum interference devices (SQUIDs); and more [3]. It is very likely that BNs will soon be applied to all these neural data types, serving an important role in future research into deciphering brain function.

9.4.4 Ecology

The newest biological discipline to see application of Bayesian network structure learning is ecology. Ecological systems consist of a vast web of interacting species and environmental characteristics, and it has been recognised that understanding these interactions is important for understanding impact of climate change and human activities on these systems [16, 67, 71]. However, revealing ecological networks has until now required detailed field data of interaction events or been limited to simple statistical methods or to small, simple systems (e.g. [44, 56]). BNs represent a way to reveal ecological network structure using species counts and environmental measures that are relatively easy to obtain.

Milns et al. [57] applied the BDe score to recover static BNs of bird and habitat interactions in the Peak District National Park. In order to handle difficulties presented by biased distributions of discrete states and inconsistent search, they developed advances in pre-processing of contingencies and in model averaging of search results. The recovered BNs corresponded to known species and habitat interactions, providing confidence for BN application in ecology [57].

Additionally, the BNs provided useful insights into the system and avenues for further research. In particular, interactions depended upon the spatial scale analysed; this suggested that the spatially explicit ecological data, which consisted of counts in different physical locations, may provide an arena for development of BNs tailored for spatial analysis [57]. Since much neural data also comes in a spatially explicit form, and many molecular processes occur in defined cellular locations (although this is not yet subject to high-throughput measurement), such BN development for ecological systems may prove synergistic for other areas of biology.

9.5 Conclusion

Bayesian network structure learning in biology has rapidly expanded from initial application in 2000, to include—in less than a decade—many types of biological data across molecular, neural, and ecological sciences. BNs are likely to continue to spread within these disciplines, as well as potentially into other areas of biology. There are now a number of tools available for BN structure learning in biology, variously tailored to a particular system or general for all BNs: two related Matlab toolboxes [36, 58], three packages for the open source statistical software R [5, 8, 10], three standalone applications [19, 32, 92], and two web interfaces [61, 92]. Easy access by biologists to such tools suggests BNs will continue to spread in biological application.

While this chapter has concentrated on the benefits that BNs have for biology, in doing so we have seen the benefits biology has had for BNs. Structure learning in BNs entered biology through the molecular realm, where limitations of available data lead to advances in dealing with low data amount, heuristic search, incorporation of prior information, and scoring metrics. BNs have only recently been applied to neural data, and already a new BN score has been developed. The single application of BNs to ecology necessitated its own advances. Thus, as BNs have found a new home in the biological sciences, research has fed back advances which can improve BN application in many domains.

Acknowledgements   I am grateful to Dr. Charles Twardy for a critical reading of the manuscript.

References

1. Auliac, C., Frouin, V., Gidrol, X., d'Alché Buc, F.: Evolutionary approaches for the reverse-engineering of gene regulatory networks: a study on a biologically realistic dataset. BMC Bioinform. **9**, 91 (2008)
2. Bach, F., Jordan, M.: Learning graphical models with Mercer kernels. In: Advances in Neural Information Processing Systems 15, pp. 1033–1040. MIT Press, Cambridge (2003)
3. Bandettini, P.: What's new in neuroimaging methods? Ann. N.Y. Acad. Sci. **1156**, 260–293 (2009)
4. Bernard, A., Hartemink, A.: Informative structure priors: joint learning of dynamic regulatory networks from multiple types of data. In: Pacific Symposium of Biocomputing 10, pp. 459–470. World Scientific, Singapore (2005)
5. Bøttcher, S., Dethlefsen, C.: DEAL: A package for learning Bayesian networks. J. Stat. Softw. **8**, 1–40 (2003)
6. Buntine, W.: Theory refinement on Bayesian networks. In: Proceedings of the 7th Conference on Uncertainty in Artificial Intelligence, pp. 52–60. Morgan Kaufmann, San Mateo (1991)
7. Burge, J., Lane, T., Link, H., Qiu, S., Clark, V.: Discrete dynamic Bayesian network analysis of fMRI data. Hum. Brain Mapp. **30**, 122–137 (2009)
8. Chavan, S.S., Bauer, M.A., Scutari, M, Nagarajan, R.: NATbox: a network analysis toolbox in R. BMC Bioinform. **10**, Suppl 11:S14 (2009)
9. Chen, X., Blanchette, M.: Prediction of tissue-specific cis-regulatory modules using Bayesian networks and regression trees. BMC Bioinform. **8**, Suppl 10:S2 (2007)
10. Chen, X., Chen, M., Ning, K.: BNArray: an R package for constructing gene regulatory networks from microarray data by using Bayesian network. Bioinformatics **22**, 2952–2954 (2006)
11. Cheng, J., Bell, D., Liu, W.: Learning belief networks from data: an information theory based approach. In: Proceedings of the 6th International Conference on Information and Knowledge Management, pp. 325–331. ACM Press, New York (1997)
12. Chickering, D.: Learning Bayesian networks is NP-complete. In: Fisher, D., Lenz, H.J. (eds.) Learning from Data: Artificial Intelligence and Statistics V. Lecture Notes in Statistics, vol. 112, pp. 121–130. Springer, Berlin (1996)
13. Cooper, G., Herskovits, E.: A Bayesian method for the induction of probabilistic networks from data. Mach. Learn. **9**, 309–347 (1992)
14. Cooper, G., Yoo, C.: Causal discovery from a mixture of experimental and observational data. In: Proceedings of the 15th Conference on Uncertainty in Artificial Intelligence, pp. 116–125. Morgan Kaufmann, San Mateo (1999)
15. Cowell, R.: Conditions under which conditional independence and scoring methods lead to identical selection of Bayesian network models. In: Proceedings of the 17th Conference in Uncertainty in Artificial Intelligence, pp. 91–97. Morgan Kaufmann, San Mateo (2001)

16. Davis, A., Jenkinson, L., Lawton, J., Shorrocks, B., Wood, S.: Making mistakes when predicting shifts in species range in response to global warming. Nature **391**, 783–786 (1998)
17. Djebbari, A., Quackenbush, J.: Seeded Bayesian networks: constructing genetic networks from microarray data. BMC Syst. Biol. **2**, 57 (2008)
18. Dojer, N., Gambin, A., Mizera, A., Wilczyński, B., Tiuryn, J.: Applying dynamic Bayesian networks to perturbed gene expression data. BMC Bioinform. **7**, 249 (2006)
19. Echtermeyer, C., Smulders, T., Smith, V.: Causal pattern recovery from neural spike train data using the Snap Shot Score. J. Comput. Neurosci. **29**, 231–252 (2010). doi:10.1007/s10827-009-0174-2
20. Eldawlatly, S., Zhou, Y., Jin, R., Oweiss, K.: Reconstructing functional neuronal circuits using dynamic Bayesian networks. In: Proceedings of the 30th Annual International Conference of the IEEE Engineering in Medicine and Biology Society, pp. 5531–5534 (2008)
21. Eldawlatly, S., Zhou, Y., Jin, R., Oweiss, K.: Inferring functional cortical networks from spike train ensembles using dynamic Bayesian networks. In: Proceedings of the 2009 IEEE International Conference on Acoustics, Speech and Signal Processing, pp. 3489–3492 (2009)
22. Eldawlatly, S., Zhou, Y., Jin, R., Oweiss, K.: On the use of dynamic Bayesian networks in reconstructing functional neuronal networks from spike train ensembles. Neural Comput. **22**, 158–189 (2010)
23. Friedman, N.: Learning belief networks in the presence of missing values and hidden variables. In: Proceedings of the 14th International Conference on Machine Learning, pp. 125–133. Morgan Kaufmann, San Mateo (1997)
24. Friedman, N.: Inferring cellular networks using probabilistic graphical models. Science **303**, 799–805 (2004)
25. Friedman, N., Koller, D.: Being Bayesian about network structure. Mach. Learn. **50**, 95–125 (2003)
26. Friedman, N., Murphy, K., Russell, S.: Learning the structure of dynamic probabilistic networks. In: Proceedings of the 14th Conference on Uncertainty in Artificial Intelligence, pp. 139–147. Morgan Kaufmann, San Mateo (1998)
27. Friedman, N., Linial, M., Nachman, I., Pe'er, D.: Using Bayesian networks to analyze expression data. J. Comput. Biol. **7**, 601–620 (2000)
28. Fusco, G.: Looking for sustainable urban mobility through Bayesian networks. Sci. Reg./Ital. J. Reg. Sci. **3**, 87–106 (2003)
29. Grewe, B., Helmchen, F.: Optical probing of neuronal ensemble activity. Curr. Opin. Neurobiol. **19**, 520–529 (2009)
30. Guha, U., Chaerkady, R., Marimuthu, A., Patterson, A., Kashyap, M., Harsha, H., Sato, M., Bader, J., Lash, A., Minna, J., Pandey, A., Varmus, H.: Comparisons of tyrosine phosphorylated proteins in cells expressing lung cancer-specific alleles of EGFR and KRAS. Proc. Natl. Acad. Sci. USA **105**, 14112–14117 (2008)
31. Hansen, A., Ott, S., Koentges, G.: Increasing feasibility of optimal gene network estimation. Genome Inform. **15**, 141–150 (2004)
32. Hartemink, A.: Banjo: Bayesian Network Inference with Java Objects (2005). http://www.cs.duke.edu/~amink/software/banjo
33. Hartemink, A., Gifford, D., Jaakkola, T., Young, R.: Using graphical models and genomic expression data to statistically validate models of genetic regulatory networks. In: Pacific Symposium of Biocomputing, vol. 6, pp. 422–433. World Scientific, Singapore (2001)
34. Hartemink, A., Gifford, D., Jaakkola, T., Young, R.: Combining location and expression data for principled discovery of genetic regulatory network models. In: Pacific Symposium on Biocomputing, vol. 7, pp. 437–449. World Scientific, Singapore (2002)
35. Heckerman, D.: A tutorial on learning with Bayesian networks. Technical Report MSR-TR-95–06, Microsoft Research (1995)
36. Husmeier, D.: Inferring dynamic Bayesian networks with MCMC (2003). http://www.bioss.ac.uk/~dirk/software/DBmcmc
37. Husmeier, D.: Sensitivity and specificity of inferring genetic regulatory interactions from microarray experiments with dynamic Bayesian networks. Bioinformatics **19**, 2271–2282 (2003)

38. Imoto, S., Goto, T., Miyano, S.: Estimation of genetic networks and functional structures between genes by using Bayesian networks and nonparametric regression. In: Pacific Symposium on Biocomputing, vol. 7, pp. 175–186. World Scientific, Singapore (2002)
39. Imoto, S., Kim, S., Goto, T., Miyano, S., Aburatani, S., Tashiro, K., Kuhara, S.: Bayesian network and nonparametric heteroscedastic regression for nonlinear modeling of genetic network. J. Bioinform. Comput. Biol. **1**, 231–252 (2003)
40. Imoto, S., Higuchi, T., Goto, T., Tashiro, K., Kuhara, S., Miyano, S.: Combining microarrays and biological knowledge for estimating gene networks via Bayesian networks. J. Bioinform. Comput. Biol. **2**, 77–98 (2004)
41. Imoto, S., Tamada, Y., Araki, H., Yasuda, K., Print, C., Charnock-Jones, S., Sanders, D., Savoie, C., Tashiro, K., Kuhara, S., Miyano, S.: Computational strategy for discovering druggable gene networks from genome-wide RNA expression profiles. In: Pacific Symposium on Biocomputing, vol. 11, pp. 559–571. World Scientific, Singapore (2006)
42. Jung, S., Nam, Y., Lee, D.: Inference of combinatorial neuronal synchrony with Bayesian networks. J. Neurosci. Methods **186**, 130–139 (2010)
43. Kiiveri, H., Speed, T., Carlin, J.: Recursive causal models. J. Aust. Math. Soc. A **36**, 30–52 (1984)
44. Knight, C., Beale, C.: Pale Rock Sparrow *Carpospiza brachydactyla* in the Mount Lebanon range: modelling breeding habitat. Ibis **147**, 324–333 (2005)
45. Kotz, S., Balakrishnan, N., Johnson, N.: Continuous Multivariate Distributions, vol. 1. Wiley-Interscience, New York (2000)
46. Lam, W., Bacchus, F.: Learning Bayesian belief networks: an approach based on the MDL principle. Comput. Intell. **10**, 269–293 (1994)
47. Lee, P., Lee, D.: Modularized learning of genetic interaction networks from biological annotations and mRNA expression data. Bioinformatics **21**, 2739–2747 (2005)
48. Li, J., Wang, Z., Eng, J., McKeown, M.: Bayesian network modeling for discovering "dependent synergies" among muscles in reaching movements. IEEE Trans. Biomed. Eng. **55**, 298–310 (2008)
49. Li, Z., Chan, C.: Inferring pathways and networks with a Bayesian framework. FASEB J. **18**, 746–748 (2004)
50. Liu, B., Jiang, T., Ma, S., Zhao, H., Li, J., Jiang, X., Zhang, J.: Exploring candidate genes for human brain diseases from a brain-specific gene network. Biochem. Biophys. Res. Commun. **349**, 1308–1314 (2006)
51. Luna, I., Huang, Y., Yin, Y., Padillo, D., Perez, M.: Uncovering gene regulatory networks from time-series microarray data with variational Bayesian structural expectation maximization. EURASIP J. Bioinform. Syst. Biol. **2007**, 71312 (2007)
52. Margaritis, D.: Distribution-free learning of Bayesian network structure in continuous domains. In: Proceedings of the 20th National Conference on Artificial Intelligence, pp. 825–830. AAAI, Washington (2005)
53. Markowetz, F., Spang, R.: Inferring cellular networks—a review. BMC Bioinform. **8**, Suppl 6:S5 (2007)
54. Matthäus, F., Smith, V.A., Fogtman, A., Sommer, W.H., Leonardi-Essmann, F., Lourdusamy, A., Reimers, M., Spanagel, R., Gebicke-Haerter, P.: Interactive molecular networks obtained by computer-aided conversion of microarray data from brains of alcohol-drinking rats. Pharmacopsychiatry **42**, 118–128 (2009)
55. McAdams, H., Arkin, A.: Stochastic mechanisms in gene expression. Proc. Natl. Acad. Sci. USA **94**, 814–819 (1997)
56. Memmott, J., Fowler, S., Paynter, Q., Sheppard, A., Syrett, P.: The invertebrate fauna on broom, *Cytisus scoparius*, in two native and two exotic habitats. Acta Oecol. **21**, 213–222 (2000)
57. Milns, I., Beale, C., Smith, V.: Revealing ecological networks using Bayesian network inference algorithms. Ecology **91**, 1892–1899 (2010). doi:10.1890/09-0731
58. Murphy, K.: The Bayes Net Toolbox for Matlab. Comput. Sci. Stat. **33**, 1024–1034 (2001)
59. Murphy, K., Mian, S.: Modelling gene expression data using dynamic Bayesian networks. Technical report, University of California, Berkeley (1999)

60. Muruzabal, J., Cotta, C.: A primer on the evolution of equivalence classes of Bayesian-network structures. In: Parallel Problem Solving from Nature VIII. Lecture Notes in Computer Science, vol. 3242, pp. 612–621. Springer, Berlin (2004)
61. Myllymaki, P., Silander, T., Tirri, H., Uronen, P.: B-Course: a web-based tool for Bayesian and causal data analysis. Int. J. Artif. Intell. Tools **11**, 369–388 (2002)
62. Nariai, N., Kim, S., Imoto, S., Miyano, S.: Using protein-protein interactions for refining gene networks estimated from microarray data by Bayesian networks. In: Pacific Symposium on Biocomputing, vol. 9, pp. 336–347. World Scientific, Singapore (2004)
63. Ong, I., Glasner, J., Page, D.: Modelling regulatory pathways in *E. coli* from time series expression profiles. Bioinformatics **18**, 241–248 (2002)
64. Pearl, J.: Bayesian networks: a model of self-activated memory for evidential reasoning. In: Proceedings of the 7th Conference of the Cognitive Science Society, pp. 329–334 (1985)
65. Pearl, J.: Probabilistic Reasoning in Intelligent Systems: Networks of Plausible Inference. Morgan Kaufmann, Cambridge (1988). 552 pp.
66. Pearl, J.: Causality. Cambridge University Press, Cambridge (2000)
67. Pearson, R., Dawson, T.: Predicting the impacts of climate change on the distribution of species: are bioclimate envelope models useful? Glob. Ecol. Biogeogr. **12**, 361–371 (2003)
68. Pe'er, D., Regev, A., Tanay, A.: Minreg: inferring an active regulator set. Bioinformatics **18**, 258–267 (2002)
69. Pe'er, D., Regev, A., Elidan, G., Friedman, N.: Inferring subnetworks from perturbed expression profiles. Bioinformatics **17**, 215–224 (2001)
70. Perrin, B.E., Ralaivola, L., Mazurie, A., Bottani, S., Mallet, J., d'Alché Buc, F.: Gene networks inference using dynamic Bayesian networks. Bioinformatics **19**, 138–148 (2003)
71. Proulx, S., Promislow, D., Phillips, P.: Network thinking in ecology and evolution. Trends Ecol. Evol. **20**, 345–353 (2005)
72. Rajapakse, J., Zhou, J.: Learning effective brain connectivity with dynamic Bayesian networks. NeuroImage **37**, 749–760 (2007)
73. Rao, R.: Bayesian computation in recurrent neural circuits. Neural Comput. **16**, 1–38 (2004)
74. Sachs, K., Perez, O., Pe'er, D., Lauffenburger, D., Nolan, G.: Causal protein-signaling networks derived from multiparameter single-cell data. Science **308**, 523–529 (2005)
75. Sameshima, K., Baccalá, L.: Using partial directed coherence to describe neuronal ensemble interactions. J. Neurosci. Methods **94**, 93–103 (1999)
76. Smith, V., Jarvis, E., Hartemink, A.: Influence of network topology and data collection on functional network influence. In: Pacific Symposium on Biocomputing, vol. 8, pp. 164–175. World Scientific, Singapore (2003)
77. Smith, V., Yu, J., Smulders, T., Hartemink, A., Jarvis, E.: Computational inference of neural information flow networks. PLoS Comput. Biol. **2**, 161 (2006)
78. Spiegelhalter, D., Dawid, A., Lauritzen, S., Cowell, R.: Bayesian analysis in expert systems. Stat. Sci. **8**, 219–247 (1993)
79. Spirtes, P., Glymour, C.: An algorithm for fast recovery of sparse causal graphs. Soc. Sci. Comput. Rev. **9**, 62–72 (1991)
80. Steck, H., Jaakkola, T.: On the Dirichlet prior and Bayesian regularization. In: Advances in Neural Information Processing Systems, vol. 15, pp. 713–720. MIT Press, Cambridge (2003)
81. Suzuki, J.: A construction of Bayesian networks from databases on an MDL principle. In: Proceedings of the 9th Conference on Uncertainty in Artificial Intelligence, pp. 266–273. Morgan Kaufmann, San Mateo (1993)
82. Tamada, Y., Kim, S., Bannai, H., Imoto, S., Tashiro, K., Kuhara, S., Miyano, S.: Estimating gene networks from gene expression data by combining Bayesian network model with promoter element detection. Bioinformatics **19**, 227–236 (2003)
83. Tamada, Y., Imoto, S., Tashiro, K., Kuhara, S., Miyano, S.: Identifying drug active pathways from gene networks estimated by gene expression data. Genome Inform. **16**, 182–191 (2005)
84. Tamada, Y., Bannai, H., Imoto, S., Katayama, T., Kanehisa, M., Miyano, S.: Utilizing evolutionary information and gene expression data for estimating gene networks with Bayesian network models. J. Bioinform. Comput. Biol. **3**, 1295–1313 (2005)

85. Truccolo, W., Eden, U., Fellows, M., Donoghue, J., Brown, E.: A point process framework for relating neural spiking activity to spiking history, neural ensemble, and extrinsic covariate effects. J. Neurophysiol. **93**, 1074–1089 (2005)
86. Twardy, C., Koester, R., Gatt, R.: Missing person behaviour: an Australian study. Final Report to the Australian National SAR Council (2006)
87. Wallace, C., Korb, K., Dai, H.: Causal discovery via MML. In: Proceedings of the 13th International Conference on Machine Learning, pp. 516–524. Morgan Kaufmann, San Mateo (1996)
88. Wang, M., Chen, Z., Cloutier, S.: A hybrid Bayesian network learning method for constructing gene networks. Comput. Biol. Chem. **31**, 361–372 (2007)
89. Wang, T., Touchman, J., Xue, G.: Applying two-level simulated annealing on Bayesian structure learning to infer genetic networks. In: Proceedings of the 2004 IEEE Computational Systems Bioinformatics Conference, pp. 647–648 (2004)
90. Werhli, A., Husmeier, D.: Reconstructing gene regulatory networks with Bayesian networks by combining expression data with multiple sources of prior knowledge. Stat. Appl. Genet. Mol. Biol. **6**, 15 (2007)
91. Wermuth, N., Lauritzen, S.: Graphical and recursive models for contingency tables. Biometrika **70**, 537–552 (1983)
92. Wilczynski, B., Dojer, N.: BNFinder: exact and efficient method for learning Bayesian networks. Bioinformatics **25**, 286–287 (2009)
93. Wright, S.: Correlation and causation. J. Agric. Res. **20**, 557–585 (1921)
94. Yoo, C., Thorsson, V., Cooper, G.: Discovery of causal relationships in a gene-regulation pathway from a mixture of experimental and observational DNA microarray data. In: Pacific Symposium of Biocomputing, vol. 10, pp. 498–509. World Scientific, Singapore (2002)
95. Yu, J.: Developing Bayesian network inference algorithms to predict causal functional pathways in biological systems. PhD thesis, Duke University (2005)
96. Yu, J., Smith, V., Wang, P., Hartemink, A., Jarvis, E.: Advances to Bayesian network inference for generating causal networks from observational biological data. Bioinformatics **20**, 3594–3603 (2004)
97. Zhang, L., Samaras, D., Alia-Klein, N., Volkow, N.: Modeling neuronal interactivity using dynamic Bayesian networks. In: Advances in Neural Information Processing Systems, vol. 18. MIT Press, Cambridge (2006)
98. Zheng, X., Rajapakse, J.: Learning functional structure from fMR images. NeuroImage **31**, 1601–1613 (2006)
99. Zhu, J., Jambhekar, A., Sarver, A., DeRisi, J.: A Bayesian network driven approach to model the transcriptional response to nitric oxide in *Saccharomyces cerevisiae*. PLoS ONE **1**, 94 (2006)

Chapter 10
Dynamics and Statistics of Extreme Events

Holger Kantz

Abstract Complex dynamics is characterized by an irregular, non-periodic time
dependence of characteristic quantities. Rare fluctuations which lead to unexpect-
edly large (or small) values are called extreme events. Since such large deviations
from the system's mean behavior have in many applications huge impact, their statistical characterization and their dynamical origin are of relevance. We discuss recent approaches, with special emphasis on dynamics on networks.

10.1 Introduction

Extreme Events as outliers in a time series have been subject to statistical analysis for more than 50 years, since Gumbel has published his book on extreme value
statistics [18] (the pioneering article by Fisher and Tippett [12] is even 30 years
older). In this context, extreme events in a sequence of independently and identi-
cally distributed random variables are either the maximal values among a block of
data (i.e. the maximum in a time window), or they are defined by overcoming a pre-
defined threshold (threshold crossing). The essential result of the statistical theory
is that the distribution of such block maxima asymptotically can be described by a
three-parameter family of *generalized extreme value distributions* (GEV) [9]. Examples where this concept of extremes has been applied are manifold: river levels
with peaks corresponding to flooding, wind speeds with peaks representing violent
gusts, seismic activity with peaks representing earthquakes.

From a more fundamental point of view, extreme events are extraordinarily large
deviations from a system's normal behavior, embedded in a background of everlast-
ing irregular fluctuations. In most systems, both the normal fluctuations and extreme
events are consequences of the complexity of a system's dynamics, as we know it

H. Kantz (✉)
Max Planck Institute for the Physics of Complex Systems, Dresden, Germany
e-mail: kantz@pks.mpg.de

E. Estrada et al. (eds.), *Network Science*,
DOI 10.1007/978-1-84996-396-1_10, © Springer-Verlag London Limited 2010

from daily weather. Only recently, attention moved from the purely statistical analysis of extreme events to the attempt of a detailed understanding of the underlying dynamical processes [1]. Which feedback loops in a system exist so that huge deviations can occur? Are there precursors of such behavior, might the occurrence of an extreme event be predictable? And what are proper scoring rules in order to evaluate the success of a prediction? This latter issue can be easily illustrated for earthquake prediction: If one predicts an earthquake of magnitude larger than six for some place where such earthquakes occur less frequently than once per 100 years, then a mis-prediction by ten days seems negligible from the physical point of view. Nonetheless, from a practical point of view, such a prediction is rather useless, since evacuating a city and not letting people back to their homes till it actually happened is impossible if it happens only ten days later, and if the prediction came ten days too late its uselessness is even more evident. So how to quantify the success or failure of such a prediction?

Scientific approaches towards extreme events currently can be sorted according to the following scheme:

- Statistical analysis such as *Extreme Value Statistics*. Since extreme events by definition are in the tail of any probability distribution, they are rare, and one of the main goals of statistical analysis is the robust estimation of these tails. A typical challenge is the extrapolation to larger observation periods: Determine the magnitude of an event which occurs on average (in the ensemble mean) once per century, given observations from a single time series of 50 years.
- *Data driven predictions* and the search for *precursors* are based on a different type of statistical analysis, which employs conditional probabilities and temporal correlations. In some sense, *data driven models* are more or less compact representations of such temporal dependencies. Such an analysis aims at understanding the dynamics behind extreme events.
- *Simplistic physical models* have been proposed for many different real world phenomena. Among the most well known are sandpile models which are inspired by landslides and which, in modified form, are supposed to have some relevance also for earthquakes. They are useful to investigate particular mechanisms leading to extreme events. Sandpile models gave rise to the concept of *self organized criticality* (SOC). An SOC system drives itself into a critical state (no fine tuning of parameters required), so that, for example, the frequency-magnitude distribution is scale free. Hence, arbitrarily large events might occur, and there are no temporal correlations between successive events.
- *Detailed disciplinary investigations*. Since extreme events are large impact events, many disciplines study "their" extremes with great care. Examples include hydrology and flooding, meteorology and extreme weather, traffic sciences and infrastructure failure.

The exchange between these different approaches should be strongly enhanced in order to make fast progress. In this article, we essentially focus on data based predictions.

10.2 Extreme Events in Networks

Extreme events are time dependent phenomena and hence require dynamics. In the context of networks, extremes can therefore occur (recurrently) if either a network with fixed topology supports some dynamics on its nodes or links (such as a static neuronal network or a traffic network), or if there is some self-regulated dynamical re-wiring of the network. Extremity in a network is related to the values of some characteristic quantity which determines the performance of the network. A typical example is network traffic and congestion. It is evident that depending on the structure of the network, the congestion of some hubs might well affect the performance of the whole network dramatically. So the network specific issue would be how the interaction of network dynamics and network topology enhance or suppress local fluctuations, and whether local network failure spreads over the whole network or not. Evident examples from real world are supply chains, transportation and information networks, and the power grid. Extreme events are congestion and black-outs. Less evident examples are epileptic seizures, which by some researchers are interpreted as a synchronization related network phenomenon [25], and perhaps civil wars, where the breakdown of network links (re-wiring) causes a fragmentation of society.

10.3 Return Times

A relevant statistical quantifier for an extreme event is its frequency. The mean relative frequency of occurrence is a number between zero and unity and describes the average probability that the event occurs at an arbitrary time instance. Its inverse is the mean return time, i.e. the mean time elapsing between two successive events. If events occur independently of each other, then the probability of occurrence is the same at every time instance, and hence the return times are exponentially distributed (a simple point process). A non-exponential return time distribution therefore contains additional information about the extremes.

Two relevant cases are known from the study of experimental data and from simple model simulations: First, return time distributions can have a single hump with a maximum at some non-zero value. This means that the time intervals between successive events tend to assume a typical value, i.e. these extremes are occurring more regularly, and in particular the occurrence a new event right after an event is quite improbable. Examples for this behavior can be found in [3, 14].

The other observed situation is that events might occur as clusters in time. One example for this behavior is the occurrence of earthquakes in earthquake catalogues [22] and models [8]. Inside such a cluster, inter-event times can be quite short, whereas the times in between two clusters can be very long: the system has episodes of activity and episodes of passivity. The return time distribution has, compared to the exponential distribution, more weight around zero and more weight in the tail at large times. It turns out that such behavior is related to long range correlations and that under suitable assumptions the corresponding return time distribution is a stretched exponential [2, 6] or a Weibull-distribution [24] (which in this context has nothing to do with GEV).

10.4 Prediction of Extreme Events

Weather forecast is sometimes a forecast of extremes: A detailed physical model which contains a relevant subset of the physical and thermodynamic processes in the atmosphere is fed with the current atmospheric state as initial condition, and a numerical solution over the following 5–10 days is computed. If this solution displays an extreme weather condition, one could thereby predict an extreme event. There are many subtleties in this process which are responsible for the fact that weather forecasts cannot be obtained by a desktop computer, using initial conditions to be downloaded from the Internet, but are instead produced with huge manpower and huge computer power by large weather services. But, in principle, one could consider applying the same scheme to the prediction of earthquakes, of stock market crashes or of epileptic seizures.

The reason that this is not always the optimal way is twofold: in many situations the physical understanding of the system is much worse than in the case of the atmosphere. This is in particular true for the three examples: earthquakes, stock market, epileptic seizure. Secondly, in most cases, one is not interested in the every-day prediction of normal short term fluctuations, so that the high effort would not pay off. The whole weather prediction business is not sustained because of the few extremes which are thereby predicted, but because the detailed knowledge of the weather itself is required. This is different in epileptic seizures or seismicity. Nobody wants to know a prediction of one's EEG as long as it does not represent an epileptic seizure. Therefore, in many situations the approach will not be to set up a detailed model of the system and to predict the details of the system's behavior. The simpler approach will be to search for a classifier which simply tells us whether at a lead time of a fixed number of hours an extreme event will happen, given the current state of the system. As an extension of this deterministic or "point prediction" one can issue probabilistic predictions, which tell us the probability that at the given time in the future an event will happen. Depending on one's own cost function, one can use the predicted probability to draw one's own conclusions.

Re-phrasing the last paragraph, a probabilistic prediction scheme for extreme events is a conditional probability of the event to take place (at a fixed time in the future) under the condition that the current state of the system is as what we know about it. It is evident that this conditional probability, in principle, is well defined but that it might be difficult to obtain it in practice. It is this latter aspect which gives rise to different schemes and different terminology.

Probabilistic predictions require also to think about scoring rules. The predictor delivers the value of a probability, whereas the observation (which in this context is called the "verification"), is a binary variable: Either there is (according to the pre-defined notion) an extreme event, or there is not. How to compare these two different types of variables?

A first relevant requirement is reliability. If we have a large set of prediction trials, then we can form a sub-sample of those where the predicted probability was x. Let us assume that this set has N members. The implicit claim is that these N cases stem from a sample where the chance for the event to follow was x, i.e. this set should contain xN cases where actually an event followed. This test has to be successful for all possible values of $x \in [0, 1]$ and in practice can only be done by suitable binning. If the prediction scheme does not pass this test, one can re-calibrate the predicted probabilities. In any case, being reliable does not mean that a probabilistic scheme is also useful. Imagine the very simple scheme which predicts a constant probability, which is identical to the rate of events. Then, all prediction trials fall into a single bin, and reliability is trivially established. But this prediction, being constant over time, might be quite useless. Imagine that our extreme event was "snowfall of more than 10 cm in 24 hours", then it is evident that taking into account the seasons would do much better than saying "this happens on average three times per year, i.e. it will happen tomorrow with a chance of $1/122$".

One test for the predictive power of a prediction is the ROC statistics [10] which, moreover, has the advantage that is has no explicit dependence on the rate of events. It therefore allows comparing the predictability of quite different phenomena. The idea behind is that prediction of extremes is a classification problem. We want to classify the current state of the system into either creating the event or not. Depending on how sensitive our prediction scheme is (i.e. depending on the value the predicted probability has to overcome in order to issue a warning), the prediction scheme produces false alarms and misses hits. Missing an event is a quite different failure than a false alarm, and it is evident that by tuning the sensitivity one can reduce one of the two failures at the cost of increasing the other one. This issue is sometimes called "sensitivity versus specificity", where sensitivity means how many of the occurring events have been correctly predicted, whereas specificity means how many of the predicted events actually took place. As a side remark, this very same issue is relevant in medical diagnostics. In a more formal setting, the ROC statistics is suitable if the variable to be predicted can assume only two values, and where the costs of a misprediction are not symmetric: if the future is "1" but one predicts "0" the costs might be different from predicting "1" when the future is "0". In contrast, other standard error measures such as the root-mean-squared prediction error, but also the *Brier score* or *Ignorance* [5, 16], are symmetric, since they rely on a distance measure between prediction and verification. The other particularity of the ROC statistics is the issue of weighting. In many error measures, one averages over a long time series as a standard time average. If, for example, the task is to predict an earthquake which takes place once in 100 years, then predicting that it will never take place leads to a single wrong prediction within 36,500 days of prediction, which seems to be an impressive hit rate (36,499 correct predictions). It will be hard to beat, but it is evidently useless. The ROC statistics therefore normalizes the number of correctly predicted extremes and of false alarms separately: It is a diagram where as a function of some parameter which controls the sensitivity

Fig. 10.1 A typical ROC
plot. The curves represent the
prediction skill of the
algorithm described in
Sect. 10.5 applied to the
sandpile model in Sect. 10.6.
The different curves represent
different magnitudes of
events to be predicted. In this
system, events are the better
predictable the larger their
magnitude m_{thres} is
(measured in percent of the
largest possible event)

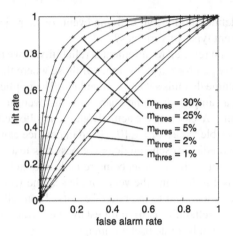

of the predictor the hit rate h is plotted versus the false alarm rate f: $h =$ (number of correctly predicted events)/(total number of events during all prediction trials) and $f =$ (number of false alarms)/(number of non-events among all prediction trials).

The benchmark for every predictor in terms of the ROC-statistics is the diagonal $h = f$: If on average every t time steps an event is predicted randomly, without any correlation to the true outcome, then the hit rate and the false alarm rate would both be $1/t$. Hence, such a useless random predictor as a function of the sensitivity parameter (which tunes t) yields the diagonal as the ROC curve. Therefore, in order to possess predictive power, a predictor's ROC curve has to be above the diagonal, and the more it is above the better it is. Depending on the specific situation one can identify the optimal working point of the predictor, i.e. the most suitable sensitivity. This will correspond to a point on the ROC curve which in some sense is close to the corner $(0, 1)$, i.e. to minimum false alarm rate and maximum hit rate. Our example from above, not predicting events at all, is zero sensitive. It does not produce false alarms, but also does not give any hits. It corresponds to $(0, 0)$ which is evidently not close to $(0, 1)$.

Depending on the structure in the input data and on the chosen prediction scheme, an ROC curve might approach the optimal point $(0, 1)$ more or less closely. Even if the approach is very good, as for the top curve in Fig. 10.1, the extreme events might be effectively unpredictable: The ROC curve does resolve the two types of prediction errors separately. But if the costs for false alarms one not negligible (as, for example, the costs to evacuate a city because of an earthquake), then there might be no working point apart from sensitivity 0 where the total costs of all false alarms are less than the avoided costs due to correct hits. Hence, we arrive at the somehow paradoxical situation that the ROC statistics guarantees that we are able to identify nontrivial prediction schemes, but that the most cost efficient strategy is to use a predictor which is optimal when weighting the costs of false alarms and of missed hits with their absolute number of occurrences.

10.5 Data Based Predictor of Extreme Events

Data based prediction relies on the fact that a stochastic process $x(t)$ is completely specified when all its joint probabilities are known. This means that in the first place we assume that the phenomenon is not necessarily deterministic, but the deterministic limit is contained in this notion. Joint probabilities are probabilities that at a couple of time instances the process assumes some specific values, $p_n(x(t_1) = x_1,$ $x(t_2) = x_2, \ldots, x(t_n) = x_n)$. Here, $x(t)$ might be a scalar or a vector, p_n is a scalar field with values between 0 and 1. The process is fully described, if we know p_n for all positive integers n and for all possible combinations of time instances t_k. From the joint probabilities, one immediately derives *conditional probabilities* or *transition probabilities*

$$P_n\big(x(t_{n+1}) = x_{n+1} | x(t_n) = x_n, x(t_{n-1}) = x_{n-1}, \ldots\big)$$
$$:= \frac{p_{n+1}(x(t_1) = x_1, \ldots, x(t_n) = x_n, x(t_{n+1}) = x_{n+1})}{p_n(x(t_1) = x_1, \ldots, x(t_n) = x_n)}.$$

These conditional probabilities denote the probability that x assumes the value x_{n+1} at time t_{n+1}, provided that the sequence of $x(t)$-values at times $t_n, t_{n-1}, \ldots$ was $x_n, x_{n-1}, \ldots$. This quantity supplies information for prediction: Having observed the values $x_n, x_{n-1}, \ldots$, we can read off the probability distribution for the future value x_{n+1}. In a general stochastic process, this probability distribution can only become sharper if we include more conditions, i.e. if we increase n. If (in discrete time) there exists a finite order n such that the conditional probabilities are all the same for $n' > n$, then this is a Markov process with finite memory. But even if a process is not Markovian (and that should be true for the majority of observed stochastic processes), then the gain of information by increasing n will decay fast in n, so that in practice one can work with a finite n. When trying to predict extreme events, it is often not suitable to predict the precise value of some observable (e.g. the magnitude of seismic activity or the water level of a river) and thereafter to decide by help of a threshold whether this is extreme or not.

It is better (and more general) to consider the following scenario: We assume to base our prediction on a time series of a *decision variable* d_t, where time t is discrete. The decision variable can be univariate or vector valued, depending on the phenomenon. Sometimes, the observable information is distributed among different quantities which are recorded as time series, and the decision variable is a function of these. In other words, passing from a series of measurements to a series of the decision variable comprises all possible steps of data processing and enhancement of the information content. It might include noise reduction by filtering of raw data, it might include reduction of dimensionality by transformation to principal components. What specifically is useful depends on the phenomenon and the available data. In any case, along with the time series of the decision variable comes an *event time series Y*. This series is a sequence of "0" and "1", and $Y_t = 1$ if and only if there is an extreme event at time t.

Two examples should illustrate this concept: (a) Flooding of a city by a river: here, the physical measurements might be the water level at some gauge in the river.

These measurements might immediately form the decision time series. The event takes place if the water level exceeds a certain threshold, i.e. the event time series is derived from the decision time series itself. (b) An epileptic seizure: the physical observations might be measurements of the electric activity of the brain, i.e. a multichannel EEG. Since this is a high dimensional vector of very noisy data, data processing might be used in order to construct a nontrivial decision variable. Noise reduction by filtering and transformation onto principal components would in this case be standard procedures. The event series, i.e. whether there is an epileptic seizure at time t or not, might be derived from very different sources of information.

In the spirit of stochastic processes, we now assume that all information which in this setting is available for prediction is contained in the knowledge of the joint probabilities $P(Y_{t+1}, d_t, d_{t-1}, \ldots)$. Therefore, a predictor should be based on this probability.

When searching for precursors of an extreme event, a commonly used scheme is to identify the pattern (which in our notation is a sequence of values of the decision variable d_t) which most probably precedes the event. If during the prediction trials a pattern similar to the precursor is observed, one would issue a warning of the event to follow. The sensitivity of this algorithm is controlled by the tolerance of what means "pattern similar to the precursor". This procedure is appealingly parsimonious in the sense that if we have a huge data set with only a few events (say, 50 years of data and 100 events), then it is easy to identify the events and to study the behavior of the decision variable prior to the event. This procedure implies to search a sequence of values in d_t such that the conditional probability $P(d_t, d_{t-1}, \ldots | Y_{t+1} = 1)$ is maximal, whereby the conditional probability is determined from the joint probability and the marginal probability $p(Y = 1)$. However, one can show that this method of prediction is not optimal [20].

When using the ROC-statistics as the measure of success, then the optimal predictor is to use the conditional probability $P(Y_{t+1} = 1 | d_t, d_{t-1}, \ldots)$, which is the probability that an event will follow, given that a specific sequence of values of d_t has been observed. Indeed, this is also the natural choice when trying to predict Y_{t+1} from $d_t, d_{t-1}, \ldots$ under the assumption that we deal with a stochastic process in d and Y. Formally, one could also include $Y_t, Y_{t-1}, \ldots$ in the condition, but in practice this is obsolete if the event rate is very small: The Y-values would be identical to zero almost always, so that this additional condition would not induce any restriction.

In summary, the optimal probabilistic predictor is to use the value of the probability $P(Y_{t+1} = 1 | d_t, d_{t-1}, \ldots)$ for the specific values of the last values of the decision variable as the prediction $\hat{P}_{t+1}$ of the probability that an event occurs at time $t + 1$. In order to assess the success of this predictor, one can either use a *skill score* as it was designed for probabilistic prediction, or one can convert the probabilistic prediction into a deterministic prediction and study the ROC statistics for the latter. The evident conversion scheme is to define a threshold probability p_0 and to predict an event to follow if and only if $\hat{P}_{t+1} > p_0$. By varying the threshold p_0, one can tune the sensitivity of the prediction scheme: For low p_0 one would predict events with a high rate, which might lead to many hits, but also to many false alarms. For hight p_0, positive predictions will be made at a low rate, resulting in much fewer false alarms, but potentially also in much fewer correct hits. Therefore, by varying p_0 from one to zero, one runs through the full ROC curve. Which p_0 is the most useful for predictions depends on the details of the prediction task, in particular on the costs of false alarms and of missed hits, and on the event rate. A plausible choice is to use such a value of p_0 that the rate at which the algorithm predicts events is identical to the event rate. There is, however, no justification that this is optimal, and it is easy to construct counter-examples.

10.6 Prediction of Extreme Avalanches in a Sandpile Model

Extreme events are usually large impact events, and the impact could be a nonlinear function of the event magnitude. Nonetheless, often extremity of the impact requires extraordinary event magnitudes, and this is best seen in the phenomenon of earthquakes: Their magnitude is measured as the logarithm of their energy release. One well studied physical mechanism which implies extraordinary event magnitudes is called *self organized criticality* (SOC). This concept was introduced by Bak, Tang, Wiesenfeld in 1987 [4] and means that a system drives itself into a critical state. Criticality implies the lack of length and time scales because of self-similarity, and the particular consequence of this is that distributions of typical observables are power laws. Hence, there is no finite upper limit to event magnitudes, and there is even no finite mean value. Very rarely, arbitrarily large events might take place. Evidently, this can be true only in an infinite system.

In order to illustrate the concepts introduced so far, we apply them to the prediction of extreme avalanches in a sandpile model of finite size. The finiteness of the system (as it is typical of systems which surround us) is responsible for correlations on which predictability is based. The sandpile model [4] mimics a growing sandpile: sand grains drop on a pile, and if locally the slope becomes too steep, a sand grain rolls down. It thereby has the potential to cause an avalanche. This process leads to a heap of sand with a well defined average slope. The model of Bak, Tang, Wiesenfeld has been shown to be critical. A particular consequence is that the frequency-magnitude distribution for avalanches is a power law, i.e. there is no "typical" avalanche size. In a finite system, the system size defines a length scale, and it has been shown that no avalanche can be larger than $L(L+1)(L+2)/6$ [14]. Therefore, the power law of the magnitude-frequency distribution has an upper cutoff. Beyond that, the finiteness of the system introduces temporal correlations between large avalanches: The distribution of time intervals in between two successive extreme avalanches (defined by their magnitude exceeding a threshold) is depleted around zero, whereas in the infinite system successive avalanches are independent of each other and the return time distribution is therefore an exponential. This "repulsion" of big avalanches allows to some degree to predict them.

Our observation time series is the sequence of magnitude values m_t of avalanches. Our event time series is derived from that. An event is an avalanche whose magnitude exceeds a threshold m_{thres}, i.e. $Y_t = 1$ iff $m_t \geq m_{\text{thres}}$. Our decision variable is constructed from the observations using the empirical fact that large avalanches repel each other. We form the weighted sum $d_t = \sum_{i=1}^{\infty} s^i m_{t-i}$ with some suitable suppression factor s, $0 < s < 1$. Thereby, the value of the decision variable is large only if very recently a very large avalanche happened. We then compute the conditional probability $P(Y_{t+1} = 1 | d_t)$ on the range of observed d-values from a part of the time series which one calls the *training set*. We then perform predictions on another part of the time series called *test set* and construct the ROC curves as explained above. From the last value d of d_t we read off the predicted probability of an avalanche to come through $\hat{P}_{t+1} = P(Y = 1 | d = d_t)$ and convert that into an alarm, if this probability exceeds some threshold. Under variation of this threshold we find the full ROC curve [15]. As a result (Fig. 10.1), avalanches are the better predictable the larger their magnitude m_{thres}. The rate of correct hits at the same rate of false alarms is larger. This phenomenon has been observed in other scenarios of extreme events as well, such as turbulent wind gusts [19]. Here, we see that the conditional probability $P(Y = 1 | d)$ is the more peaked the larger the magnitude of the target avalanches. In view of practical applicability, we must confess that in this case the ROC statistics is a bit misleading. The number of avalanches of magnitude larger than m_{thres} decreases when increasing m_{thres} so much that the higher hit rate for larger m_{thres} at fixed false alarm rate actually leads to *less hits* for about the same absolute number of false alarms. Hence, the number of false alarms per hit increases with increasing m_t, which is not what one would call improving the predictability. In particular, if one considers that humans tend to ignore alarms when there are too many false alarms, the prediction of very large avalanches in the SOC sandpile model would be a complete failure. Despite the fact that the predictor is optimal in the ROC sense, one cannot know whether different decision variables would lead to better predictability. Hence, the predictive skill which one obtains empirically is always a lower bound to what might be possible.

10.7 Back to Networks

Indeed, a few authors consider avalanches and similar phenomena in networks, e.g. [11, 21]. The sandpile model lives on a square lattice with nearest neighbor coupling. A straightforward generalization would be to define it on an arbitrary network. Indeed, this has been done, where various motivations and applications for sandpile-like dynamics on networks has been given. Generally speaking, the sandpile-dynamics is a re-distribution of load from one node onto the others and thereby a typical effect of the temporary knock-out of one node. Several authors study how the exponents of the power law for the frequency-magnitude-distribution depend on the network structure [17]. Also, dynamical re-wiring of the nodes according to avalanches has been proposed [13]. It seems, however, that currently there is no work which emphasizes the properties of *extreme* avalanches as a function of the network structure, and, in particular, no work on their prediction. However, a different SOC system, namely the Olami–Feder–Christensen (OFC) [23] model for earthquakes, has been simulated on small world networks, and the predictability of extreme avalanches was qualitatively the same as in the sandpile model: Since due to the finiteness of the system large avalanches repel each other, very large avalanches are better predictable than just by chance [7]. However, the actual effect of the small world property on the predictability has not yet been fully quantified and understood.

10.8 Conclusion

Extreme events are very large deviations of a system's behavior from normality. Extreme events occur in all systems with complex dynamics, also in dynamical networks. Details of the creation of these large fluctuations are still rarely understood, so that their prediction remains a challenge. We have presented a universal prediction scheme for data based predictions (as opposed to model based predictions, which evidently depend on the system specific model), but we have also outlined the limits of predictability, which are the more relevant the rarer the events are.

References

1. Albeverio, S., Jentsch, V., Kantz, H. (eds.): Extreme Events in Nature and Society. Springer, Berlin (2006)
2. Altmann, E., Kantz, H.: Recurrence time analysis, long-term correlations, and extreme events. Phys. Rev. E **71**, 056106 (2005)
3. Altmann, E., Hallerberg, S., Kantz, H.: Reactions to extreme events: Moving threshold model. Physica A **364**, 435–444 (2006)
4. Bak, P., Tang, C., Wiesenfeld, K.: Self-organized criticality: an explanation of $1/f$ noise. Phys. Rev. Lett. **59**, 381–384 (1987)
5. Brier, G.: Verification of forecasts expressed in terms of probability. Mon. Weather Rev. **78**, 1–3 (1950)
6. Bunde, A., Eichner, J., Kantelhardt, J., Havlin, S.: Long-term memory: A natural mechanism for the clustering of extreme events and anomalous residual times in climate records. Phys. Rev. Lett. **94**, 048701 (2005)
7. Caruso, F., Kantz, H.: Prediction of extreme events in the OFC model on a small world network (2010, in review). arXiv:1004.4774v1
8. Christensen, K., Olami, Z.: Variation of the Gutenberg–Richter b values and nontrivial temporal correlations in a spring-block model for earthquakes. J. Geophys. Res. **97**, 8729–8735 (1992)
9. Coles, S.: An Introduction to Statistical Modeling of Extreme Values. Springer, London (2001)
10. Egan, J.: Signal Detection Theory and ROC Analysis. Academic Press, New York (1975)
11. Eurich, C., Ernst, U.: Avalanches of activity in a network of integrate-and-fire neurons with stochastic input. In: Proc. of Int. Conf. on Artificial Neural Networks, ICANN 1999, vol. 2, pp. 545–550 (1999)
12. Fisher, R., Tippett, L.: Limiting forms of the frequency distribution of the largest and smallest member of a sample. Proc. Camb. Philos. Soc. **24**, 180–190 (1928)
13. Fronczak, P., Fronczak, A., Holyst, J.: Self-organized criticality and coevolution of network structure and dynamics. Phys. Rev. E **73**, 046117 (2006)

14. Garber, A., Kantz, H.: Finite size effects on the statistics of extreme events in the BTW model. Eur. Phys. J. B **67**, 437–443 (2009)
15. Garber, A., Hallerberg, S., Kantz, H.: Predicting extreme avalanches in self-organized critical sandpiles. Phys. Rev. E **80**, 026124 (2009)
16. Gneiting, T., Raftery, A.: Strictly proper scoring rules, prediction, and estimation. Tech. Rep. 436, Department of Statistics (2004)
17. Goh, K., Lee, D., Kahng, B., Kim, D.: Sandpile on scale-free networks. Phys. Rev. Lett. **91**, 148701 (2003)
18. Gumbel, E.: Statistics of Extremes. Columbia University Press, New York (1958)
19. Hallerberg, S., Kantz, H.: How does the quality of a prediction depend on the magnitude of the events under study? Nonlinear Process. Geophys. **15**, 321–331 (2008)
20. Hallerberg, S., Altmann, E., Holstein, D., Kantz, H.: Precursors of extreme increments. Phys. Rev. E **75**, 016706 (2007)
21. Hughes, D., Paczuski, M., Dendy, R., Helander, P., McClements, K.: Solar flares as cascades of reconnecting magnetic loops. Phys. Rev. Lett. **90**, 131101 (2003)
22. Kagan, Y., Jackson, D.: Long-term earthquake clustering. Geophys. J. Int. **104**, 117–133 (1991)
23. Olami, Z., Feder, H., Christensen, K.: Self-organized criticality in a continuous, nonconservative cellular automaton modeling earthquakes. Phys. Rev. Lett. **68**, 1244–1247 (1992)
24. Santhanam, M., Kantz, H.: Return interval distribution of extreme events and long-term memory. Phys. Rev. E **78**, 051113 (2008)
25. Sutula, T.: Mechanisms of epilepsy progression: current theories and perspectives from neuroplasticity in adulthood and development. Epilepsy Res. **60**, 161–171 (2004)

Chapter 11
Dynamics of Networks
of Leaky-Integrate-and-Fire Neurons

Antonio Politi and Stefano Luccioli

Abstract   The dynamics of pulse-coupled leaky-integrate-and-fire neurons is discussed in networks with arbitrary structure and in the presence of delayed interactions. The evolution equations are formally recasted as an event-driven map in a general context where the pulses are assumed to have a finite width. The final structure of the mathematical model is simple enough to allow for an easy implementation of standard nonlinear dynamics tools. We also discuss the properties of the transient dynamics in the presence of quenched disorder (and δ-like pulses). We find that the length of the transient depends strongly on the number N of neurons. It can be as long as 10^6–10^7 inter-spike intervals for relatively small networks, but it decreases upon increasing N because of the presence of stable clustered states. Finally, we discuss the same problem in the presence of randomly fluctuating synaptic connections (annealed disorder). The stationary state turns out to be strongly affected by finite-size corrections, to the extent that the number of clusters depends on the network size even for $N \approx 20,000$.

11.1 Introduction

Among all kinds of networks that play some role in the physical, biological, and social world [37], neuronal systems are presumably the most complex ones, as they store and process a huge amount of information and are able to do that by simultaneously performing many different tasks [25, 35]. The remarkable robustness of the mammalian brain against relevant damages hints at the general nature of the underlying mechanisms that are responsible for its functioning [2, 13, 23, 26]. As a

A. Politi (✉) · S. Luccioli
Consiglio Nazionale delle Ricerche, Istituto dei Sistemi Complessi, 50019 Sesto Fiorentino, Italy
e-mail: antonio.politi@isc.cnr.it

A. Politi · S. Luccioli
Centro Studi Dinamiche Complesse, Sesto Fiorentino, Italy

E. Estrada et al. (eds.), *Network Science*,
DOI 10.1007/978-1-84996-396-1_11, © Springer-Verlag London Limited 2010

result, even though accurate mathematical models have been developed, which describe the activity of single neurons and of their synaptic connections [15, 36, 40], it is convenient to analyze relatively simple systems under the assumption that they are able to reproduce (most of) the relevant phenomena exhibited by more realistic systems. This does not dispense with testing whether and to what extent the collective behavior exhibited by such simple networks does mimic the evolution of real brains. However, the efforts made in the last years to characterize networks of simple neurons have revealed that this is already a difficult task and it is worth studying them also as a testbed for the development and tuning of appropriate mathematical tools.

In this paper, we focus our attention on a class of simple neuron models that exhibit a periodic spiking behavior in the absence of coupling. The single element is schematically described as a so-called leaky-integrate-and-fire neuron [15] (LIF): a dynamical system characterized by a single phase-like variable. The coupling is the result of (inhibitory/excitatory) pulses that are sent across the system. In the last 20 years, a large amount of literature has accumulated on this subject [1, 3, 4, 6–8, 11, 30, 41]. To this literature one should also add papers devoted to the substantially equivalent class of pulse coupled phase oscillators [17, 19].

In spite of the simplicity of the equation describing the single neuron, many ingredients can be naturally included which make the network evolution not so trivial. We have in mind: (i) the shape of the pulses that can be assumed to be either δ-like [30] or to have, for example, an exponential tail [1, 41]; (ii) the presence of delay in the synaptic connections [11]; (iii) the topological structure of the network (leaving aside the question of the synaptic dynamics) [9, 14, 24, 39]; (iv) the diversity of the single neurons [28]. Altogether, the four ingredients contribute to generate a wealth of different phenomena, and it is necessary to identify those which are truly general and robust. The attention of the first studies was focused on perfectly synchronized states, where all neurons follow exactly the same trajectory [30, 39]. A complementary class of dynamical regimes, later uncovered is that of splay states, that are characterized by a uniform distribution of the single oscillator phases [32, 38].

A further ubiquitous regime that has been repeatedly analyzed is the spontaneous grouping of neurons into clusters [1, 7, 11, 12, 28, 47]. It is typically induced by the presence of delay, but it appears also for pulses of finite width. Another regime that has attracted a considerable interest are the so-called balanced states. They have been identified as the most appropriate candidates to reproduce the irregular background activity affecting the cerebral cortex [5, 6, 21, 42, 43]. The irregular dynamics is the result of a careful "balance" between excitatory and inhibitory synapses. Collective oscillations represent perhaps the least trivial phenomenon: the coarsegrained evolution as revealed by, for example, the electric activity, is qualitatively different from the microscopic dynamics of the single neurons [31, 41]. The behavior is robust against the addition of noise [6, 31] and disorder [33]. Finally, given the evidence that transient dynamics plays an important role in odor recognition [29], some efforts have been devoted to the characterization of long lasting transients [45, 47].

In this paper, we first focus our attention on the introduction of a sufficiently general formalism to describe and analyze a rather broad class networks of LIF neurons, namely in the presence of (equal) delays, finite pulse-widths and disorder (either of quenched or annealed type). In fact, too often different notations are adopted by different groups of researchers, and this makes it difficult to compare the conditions under which the various results have been obtained. Additionally, with reference to the standard formalism, it is not always obvious to infer the relative strength of the resulting coupling. Addressing this questions is the goal of the second section, where we first define the model and introduce an appropriate parametrization of the evolution equations (the technical details are presented in the appendix at the end of the paper).

In Sect. 11.3, the set of differential equations is transformed into an event-driven discrete-time mapping with reference to a rather general setup which, incidentally, allows appreciating the implications of dealing with disorder, delay and pulses of finite width. The reformulation of the original problem solves also once for all the practical problems that are sometime encountered in the implementation of standard dynamical-systems tools (such as the computation of Lyapunov exponents) in the context of pulse coupled oscillators.

The rest of the paper deals with δ-like pulses. This choice is mostly dictated by the simplicity of the corresponding model, combined with the past evidence that the resulting phenomenology is substantially equivalent to that obtained in more realistic setups. However, it is wise to recall that the δ-like case is a singular limit which does not always coincide (for the stability properties) with the behavior of networks with pulse-width of arbitrarily small but finite width [46]. Thus a word of caution is needed to stress on the need to check a posteriori the general validity of resulting scenario. More precisely, in Sect. 11.4, we investigate the role of delay in the (transient) irregular dynamics. The seminal paper [45] revealed that, in the absence of delay, there is a finite parameter region where exponentially (with the number of neurons) long and yet stable transients can be observed. This peculiar regime is a specific instance of a more general phenomenon, the so-called stable chaos [34]. The validity of this scenario in the presence of delay has been preliminarily investigated in [20, 21, 44]. In Sect. 11.5, we pass to analyze the, in principle, simpler setup of annealed disorder with the goal of investigating the stability properties of the clustered states in the presence of an additional dynamical noise.

11.2 Model Definition

Networks of LIF neurons have been repeatedly investigated in the literature. In spite of the simplicity of the single-neuron model, this choice allows exploring a rich variety of setups and reproducing many different phenomena. Unfortunately, different notations are often adopted in the literature, thus making it difficult to organize the various results into a coherent picture. It is therefore useful to introduce suitably rescaled variables and parameters both to single out the minimal set of relevant parameters and to discuss their physical role. As a result, the evolution equation for the membrane potential v_i, is written as (see the appendix for the mapping between our notations and those adopted in [20, 44])

$$\dot{v}_i = a - v_i + \frac{g}{N} \sum_{n:t_n<t} S_{i,l(n)} F(t - t_n - \tau), \quad i = 1, \ldots, N. \tag{11.1}$$

When the potential v_i reaches the threshold $v_i = 1$, it is instantaneously reset to the value $v_i = 0$. The parameter a, which corresponds to the rescaled external current, sets the time scale for the Inter Spike Interval (ISI), relative to the relaxation time of the membrane potential. The function $F(t)$ describes the shape of the single pulse (starting at time $t = 0$ and with unit area), t_n's are the firing times of the neurons connected to neuron i, while τ is the delay time with which the pulse is received. The parameter g measures the average pulse strength: $g > 0$ ($g < 0$) corresponds to excitatory (inhibitory) coupling. Moreover, the matrix $S_{i,l}$ describes the relative strength of the synaptic connection from neuron l to neuron i (notice that there is no reason to expect any symmetry). As the average coupling strength is determined by g, the connectivity matrix is normalized in such a way that $\langle S \rangle = 1$. Finally, the variance σ^2 of $S_{i,l}$ measures the strength of the disorder.

Besides the ingredients introduced so far, one may wish to include a stochastic term to account for the uncontrollable interactions with the environment. This is the setup often studied by Brunel et al. and can be studied with the help of mean field approach. Here we limit ourselves to consider random connections and suggest the interested reader to look at [7].

Often disorder is introduced by assuming that the synaptic connection from neuron l to neuron i is present with a probability f. In this case, as shown in the appendix, $S_{i,l} = \{1/f, 0\}$ so that $\langle S \rangle = 1$ and $\sigma^2 = (1 - f)/f$. It is easy to check that the highest degree of randomness is obtained in the limit of $f \to 0$; σ^2 is a better parameter to characterize the amount of disorder and compare different forms of randomness.

In order to clarify the coupling mechanism and to allow for a comparison with the standard mean-field coupling, it is necessary to understand the meaning of the various parameters and in particular of a and g. We do so by referring to homogeneous networks ($\sigma^2 = 0$) in the presence of δ-like pulses. According to model (11.1), the membrane potential of each neuron evolves independently until when a pulse is emitted. The coupling is the indirect consequence of the dependence of the velocity $\dot{v}_i$ on v_i itself. This is better appreciated by focusing our attention on the evolution of the *time distance* between any two neurons. As long as no pulses are received, such a distance stays constant. When a pulse is received, v_i is pushed back (we assume an inhibitory coupling, i.e. $g < 0$) by a fixed amount g/N. This implies that the temporal distance shrinks (increases) if the potential lies in a region of decreasing (increasing) velocity. As a result, the strength of the mutual interaction is not related to the amplitude of the (backward) kick, but rather to its variability as a function of v_i. The discussion can be put on a more quantitative ground by transforming the variable v into a "time-like" variable ϕ. In practice, it is sufficient to integrate the equation of motion (11.1) to determine $v(t)$ (with initial condition

$v(0) = 0$) and thereby rescale the time variable in such a way that the ISI—identified by the condition $v(T) = 1$—is normalized to 1 ($\phi(v) = t/T$),

$$\phi(v) := \frac{t}{T} = \frac{1}{T} \ln \frac{a}{a-v} \tag{11.2}$$

where the phase $\phi \in [0, 1]$ and

$$T = \ln \frac{a}{a-1}. \tag{11.3}$$

The phase jump due to the an incoming pulse is

$$\Delta\phi \equiv \phi(v - g/N) - \phi(v). \tag{11.4}$$

In the large N limit,

$$\Delta\phi = \frac{g\phi'(v)}{N} = \frac{ge^{\phi T}}{aNT}. \tag{11.5}$$

In the context of pulse-coupled phase oscillators [17, 19], all of this comes naturally, as they are defined by assuming that the phase increases linearly in between spikes ($\dot{\phi} = 1$) and by introducing directly a phase-dependent shift $\Delta\phi$ (the so-called phase response curve [16]). This way, one can immediately recognize the two leading effects of receiving a spike. On the one hand, the neuron undergoes a relative average slowing down,

$$\overline{\Delta\phi} = \frac{g(e^T - 1)}{aNT^2} = \frac{g}{aN(a-1)\ln^2(1-1/a)} \equiv \frac{\chi}{N} \tag{11.6}$$

where the last equality can be seen as the definition of the slowness parameter χ.

A second relevant parameter is the variation of $\Delta\phi$, which according to the previous arguments, can be considered as more meaningful measurement of the effective coupling strength. We propose to quantify the variation in terms of $\Delta\phi_{max} - \Delta\phi_{min}$. In the large N limit, we find

$$G \equiv (\Delta\phi_{max} - \Delta\phi_{min})N = \frac{g}{a(a-1)\ln(1-1/a)}. \tag{11.7}$$

χ and G are the most appropriate parameters for the characterization of networks of pulse coupled neurons. In particular, we claim that they prove useful when functionally different velocity fields have to be compared.

In Fig. 11.1, we have plotted the isolines identified by constant a and g values in the (χ, G)-plane. By comparing the straight lines (which correspond to different a values), one can appreciate how an increase in the external current a contributes to decrease the effective coupling strength. The crucial role of a in determining the effective coupling strength is further confirmed by the shape of the isolines with constant g. In the diagram, we have inserted the two points which correspond to the parameter values selected in [44] (diamond) and [20] (circle), respectively. One can notice that the former choice corresponds to a rather strong coupling regime.

Fig. 11.1 The parameter plane as identified by the effective coupling strength G and the slowness parameter χ. The *solid straight lines* parameterize LIF neurons with constant a ($a = 1.1, 1.5, 2$ and 3, by moving counter-clockwise). The *dashed lines* correspond to $g = 1, 2, 3, 4$, and 5 (from bottom to top). The *diamond* corresponds to the parameter values adopted in [44]; the *circle* corresponds to [20]

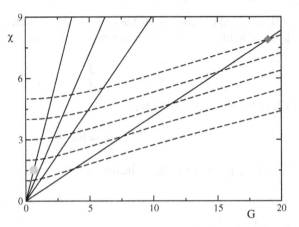

11.3 Model Implementation

A simple inspection of (11.1) reveals that they are piecewise linear. Therefore, it is convenient to transform the model into a discrete-time map by integrating the differential equation between two consecutive times when discontinuities are encountered. There are two different types of such events: (i) the times t_n when a neuron crosses the threshold; (ii) the times $t_n + \tau$ when the pulses are received. Let us then order all such times and call t'_n the nth discontinuity which can be of either the former or latter type.

Before going on, it is necessary to focus our attention on the field resulting from the collection of pulses received by each single neuron. In fact, the dynamical system as defined by the differential equations (11.1) is highly non-standard: it looks like a non-autonomous system, although the model is autonomous (no external modulation is involved). In fact, the optimal strategy consists in formally introducing the variable E_i which describes the field seen by neuron i,

$$E_i(t) = \frac{1}{N} \sum_{n:t_n < t} S_{i,l(n)} F(t - t_n - \tau). \tag{11.8}$$

Under the assumption that the shape $F(t)$ of the single pulse is the Green's function of a linear differential equation of order d, we can turn the above explicit definition into

$$E_i^{(d)} = \sum_{j=1}^{d} b_{i,j} E_i^{(j-1)} + \frac{k}{N} \sum_{n:t_n < t} S_{i,l(n)} \delta(t - t_n - \tau) \tag{11.9}$$

where $E_i^{(d)}$ denotes the dth time derivative of E_i and k is a suitable constant introduced to normalize the area of the single pulse. Equations (11.1), complemented by (11.9), identify a standard dynamical system: each neuron is described by the membrane potential plus d variables to characterize the field. From now on, we proceed in a formal way to unravel the dynamical complexity of a generic model, while presenting the technical details for a specific example.

We can construct a map by integrating (11.9) from the initial condition $E_i^{(j)}(t_n') = E_i^{(j)}(n)$ (with $0 \le j < d$), $v_i(t_n') = v_i(n)$ for a time $\Delta t(n)$ that we leave for the moment unspecified. The field equation can be formally solved, yielding

$$E_i(t_n' + \Delta t) = E_i(n) + \sum_{j=1}^{d} c_{i,j} e^{\lambda_j \Delta t} \tag{11.10}$$

where λ_j's are the eigenvalues of the linear equation (for the sake of simplicity, we assume no degeneracy) and the coefficients $c_{i,j}$ are linear combinations of $E_i^{(j)}(n)$'s. Upon replacing such an expression in (11.1), we obtain a linear differential equation with time-dependent coefficients that can be explicitly solved.

Now, it comes the problem of determining $\Delta t(n)$. We start by computing the time $\Delta t_i(n)$ needed by each neuron to reach its threshold. Such a time is a function only of the ith variables, $\Delta t_i(n)(v_i(n), \{E_i^{(j)}\})$. Moreover, at all times there exists a list of times $t_m + \tau$ with $m \in \{m_1, \ldots, m_2\}$ such that $t_m < t_n'$ and $t_m + \tau > t_n'$. This is the list of the pulses that have not yet been received. It may be empty, but it cannot contain more than N items, as the delay is assumed to be (much) smaller than the ISI, in accordance with physiological measurements, so that there cannot be more than one *pending* pulse per neuron. By combining all such information, it turns out that

$$\Delta t = \min\{(\Delta t)_i; t_m + \tau\}, \quad i \in \{1, \ldots, N\}, \ m \in \{m_1, \ldots, m_2\}. \tag{11.11}$$

If the minimum belongs to the first group, we are in front of a typical Poincaré section: one variable is determined by the constraint identifying the surface of section, the potential of the neuron which reaches threshold and which is reset to 0. All the other $N(d+1) - 1$ variables can be updated by implementing the above mentioned integration schemes. If the minimum belongs to the second group, it means that a pulse is received and the variables of the neurons that are supposed to receive it (as dictated by the connectivity matrix) must be updated. It is here that the δ function in (11.9) comes into play: the $(d-1)$th derivative of the field is incremented by an amount that depends on the coupling strength. Moreover, as the label of the neuron that has emitted the spike to be received at time $t_m + \tau$ can be any $l \in \{1, \ldots, N\}$ and since t_m depends on all the $d+1$ variables associated to the lth neuron, this seems to suggest that the effective phase-space dimension is $2N(d+1)$, but this would be a wrong conclusion. To understand why this is so, consider the simple delayed map

$$u_{n+1} = \gamma_{uu} u_n + \gamma_{uv} v_n + \beta_u u_{n-N+1} v_{n-N+1},$$

$$v_{n+1} = \gamma_{vu} u_n + \gamma_{vv} v_n + \beta_v u_{n-N+1} v_{n-N+1}.$$

At the first sight, one is tempted to conclude that the evolution of such a map requires knowing both u and v for N consecutive time steps in the past, and that the phase-space dimension is $2N$. However, this is not the case, since the only information on the delayed state that is required is contained in the variable $x_n = u_n v_n$. In other words, a simple change of variable from u_n and v_n to, for example, u_n and

x_n would reveal that the true phase-space dimension is $N + 1$. The same is true in our neural network, since the only past information that is required is contained in the variables t_m. Therefore, we can conclude that the "delayed" arrival of the pulses increases the dimension only by N (the maximal number of possible pending pulses), so that the phase-space dimension is $D = N(d + 2) - 1$ (having taken into account that one is eliminated because of taking the Poincaré section). It is quite interesting to notice that, contrary to standard models of continuous-time dynamical systems with delayed feedback where the delay induces an infinite-dimensional phase space [18], here the dimension stays finite and there are no conceptual difficulties in simulating the model on a digital computer. From a practical point of view, the correct dimensionality manifests itself as soon as the variable v_n is replaced by a time-like variable corresponding to the expected crossing time (given the current shape of the field E). Such a variable is nothing but the generalization of the variable ϕ mentioned in the previous section to the case of nonsingular pulses (except for a sign and a scaling factor).

Altogether the above outlined approach has allowed transforming the initial set of ordinary differential equations into an event-driven map which can be easily simulated numerically and studied analytically. In the last part of this section, we illustrate the method with reference to a specific example.

11.3.1 An Example

In this subsection we consider a pulse shape that has been repeatedly investigated in the literature [1]

$$F(t) = \alpha^2 t\theta(t)e^{-\alpha t} \tag{11.12}$$

where $\theta(x)$ is the Heavyside θ function and α is the inverse pulse-width. The corresponding field equation is two dimensional [33]

$$\ddot{E}_i(t) = -2\alpha\dot{E}_i(t) - \alpha^2 E_i(t) + \frac{\alpha^2}{N}\sum_{n:t_n<t} S_{i,l(n)}\delta(t - t_n - \tau). \tag{11.13}$$

Notice that this is an example of a degenerate spectrum, as the two eigenvalues are equal to one another. Since the differential equation is of second order ($d = 2$), we need two variables, namely the field E_i and its first time derivative $\dot{E}_i$. For the sake of simplicity, we replace the latter with $Q_i := \alpha E_i + \dot{E}_i$. The resulting map for the field variables reads

$$E_i(n+1) = E_i(n)e^{-\alpha\eta} + Q_i(n)\eta e^{-\alpha\eta}, \tag{11.14a}$$

$$Q_i^-(n+1) = Q_i(n)e^{-\alpha\eta} \tag{11.14b}$$

where η denotes the yet unspecified integration time and the minus superscript means that we have still to include the possible effect of a pulse arrival at the end of the time interval. At the same time, the updating rule for the membrane potential is

$$v_i(n+1) = v_i(n)e^{-\eta} + a(1 - e^{-\eta}) + gH[\eta, E_i(n), Q_i(n)] \tag{11.15}$$

where

$$H[\eta, E, Q] = \frac{e^{-\eta} - e^{-\alpha\eta}}{\alpha - 1}\left(E + \frac{Q}{\alpha - 1}\right) - \frac{\eta e^{-\alpha\eta}}{\alpha - 1}Q, \tag{11.16}$$

(there is no need to mention the dependences on i and n here). These two equations can be used to introduce the above mentioned phase-like variable and define its updating rule. The phase-like variable $\eta_i(n)$ is nothing but the time needed by the neuron i to reach the threshold, given the current field dynamics. This can be determined by setting $v_i(n+1) = 1$ in (11.15). The resulting relationship between η and v (for a given pair of E, Q values) is

$$v_i(n) = a - e^{\eta}(a + gH[\eta, E, Q] - 1) = R[\eta, E, Q]. \tag{11.17}$$

The corresponding updating rule is the trivial equation

$$\eta_i^-(n+1) = \eta_i(n) - \eta \tag{11.18}$$

where the superscript again warns us that the "last minute" corrections have not been included and where the value of η is still to be determined. In order to do so, we have to introduce another set of variables, the arrival time $\overline{\eta}_i$ of the last pulse emitted by the ith neuron (this time is infinite, if there is no pending pulse). Their evolution rule is, obviously,

$$\overline{\eta}_i^-(n+1) = \overline{\eta}_i(n) - \eta. \tag{11.19}$$

Now, we are in the position to determine the time η which is nothing but

$$\eta = \min\{\eta_i^-(n), \overline{\eta}_i^-\}. \tag{11.20}$$

The knowledge of η allows completing the transformation equation. In the case η belongs to the first set of variables, it means that the end of the time interval corresponds to the threshold crossing of, say, the neuron m, i.e. $\eta_m(n) = \eta$. In this case, the evolution equation completes as (unless stated otherwise, the index i ranges in the whole $\{1, N\}$ interval)

$$\begin{aligned}
Q_i(n+1) &= Q_i^-(n+1), \\
\eta_i(n+1) &= \eta_i^-(n+1), \quad i \neq m, \\
\eta_m(n+1) &= R^{-1}[0, E_m(n+1), Q_m(n+1)], \\
\overline{\eta}_i(n+1) &= \overline{\eta}_i^-(n+1), \quad i \neq m, \\
\overline{\eta}_m(n+1) &= \tau.
\end{aligned} \tag{11.21}$$

In the case η belongs to the second set of variables, it means that the pulse sent by the neuron $l(n)$ is received by the connected neurons. With the same convention as before,

$$Q_i(n+1) = Q_i^- + S_{i,l}\frac{\alpha^2}{N},$$
$$\eta_i(n+1) = R^{-1}[R(\eta_i^-, Q_i^-, E_i), E_i, Q_i],$$
$$\overline{\eta}_i(n+1) = \overline{\eta}_i^-(n+1), \quad i \neq l,$$
$$\overline{\eta}_l(n+1) = +\infty.$$

(11.22)

The equation for η_i (where, for the sake of clarity, we have dropped the $n + 1$ dependence in the r.h.s.) states that the estimated crossing time has to be readjusted after the variable Q has been affected by the pulse arrival.

The whole dynamical model consists of (11.14a), (11.14b) and (11.17)–(11.22). It involves $4N - 1$ variables. In the case of fully homogeneous networks (all-to-all identical couplings), there is no need to attach a different field to each neuron. Accordingly, the number of variables reduces to $2N + 1$.

This model is often studied in the limit of δ-like pulses. It is instructive to recall that the stability property of the resulting solutions do not connect smoothly to those of the above model in the limit $\alpha \to \infty$ [46]. In other words, the zero-width is a singular limit that has to be carefully considered, especially since real pulses in the brain have a finite width. With these words of caution, we nevertheless restrict ourselves to neurons coupled via inhibitory δ-like pulses. In fact, in spite of its simplicity, the corresponding setup provides a wealth of nontrivial phenomena that need be understood.

11.4 Quenched Disorder

In this section, we study the network behavior in the presence of *quenched* disorder, i.e. we assume that the geometry of the connections, as well as the synaptic strength, does not change during the evolution.

In the case of *inhibitory* coupling ($g < 0$) and δ-like pulses, it is known that the network exhibits a *non-chaotic* dynamics (the maximum Lyapunov exponent is negative) both with and without synaptic delay [20–22, 44, 45].[1] This means that any trajectory eventually converges towards a *periodic orbit*. It is convenient to introduce the recurrence time

$$T_r = \min\{n \mid \text{dist}(C(n), C(m)) < \rho, \ 1 \leq m < n\}$$

(11.23)

where $C(n) \equiv \{\eta_i, \overline{\eta}_i\}$ denotes the time-n generic configuration,[2] *dist* is a measure of the distance between any two configurations, and finally ρ is some fixed resolution.

---

[1] Jahnke et al. [20, 21] showed that the same holds also in the case of heterogeneity in the single oscillator parameters and in the synaptic delays.

[2] As we refer to δ-like pulses, it is not necessary to invoke E and Q variables.

T_r is the first time that the current configuration $\mathcal{C}(n)$ is ρ-close to a previous one $\mathcal{C}(m^*)$ (where m^* is the value of m for which the minimum is achieved in (11.23)) and $T := T_r - m^*$ is the period of the asymptotic orbit $\mathcal{O}_T$. A condition for the above formula to be meaningful is that ρ must be smaller than the radius of the largest ball entirely contained in the basin of attraction of $\mathcal{O}_T$. Numerical simulations indicate that it is typically sufficient to set $\rho \leq 0.01$. Finally, in order to define a statistically reliable observables, it is necessary to average T_r and T both on a set of different initial conditions and different realizations of the connectivity matrix.

With reference to a *diluted* ($f < 1$) network without delay, Zillmer et al. [45] found that when the coupling strength g is small enough, the transient time needed to approach the asymptotic orbit increases linearly with the number N of neurons. On the other hand, above some critical value, the transient becomes *exponentially* long in N and turns out to be effectively stationary (with the exception of an initial time-interval of length independent of the system size). More important, the "transient" dynamics turns out to be irregular, as testified by a non zero coefficient of variation of the ISI.[3] This dynamical behavior is often referred to as *stable chaos* [34]; it is akin to the irregular evolution exhibited by some cellular automata. Stable chaos has raised an increasing interest in the context of neuroscience, as a possible mechanism to give rise to highly irregular spike-train patterns without the need to involve standard deterministic chaos [10].

In order to investigate the robustness of this scenario against the introduction of delayed spikes, Zillmer et al. [44] studied the setup A defined in the appendix with the additional constraint that each neuron has *exactly* the same number $K = fN$ of incoming connections. The typical scenario is illustrated in Fig. 11.2, where one can see that an initial exponential growth (see small circles) of the average transient time is followed by a rapid decrease. In the same figure, one can see that qualitatively similar results are found once the constraint on the number of incoming links is released. As a matter of fact, the only difference is that the initial exponential growth extends to larger network sizes. This is coherent with the naive idea that removing such a constraints is equivalent to slightly increasing the disorder in the network.

Moreover, in Fig. 11.2, one can follow the dependence of the average asymptotic period $\langle T \rangle$ on the system size. For this choice of the parameters, $\langle T \rangle$ follows the same trend exhibited by the transient. This implies that the complexity of the transient dynamics mirrors the complexity of the recurrent orbits. This is illustrated in Fig. 11.3, where we show the raster plots of two typical periodic orbits, after labelling the neurons according to their first firing time. The periodic orbit shown in Fig. 11.3(a) does not reveal any special regularity, except for the ordering which must manifest itself whenever a period is completed. A very different structure is seen in Fig. 11.3(b), where the neurons are clearly organized in two groups (clusters) which fire almost synchronously. The enlarged view plotted in the inset of Fig. 11.3(b) allows appreciating the fine structure and the width w of each cluster.

---

[3]The coefficient of variation of a stochastic variable is nothing but the normalized standard deviation.

Fig. 11.2 Average transient lengths $\langle T_r \rangle$ (*circle*) and average periods $\langle T \rangle$ (*open squares*) as a function of the size of the network N. The *dashed line* is an exponential fit on $\langle T_r \rangle$. The parameters used are reported in Table 11.1, setup A. The *small circles* represent $\langle T_r \rangle$ in the presence of the constraint discussed in the text: the *dotted vertical line* indicates the position of the peak

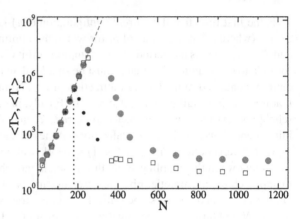

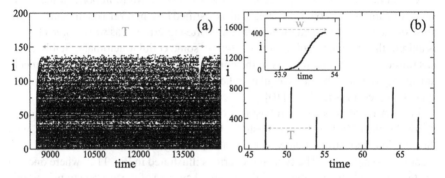

Fig. 11.3 Typical periodic solutions for small ($N = 138$) (**a**), and large ($N = 805$) (**b**), network size (an enlargement in (**b**) shows the broadness, w, of the smeared clusters). The *dashed lines* represent the periods T of the solutions. The neurons (i index) are sorted according to their firing times. The parameters used are reported in Table 11.1, setup A

On the other hand, very recently, Jahnke et al. [21], with reference to the setup B defined in the appendix, found a seemingly steady exponential increase of the transient time. A priori, it is not obvious whether the different scenario can be attributed to the choice of substantially different parameter values. Indeed, from Table 11.1, one can see that the setup B refers to a much weaker coupling and a stronger disorder. In order to clarify the issue, we have investigated this model [27] for significantly larger system sizes than those analyzed in [21], discovering that stable clusters exist also in this latter case and rapidly attract generic initial conditions.

In order to shed some light on the observed behavior, it is convenient to consider the large N limit. We may think that two neurons belonging to the same cluster are characterized by independent sets of connections, so that their initial (just after having been reset) distance diffuses. After one ISI, i.e. after receiving a number of order N of spikes of amplitude $\approx 1/N$, it is reasonable to conjecture that their positions diffuse away by an amount of order $1/\sqrt{N}$ that can be considered as a rough estimate of the cluster width. As a result we can conclude that the fluctuations due to the disorder are increasingly negligible. In other words, it is reasonable to assume that for $N \to \infty$, the dynamics coincides with that of a homogeneous network with all parameters set as in the original model except for a zero variance σ^2.

The analysis of regular networks can therefore serve as a reference to have a first order approximation of the phenomena expected in large disordered networks. Ernst et al. [11, 12] have shown that in large such networks, when the delay is small compared to the ISI of the single neuron T_{ISI}, the attractors are states composed of clusters of *synchronized* oscillators, which fire exactly at the same time. In fact, the delay typically breaks the very existence of a splay state as soon as $\tau < T_{\text{ISI}}/N$; this is because the symmetry among all neurons is broken and one must distinguish between those which are waiting for the arrival of an incoming spike and those which are not. By replacing N with the number n_c of distinct clusters, one can turn the above inequality into a relation for the maximal number of clusters as a function of τ, $n_c = T_{\text{ISI}}/\tau$. As discussed in [11, 12], the larger the delay, the smaller is the expected number of clusters. Depending on the initial condition, the dynamics can converge towards different states characterized by both different numbers of clusters and different populations of neurons within the clusters. Here we briefly elucidate the interaction mechanisms. Let us consider a state where the neuron of a given cluster is slightly perturbed. The effect of receiving a spike is to push back the potential by some fixed amount, irrespective of the actual value. Since the velocity field steadily decreases upon increasing v, the push-back effect turns into a small decrease of the time distance and thus into an effective attraction. A different scenario may emerge in the case of the spikes sent by the neurons belonging to the same cluster. As long as the distance of the perturbed neuron from the reference cluster (transformed into a time-distance δt) is smaller than τ, all neurons receive the spikes after having been reset, and the above described stabilizing mechanism is again at work. This mechanism accounts for the transversal stability of such states.[4] If $|\delta t| > \tau$ and, let's say, the single neuron lags behind, it receives the "self-spikes", when it is still in the low velocity region (below threshold), so that it is significantly slowed down, i.e. it is pushed away. This asymmetric mechanism induces a cluster destabilization for perturbations that are sufficiently large.

According to the previous argument, which predicts the perturbation induced by the disorder to be of amplitude $1/\sqrt{N}$, we can conclude that as long as $N < \tau^{-2}$, no stable clusters exist and generic trajectories are obliged to wander across the phase space until peculiar periodic orbits are found which attract them (the one reported in Fig. 11.3(a) being one example). This explains why long transients are observed in relatively small networks. On the other hand, for large N, many clustered states exist, which facilitate the convergence of generic trajectories, thus contributing to shorten the transient length as reported in Fig. 11.2.

However, we have not yet touched the most tricky point. The very existence of a clustered state means that all the neurons are characterized by the same Inter

---

[4]The stability against perturbations of the cluster positions is a different story and requires a more detailed analysis.

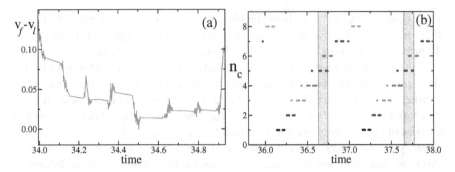

Fig. 11.4 (a) Difference between the membrane potential of the first, v_f, and last, v_l, neuron within the same cluster. Data refers to a periodic orbit composed of eight clusters in a network with $N = 5,000$ neurons. (b) Raster plot of the crossing times of the threshold $v = 0.3$ in a network of $N = 10,000$ neurons. Neurons are labelled according to their corresponding cluster (as determined when the physical threshold $v = 1$ is crossed). In both figures, the parameters are as reported in Table 11.1, setup B

Spike Interval, T_{ISI}. It is amazing that neurons self-organize in such states irrespective whether they receive stronger/weaker, more/less inhibitory spikes. The fluctuations of the mutual distance are better appreciated in the setup B since there is a larger number of clusters (eight, nine). With reference to this latter setup, we see in Fig. 11.4(a), how the difference between the membrane potential of the first (v_f) and the last (v_l) neuron (within the same cluster) fluctuates in between two consecutive spikes.

In some case the inter-spike fluctuations may be so large that single clusters mix themselves, making almost impossible their identification far from the threshold. This behavior can be appreciated in Fig. 11.4(b), where the crossing times of an intermediate threshold ($v = 0.3$) are reported for the neurons of the different clusters. From the shadowed regions we see that some neurons of the sixth cluster cross the threshold before all neurons of the fifth cluster have done so.

Some evidence of correlations spontaneously arising among the different neurons, can be discovered by studying the following indicator. Given any two clusters I, J composed respectively of N_I, and N_J neurons, let us introduce

$$\overline{\delta t}_J^I(j) = \sum_{i=1}^{N_I} \delta t_j^i, \quad j = 1, \ldots, N_J \qquad (11.24)$$

where δt_j^i are the temporal slowing down of the jth neuron (within cluster J) as a result of the spikes coming from the neurons of cluster I.

In Fig. 11.5(a), $\overline{\delta t}_J^I(j)$ is plotted as a function of the firing time t_j, for the pair of clusters $I = 2$, $J = 3$. There we see that the first neurons in the cluster (those with a smaller abscissa) are slowed down less than the last neurons. This "destabilizing" effect can be effectively described by approximating the cloud of points with a straight line of slope $s(I, J)$ which, in this case, turns out to be $s = -0.51$. Quite remarkably, $s(I, J) \approx s(I', J')$ when $I - J = I' - J'$. After averaging over pairs of

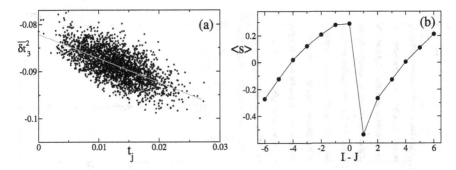

Fig. 11.5 Measure of correlations between clusters. (**a**) $\overline{\delta t_3^2}$ as a function of the firing times t_j, $j = 1, \ldots, N_J$ for clusters $I = 2$, $J = 3$; the straight line is a linear fit. (**b**) The average slope $\langle s \rangle$ defined as in the text as a function of the distance $(I - J) \mod n_c$. Data refers to a network size of $N = 20{,}000$ with a periodic orbit composed of $n_c = 8$ clusters; the other parameters are as in Table 11.1, setup B

clusters sitting at the same distance, we obtain the data plotted in Fig. 11.5(b). One can see that the spikes of neurons of the previous cluster have a destabilizing effect, while the contrary happens for the following cluster. The origin of this organization has yet to be understood.

11.5 Annealed Disorder

Networks of LIF neurons can be studied in a different framework where the strength of the connections between any two nodes, or the *topology* of the network, is not fixed, but changes in a stochastic way during the dynamics evolution (the so-called *annealed* connections). The biological motivation for referring to this kind of connections relies on the fact that the synaptic transmission of a signal is a stochastic, or *unreliable* [14], process. The mathematical motivation is that this setup can help us to understand the dynamics in the presence of quenched disorder. Obviously, in this case there are no longer periodic orbits, as the system is not deterministic.

At variance with other authors [14], who consider the synaptic strengths to be dichotomic variables, here they can assume a whole range of different values (see (11.28)). Accordingly, $P(S)$ represents the probability for a generic neuron to receive a spike of strength S whenever any other neuron reaches its threshold.

Also in the annealed case, when the delay is much smaller than the ISI of the single neuron, the typical stationary state is composed of *clusters* of neurons firing within a narrow time window of the order of magnitude of the delay τ. However, at variance with *quenched* disorder, where many stable cluster states co-exist that are characterized by different populations of neurons, here the fluctuating connections induce a continuous exchange of neurons between neighboring clusters [14]. As a result, the dynamics relaxes towards a maximum entropy state, characterized by evenly spaced clusters of equal sizes. One instance of the dynamics is illustrated

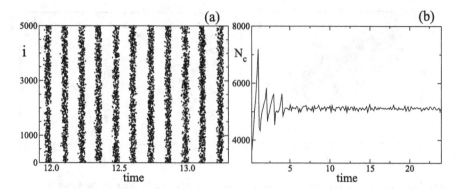

Fig. 11.6 Networks of LIF with annealed connections. (**a**) Firing neuron, labelled with index i, as a function of the time in the stationary state for $N = 5,000$. (**b**) Number of neurons within clusters, N_c, as a function of the time in approaching the stationary state for $N = 40,000$. If the neurons are sorted according to their firing times, as in Fig. 11.10, one gets in both cases that the stationary state is composed of eight clusters

in Fig. 11.6(a), where the raster plot refers to the stationary state of a network with $N = 5,000$ neurons, in the presence of eight clusters. In other words, the average ISI corresponds to the distance between a given cluster and the eighth successive one. The convergence towards the asymptotic state can be appreciated in Fig. 11.6(b), where the population of each cluster is plotted as a function of time.[5] There, we see that after some oscillations, the populations of the eight clusters become soon equal to one another (apart from unavoidable statistical fluctuations).

11.5.1 Cluster Width

In order to compare the behavior of *quenched* and *annealed* systems for different network sizes, it is convenient to focus our attention on the spreading of each cluster. We do that by introducing two indicators: the width w, equal to the time distance between the first and the last firing event, and the standard deviation Σ of the firing times inside a cluster. In both cases, it is first necessary to identify all the spikes which belong to the same cluster. As shown in Fig. 11.7, this is not a difficult task: the only problem may be the isolated spikes coming from neurons that are occasionally travelling across different clusters, that must be carefully identified and removed from the counting.

In Fig. 11.8, the two indicators are plotted versus the system size for both quenched and annealed disorder. There, we see that quenched disorder is always characterized by a smaller spreading. Moreover, we see that up to $N \approx 5,000$ both

---

[5]The simulation is started from a random uniform distribution of the membrane potentials in a network of $N = 40,000$ neurons.

Fig. 11.7 Enlarged view of the spiking times in two consecutive clusters for a network of $N = 10,000$: w represents the distance between the first and the last firing event within a cluster (i labels the firing neuron)

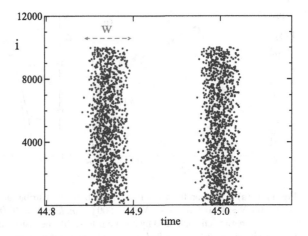

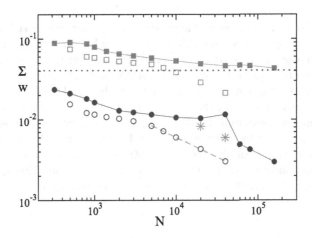

Fig. 11.8 Broadness of clusters as a function of the size of the network for *quenched* (*open symbols*) and *annealed* (*full symbols*) connections; circles and squares refer respectively to Σ and w. The *horizontal dotted line* indicates the value of the synaptic delay; the *dashed line* is a power-law fit giving an exponent of ≈ -0.49. The *stars* represent the standard deviation Σ in the *annealed* framework for a seven-clusters state (see the text and Fig. 11.9). Data corresponding to the quenched case have been averaged over about hundred different realizations of the disorder

setups are characterized by a similar decreasing trend. For quenched disorder, the decreasing trend continues smoothly for larger network sizes and appears to be consistent with a standard $1/\sqrt{N}$ statistical law (see the dashed line with slope -0.49, which is the result of a power-law fit of the last five points). On the other hand, in the annealed case, in between $N = 10,000$ and $N = 40,000$, the standard deviation Σ does even exhibit a small increase!

A first indication that something anomalous is happening comes from the number of clusters which, for $N > \approx 60,000$ passes from eight to seven, suggesting a sort of

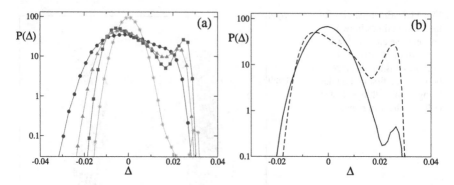

Fig. 11.9 (**a**) Transition from a unimodal to a bimodal distribution $P(\Delta)$ of firing times within a cluster, for $N = 10,000$ (*circles*), $N = 20,000$ (*triangles*), $N = 40,000$ (*squares*), and $N = 80,000$ (*stars*), in a regime characterized by eight clusters. (**b**) The distribution $P(\Delta)$ for $N = 40,000$ in a regime with eight clusters (*dashed curve*) and seven clusters (*solid curve*)

transition.[6] To gain further insight about this phenomenon, we looked at the distribution of the firing times within a cluster. We do so by referring the generic firing time t_j to an origin t_o, defined as the median of the spiking times within the cluster the jth neuron belongs to. Thereby, we construct the distribution of the differences $\Delta = t_j - t_o$ for all spiking events in all clusters. In Fig. 11.9(a), we see a qualitative change upon increasing the network size from $N = 10,000$ to $N = 20,000$: the distribution becomes bimodal. The presence of two peaks is responsible for the anomalous increase of the standard deviation. For larger networks, the second peak in $P(\Delta)$ becomes so small that for $N > 40,000$ it does no longer appreciably contribute to the standard deviation (see Fig. 11.9(a)). On the other hand, the second peak contributes to keep the value of w above the synaptic delay τ.

11.5.2 Bistability and Inter-Cluster Fluxes

The spontaneous onset of a bimodal distribution further confirms the existence of qualitative changes for $N \approx 40,000$. In order to further clarify this issue, we have changed the protocol used to prepare the initial conditions. Instead of choosing randomly $\{v_i(0)\}_N$ for a given size N, we prepare the initial conditions directly in a state with a fixed number n_c of clusters, by referring to the stationary state $\{u_i\}_M$ generated with a different number M of neurons. More precisely, we set $\{v_i(0)\}_N = \{u_i\}_M$. If $N < M$, the u variables are pruned, removing $(M - N)/n_c$ elements from each cluster. When $N > M$, a number $(N - M)/n_c$ of new variables is added to each cluster, by randomly setting them equal to some of the existing values.

---

[6]Unfortunately, testing whether this phenomenon occurs for quenched disorder, too, is beyond our computational capability.

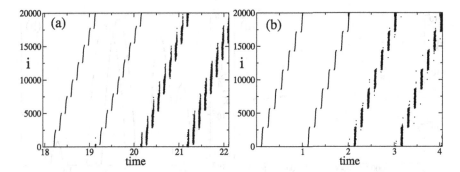

Fig. 11.10 Bistability for $N = 20,000$: eight-clusters (**a**) and seven-clusters (**b**) state. The neurons (i index) are sorted according to their firing times

Starting from a seven-cluster state typically obtained for $M = 80,000$, and decreasing the number of neurons, we have found that seven-cluster states exist and are stable for $N = 40,000$ as well as for $N = 20,000$. The corresponding standard deviations are plotted in Fig. 11.8 (see the stars); they exhibit a more natural decrease with the system size. If the system size is further decreased to $N = 10,000$, the seven-cluster state destabilizes and the dynamics converges to the eight-cluster state. Analogously, we have verified that the eight-cluster state is no longer supported for $N = 80,000$. Therefore, we conclude that in between 10,000 and 80,000 there exists a bistability between the two regimes. In that range of sizes, one should occasionally observe jumps between the two metastable regimes. However, on the time scales numerically accessible, we have not been able to see any switch. It would be extremely important to develop some theory to estimate the order of magnitude of the dwelling times.

A more detailed comparison between the two regimes can be made by looking at the distribution of the firing-times (suitably shifted as discussed above). In Fig. 11.9, we see that the bimodal distribution clearly visible in the eight-cluster regime, is strongly depressed in the seven-cluster regime, but it does not disappear. In other words, the bimodality does not seem to be associated with an incipient loss of stability.

Another method to compare the two regimes is by plotting the firing times in a raster plot where the neurons are labelled (once for all) according to the ordering of their first firing times. The plots obtained for $N = 20,000$ are presented in Fig. 11.10, where we see that in both cases the clusters, initially well separated, become increasingly blurred over time as a result of jumps between neighboring clusters. Moreover, we see that this phenomenon is definitely more relevant in the eight-cluster regime.

The inter-cluster fluxes can be studied more quantitatively in the following way. We start labelling the clusters according to their firing order (modulus n_c) and thereby assign to each neuron the label ℓ of the corresponding cluster. By then letting the system evolve, each time a neuron fires we compute the difference $\delta\ell = \ell' - \ell$ between the previous and the new label; $\delta\ell = +1$ ($\delta\ell = -1$) corresponds to a *forward* (resp., *backward*) jump. We found that $\delta\ell$ assumes only the values, -1, 0,

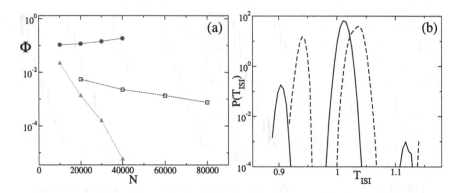

Fig. 11.11 (**a**) Fluxes of neurons between clusters: *circles* and *triangles* represent the forward (Φ^+) (resp., backward ($-\Phi^-$)) flux in the eight-clusters regime; *open squares* represent the forward flux in the seven-clusters regime. (**b**) Comparison of the distributions of T_{ISI} for $N = 40{,}000$ for eight-clusters (*dashed curve*) and seven-clusters (*solid curve*) state

and 1, which means that jumps occur only between neighboring clusters. Finally, the relevant fluxes are defined as

$$\Phi^+(n) = \frac{\#(\delta\ell = +1)}{n}, \qquad \Phi^-(n) = \frac{\#(\delta\ell = -1)}{n} \qquad (11.25)$$

where the symbol # denotes the cardinality of the set of events identified by the condition expressed in parentheses and we recall that the time n coincides with the number of firing events.

In Fig. 11.11(a), the two fluxes are compared for different system sizes in the eight-cluster regime. It is transparent that the positive flux is larger than the negative one. This means that the average ISI of the single neuron is slightly smaller than the (macroscopic) period of the clustered regime. This is reminiscent of the self-organized quasi periodic regime observed in networks of identical neurons in the presence of spikes of the type (11.12) [31, 41], although in the present case both fluxes vanish in the thermodynamic limit. In the same figure, we have plotted also the forward flux for the seven-cluster state (the backward flux being too small to be reliably quantified) which confirms the earlier impression that this regime is characterized by smaller fluxes.

In order to further refine the analysis of the clustered regime, we have analyzed the distribution $P(T_{\mathrm{ISI}})$ of the single neuron ISIs. The results for $N = 40{,}000$ are plotted in Fig. 11.11(b) both for the eight- and seven-cluster states (please note the logarithmic scale on y-axis). Both distributions show three well separated peaks. Having noticed that the dynamics is characterized by forward and backward jumps, it is tempting to associate such peaks with the jumps. In order to test this natural idea, we have plotted the relative firing time Δ (within the cluster) versus the last ISI T_{ISI}. The results plotted in Fig. 11.12 for $N = 20{,}000$ show a clear correlation between Δ and T_{ISI}: the small peak in the distribution $P(\Delta)$, occurring for positive Δ values, is due to the presence of neurons with a smaller-than-average last T_{ISI} (*fast neurons*). The smaller spot noticeable in the lower right corner of Fig. 11.12 suggests

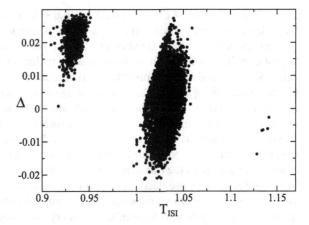

Fig. 11.12 Time position Δ of the neurons within the cluster plotted versus the last T_{ISI} for a network of $N = 20,000$ neurons in the eight-cluster regime

that a similar correlations occurs for *slow* neurons. The picture is completed once we realize that the two spots contain all neurons that have just exhibited plus and minus jumps, respectively. In other words, the multimodality in the spike times is due to a memory effect of the inter-cluster jumps.

11.6 Summary and Perspectives

In this paper, we have discussed the behavior of networks of pulse coupled LIF neurons. We have developed a formalism that allows studying such networks in the wide context of generic pulse-shapes in the presence of both disorder and delay. More precisely, we have found that the evolution of such networks can be described by an event-driven map which involves $(2 + d)N - 1$ variables, where N is the number of neurons and d the number of variables needed to describe the field seen by each single neuron. This is at variance with standard dynamical systems with delayed feedback, that are characterized by an infinite dimensional phase-space. Moreover, we have suitably rescaled the equations and introduced two adimensional parameters G and χ which quantify the effective coupling strength and the slowing down induced by the (inhibitory) coupling. Such parameters provide a direct and instructive characterization of the system dynamics and allow for a qualitative comparison between networks characterized by different force fields.

Next, we have extensively discussed the case of δ-like inhibitory pulses both in the presence of quenched and annealed disorder. In the quenched case, we have verified that the dynamics always converges towards a periodic orbit. This is in agreement with the known stability of such networks. Less obvious is that the convergence time initially grows exponentially with the number N of neurons, becoming as long as 10^6–10^7 time units, before decreasing down to a few hundreds of time units. This is because upon increasing N, neuron-to-neuron fluctuations (due to the presence of disorder) progressively decrease and the network dynamics becomes increasingly akin to that of homogeneous networks. In homogeneous networks, there exists a huge number of clustered states that are simultaneously stable. Part of the large degree of multistability may be ascribed to the variability of the number of clusters, as well as of the number of neurons within each cluster. However, the largest contribution arises from the invariance under permutation of the (identical) neurons. The introduction of disorder breaks the invariance: some solutions are simply perturbed, giving rise to clusters of finite width, while others are destroyed. For the parameter values that we have selected, and N-values smaller than a few hundreds, the effective amplitude of the noise is such that very few clustered solutions survive. As a result, most of the trajectories wander in a phase-space whose dimension is proportional to N and this, we believe, is the mechanism responsible for the exponential growth of the transient dynamics. On the other hand, by further increasing N, the effective noise decreases, so that the number of clustered states increases and they can rapidly attract the transient dynamics. It would be useful to turn these qualitative arguments into a quantitative theory, but many subtle effects enter the game, making the development of even approximate arguments quite a difficult task.

In fact, we have preferred to turn our attention to the simpler case of networks with annealed disorder. Because of the noise, the dynamics wanders among the different clustered states and one can thereby focus the attention onto the structure of the stationary state. As already noticed in [14], the asymptotic state is characterized by an even distribution of neurons among the various clusters. However, the number of clusters, as well as their width appears to be strongly affected by finite-size corrections. For instance, we have seen that the typical number of clusters decreases from eight to seven, in the N range $[10^4, 10^5]$ where it is accompanied by a bistability region, where the number of clusters depends on the initial preparation, and is characterized by a strong stability: we have never seen a switch in our simulations. We have also discovered that the clusters are characterized by a multimodal structure, that reflects inter-cluster fluxes. Such fluxes are presumably the key point to understand the overall loss of stability of the corresponding macroscopic solutions.

Finally, it is at least curious to notice that these qualitative changes occur in a range of connectivity values that are similar if not even larger than that of the cerebral cortex (10^4). This suggests, that although it is certainly important to understand the behavior of neural networks in the "thermodynamic limit", as this represents a 0th-order approximation of the dynamics, finite-size corrections may be nonnegligible.

Acknowledgements We wish to thank A. Torcini for enlightening discussions. This work has been partly carried out with the support of the EU project NEST-PATH-043309 and of the Italian project "Struttura e dinamica di reti complesse" N. 3001 within the CNR programme "Ricerca spontanea a tema libero".

Appendix: Rescaling the Equations of Motion

Models of LIF neurons are often introduced by referring to different normalizations. In order to facilitate the comparison of the results obtained by different groups, in the following we illustrate the rescaling needed to express the equations in the adimensional setting adopted in (11.1).

A.1 Setup A

Zillmer et al. [44] analyze a network of N LIF neurons by referring to the equations

$$\beta \dot{V}_i = I_{ext} - V_i + \beta \frac{J}{K} \sum_{l=1}^{N} \mu_{i,l} \sum_{m} F\left(t - t_l^{(m)} - D\right), \quad i = 1, \ldots, N \quad (11.26)$$

(some variable names have been changed to avoid the confusion arising from the overlap between symbols which denote different quantities), where K is the number of incoming links to each neuron ($f = K/N$ is the dilution of the network); β is the membrane time constant of the neuron; I_{ext} is an external current and D is the synaptic delay. Moreover, the model definition includes the reset potential V_r and the firing threshold V_t. The parameter J with $J < 0$ (resp., $J > 0$) for *inhibitory* (resp., *excitatory*) coupling represents the coupling strength, while the topology of the network is defined by the connectivity matrix $\mu_{i,l}$. The distribution $P(\mu)$ is chosen to be dichotomic, i.e. $P(\mu) = (1 - f)\delta(\mu) + f\delta(\mu - 1)$, which implies that the average is $\langle \mu \rangle = f$, while the variance is $\sigma^2(\mu) = f(1 - f)$. Finally, the function $F(t)$ (that becomes a Dirac's δ-function in the case of *zero-width* pulses) describes the shape of the single pulse, while $t_l^{(m)}$ represents the mth firing time of the lth neuron.

The above equations transform into (11.1), once the following changes of variables are introduced,

- $t \rightarrow t/\beta$,
- $D \rightarrow \tau = D/\beta$,
- $V \rightarrow v = (V - V_r)/(V_t - V_r)$,
- $I_{ext} \rightarrow a = (I_{ext} - V_r)/(V_t - V_r)$,
- $J \rightarrow g = J/(V_t - V_r)$,
- $\mu_{i,j} \rightarrow S_{i,j} = \mu_{i,j}/\langle \mu \rangle = \mu_{i,j}/f$,

where the new distribution $P(S)$ of connections strengths writes $P(S) = (1 - f)\delta(S) + f\delta(S - 1/f)$, so that its average is equal to one as required, while the variance is $\sigma^2(S) = (1 - f)/f$. The parameter values corresponding to this setup are summarized in Table 11.1.

A.2 Setup B

In Jahnke et al. [20, 21] the model is defined as

$$\dot{V}_i = I_{ext} - \gamma V_i + \sum_{j=1}^{N} \epsilon_{i,j} \sum_{m} F\left(t - t_j^{(m)} - D\right), \quad i = 1, \ldots, N, \quad (11.27)$$

Table 11.1 Parameters used with the two different setups. The parameter a, representing an external input current is always larger than the firing threshold ($a > 1$): in this regime, non-interacting neurons exhibit a periodic firing with a period $T = \ln(a/(a - 1))$

	a	τ	τ/T	g	f	σ^2
Setup A	1.1	0.1	0.041	-5	0.869	0.15
Setup B	3.0	0.04054	0.1	-1.5	0.25	4.33

where $V_r = 0$, $V_t = 1$ and $\sum_{j=1}^{N} \epsilon_{i,j} = J_T$. The coupling strengths $\epsilon_{i,j}$ are randomly chosen according to the distribution

$$P(\epsilon) = (1 - f)\delta(\epsilon) + \frac{f^3 N}{2J_T} H(\epsilon) H\left(\frac{2J_T}{Nf^2} - \epsilon\right) \tag{11.28}$$

where $H(x)$ is the Heaviside step function.

By performing the transformations,

- $t \to t\gamma$,
- $D \to \tau = D\gamma$,
- $I_{\text{ext}} \to a = I_{\text{ext}}/\gamma$,
- $J_T \to g = J_T$,
- $\epsilon_{i,j} \to S_{i,j} = \epsilon_{i,j}/\langle\epsilon\rangle = \epsilon_{i,j}Nf/J_T$,

the model (11.27) can be rewritten in the form (11.1). The probability of connections strengths becomes

$$P(S) = (1 - f)\delta(S) + \frac{f^2}{2} H(S) H(2/f - S)$$

so that $\langle S \rangle = 1$, and $\sigma^2(S) = 4/(3f) - 1$. The parameter values corresponding to this setup are summarized in Table 11.1.

References

1. Abbott, L.F., van Vreeswijk, C.: Asynchronous states in networks of pulse-coupled oscillators. Phys. Rev. E **48**(2), 1483–1490 (1993). doi:10.1103/PhysRevE.48.1483
2. Amit, D.: Modelling Brain Function: The World of Attractor Neural Networks. Cambridge University Press, New York (1990)
3. Bressloff, P.C., Coombes, S.: A dynamical theory of spike train transitions in networks of integrate-and-fire oscillators. SIAM J. Appl. Math. **60**(3), 820–841 (2000)
4. Bressloff, P.: Mean-field theory of globally coupled integrate-and-fire neural oscillators with dynamic synapses. Phys. Rev. E **60**(2), 2160–2170 (1999). doi:10.1103/PhysRevE.60.2160
5. Brunel, N.: Dynamics of sparsely connected networks of excitatory and inhibitory spiking neurons. J. Comput. Neurosci. **8**(3), 183–208 (2000)
6. Brunel, N., Hakim, V.: Fast global oscillations in networks of integrate-and-fire neurons with low firing rates. Neural Comput. **11**(7), 1621–1671 (1999)
7. Brunel, N., Hansel, D.: How noise affects the synchronization properties of recurrent networks of inhibitory neurons. Neural Comput. **18**(5), 1066–1110 (2006)

8. Cessac, B., Viéville, T.: On dynamics of integrate-and-fire neural networks with conductance based synapses. Front. Comput. Neurosci. **2**, 2–20 (2008). doi:10.3389/neuro.10.002.2008
9. Denker, M., Timme, M., Diesmann, M., Wolf, F., Geisel, T.: Breaking synchrony by heterogeneity in complex networks. Phys. Rev. Lett. **92**(7), 074103 (2004). doi:10.1103/ PhysRevLett.92.074103
10. Destexhe, A.: Self-sustained asynchronous irregular states and Up–Down states in thalamic, cortical and thalamocortical networks of nonlinear integrate-and-fire neurons. J. Comput. Neurosci. **27**(3), 493–506 (2009). doi:10.1007/s10827-009-0164-4
11. Ernst, U., Pawelzik, K., Geisel, T.: Synchronization induced by temporal delays in pulse-coupled oscillators. Phys. Rev. Lett. **74**(9), 1570–1573 (1995). doi:10.1103/PhysRevLett.74. 1570
12. Ernst, U., Pawelzik, K., Geisel, T.: Delay-induced multistable synchronization of biological oscillators. Phys. Rev. E **57**(2), 2150–2162 (1998). doi:10.1103/PhysRevE.57.2150
13. Fell, D.: Understanding the Control of Metabolism. Portland Press, London (1997)
14. Friedrich, J., Kinzel, W.: Dynamics of recurrent neural networks with delayed unreliable synapses: metastable clustering. J. Comput. Neurosci. **27**(1), 65–80 (2009). doi:10.1007/ s10827-008-0127-1
15. Gerstner, W., Kistler, W.: Spiking Neuron Models: Single Neurons, Populations, Plasticity. Cambridge University Press, Cambridge (2002)
16. Glass, L., Mackey, M.: From Clocks to Chaos: The Rhythms of Life. Princeton University Press, Princeton (1988)
17. Golomb, D., Hansel, D., Shraiman, B., Sompolinsky, H.: Clustering in globally coupled phase oscillators. Phys. Rev. A **45**(6), 3516–3530 (1992). doi:10.1103/PhysRevA.45.3516
18. Hale, J.: Delay Differential Equations and Dynamical Systems. Springer, New York (1991)
19. Hansel, D., Mato, G., Meunier, C.: Clustering and slow switching in globally coupled phase oscillators. Phys. Rev. E **48**(5), 3470–3477 (1993). doi:10.1103/PhysRevE.48.3470
20. Jahnke, S., Memmesheimer, R., Timme, M.: Stable irregular dynamics in complex neural networks. Phys. Rev. Lett. **100**(4), 048102 (2008). doi:10.1103/PhysRevLett.100.048102
21. Jahnke, S., Memmesheimer, R., Timme, M.: How chaotic is the balanced state? Front. Comput. Neurosci. (2009). doi:10.3389/neuro.10/013.2009. www.frontiersin.org/neuroscience/ computationalneuroscience/paper/10.3389/neuro.10/013.2009/html/
22. Jin, D.: Fast convergence of spike sequences to periodic patterns in recurrent networks. Phys. Rev. Lett. **89**(20), 208102 (2002). doi:10.1103/PhysRevLett.89.208102
23. Kandel, E., Schwartz, J., Jessell, T.: Principles of Neural Science. McGraw-Hill, New York (2000)
24. Kinzel, W.: On the stationary state of a network of inhibitory spiking neurons. J. Comput. Neurosci. **24**(1), 105–112 (2008). doi:10.1007/s10827-007-0049-3
25. Koch, C.: Biophysics of Computation. Oxford University Press, New York (1999)
26. Kuramoto, Y.: Chemical Oscillations, Waves, and Turbulence. Springer, Berlin (1984)
27. Luccioli, S., Politi, A.: Paper in preparation
28. Mauroy, A., Sepulchre, R.: Clustering behaviors in networks of integrate-and-fire oscillators. Chaos **18**, 037122 (2008). doi:10.1063/1.2967806
29. Mazor, O., Laurent, G.: Transient dynamics versus fixed points in odor representations by locust antennal lobe projection neurons. Neuron **48**(4), 661–673 (2005). doi:10.1016/j.neuron. 2005.09.032
30. Mirollo, R., Strogatz, S.: Synchronization of pulse-coupled biological oscillators. SIAM J. Appl. Math. **50**(6), 1645–1662 (1990)
31. Mohanty, P., Politi, A.: A new approach to partial synchronization in globally coupled rotators. J. Phys. A, Math. Gen. **39**(26), L415–L421 (2006). http://stacks.iop.org/0305-4470/39/i=26/ a=L01
32. Nichols, S., Wiesenfeld, K.: Ubiquitous neutral stability of splay-phase states. Phys. Rev. A **45**(12), 8430–8435 (1992). doi:10.1103/PhysRevA.45.8430
33. Olmi, S., Livi, R., Politi, A., Torcini, A.: Collective oscillations in disordered neural networks. Phys. Rev. E **81**(4), 046119 (2010). doi:10.1103/PhysRevE.81.046119

34. Politi, A., Torcini, A.: Stable chaos. In: Nonlinear Dynamics and Chaos: Advances and Perspectives, Understanding Complex Systems. Springer, Heidelberg (2010)
35. Rieke, F., Warland, D., de Ruyter van Steveninck, R., Bialek, W.: Spikes: Exploring the Neural Code. MIT Press, Cambridge (1996)
36. Sheperd, G. (ed.): The Synaptic Organization of the Brain. Oxford University Press, New York (2004)
37. Strogatz, S.H.: Exploring complex networks. Nature **410**, 268–276 (2001)
38. Strogatz, S., Mirollo, R.: Splay states in globally coupled Josephson arrays: Analytical prediction of Floquet multipliers. Phys. Rev. E **47**(1), 220–227 (1993). doi:10.1103/PhysRevE.47.220
39. Timme, M., Wolf, F., Geisel, T.: Coexistence of regular and irregular dynamics in complex networks of pulse-coupled oscillators. Phys. Rev. Lett. **89**(25), 258701 (2002). doi:10.1103/PhysRevLett.89.258701
40. Tuckwell, H.: Introduction to Theoretical Neurobiology. Cambridge University Press, New York (1988)
41. van Vreeswijk, C.: Partial synchronization in populations of pulse-coupled oscillators. Phys. Rev. E **54**(5), 5522–5537 (1996). doi:10.1103/PhysRevE.54.5522
42. van Vreeswijk, C., Sompolinsky, H.: Chaos in neuronal networks with balanced excitatory and inhibitory activity. Science **274**(5293), 1724–1726 (1996)
43. van Vreeswijk, C., Sompolinsky, H.: Chaotic balanced state in a model of cortical circuits. Neural Comput. **10**(6), 1321–1371 (1998)
44. Zillmer, R., Brunel, N., Hansel, D.: Very long transients, irregular firing, and chaotic dynamics in networks of randomly connected inhibitory integrate-and-fire neurons. Phys. Rev. E **79**(3), 031909 (2009). doi:10.1103/PhysRevE.79.031909
45. Zillmer, R., Livi, R., Politi, A., Torcini, A.: Desynchronization in diluted neural networks. Phys. Rev. E **74**(3), 036203 (2006). doi:10.1103/PhysRevE.74.036203
46. Zillmer, R., Livi, R., Politi, A., Torcini, A.: Stability of the splay state in pulse-coupled networks. Phys. Rev. E **76**(4), 046102 (2007). doi:10.1103/PhysRevE.76.046102
47. Zumdieck, A., Timme, M., Geisel, T., Wolf, F.: Long chaotic transients in complex networks. Phys. Rev. Lett. **93**(24), 244103 (2004). doi:10.1103/PhysRevLett.93.244103

Index

E. Estrada et al. (eds.), *Network Science*,
DOI 10.1007/978-1-84996-396-1, © Springer-Verlag London Limited 2010